New Insights into Metabolic Dysfunction

New Insights into Metabolic Dysfunction

Editor: Hudson Cole

hayle medical

New York

Hayle Medical,
750 Third Avenue, 9th Floor,
New York, NY 10017, USA

Visit us on the World Wide Web at:
www.haylemedical.com

ISBN 978-1-64647-561-2 (Hardback)

Cataloging-in-Publication Data

New insights into metabolic dysfunction / edited by Hudson Cole.
p. cm.
Includes bibliographical references and index.
ISBN 978-1-64647-561-2
1. Metabolic syndrome. 2. Metabolism--Disorders. 3. Insulin resistance. I. Cole, Hudson.
RC662.4 .N49 2023
616.399--dc23

Contents

Preface

I am honored to present to you this unique book which encompasses the most up-to-date data in the field. I was extremely pleased to get this opportunity of editing the work of experts from across the globe. I have also written papers in this field and researched the various aspects revolving around the progress of the discipline. I have tried to unify my knowledge along with that of stalwarts from every corner of the world, to produce a text which not only benefits the readers but also facilitates the growth of the field.

Metabolism refers to a range of chemical processes that occur when the body converts the food consumed by a person into energy. A metabolic disorder occurs when abnormal chemical reactions disrupt the metabolism of the body. Genetics, mitochondrial dysfunction, and organ dysfunction are some of its common causes. There are various kinds of metabolic disorders including Gaucher's disease, diabetes, hemochromatosis, phenylketonuria, and mitochondrial disorders. Some common symptoms of these disorders include reduced appetite, stomach pain, muscle weakness, tiredness, changes in skin color, unexpected weight gain or loss, and developmental problems in babies and infants. Metabolic syndrome comprises a group of five medical conditions which can lead to various health problems such as diabetes, heart disease and stroke. These conditions are high blood glucose, high levels of triglycerides in the blood, large waist circumference, low levels of HDL cholesterol and high blood pressure. The topics covered in this book offer the readers new insights into metabolic dysfunction. It includes contributions of experts and scientists, which will provide innovative insights into these disorders. The book will greatly assist the researchers and students associated with the diagnosis and management of metabolic dysfunction.

Finally, I would like to thank all the contributing authors for their valuable time and contributions. This book would not have been possible without their efforts. I would also like to thank my friends and family for their constant support.

Editor

1

Effects of High-Fat Diet Induced Obesity and Fructooligosaccharide Supplementation on Cardiac Protein Expression

Sidra Sarfaraz [1], Shamjeet Singh [2], Aileen Hawke [1], Sandra T. Clarke [3] and D. Dan Ramdath [1,*]

1 Guelph Research and Development Centre, Agriculture and Agri-Food Canada, Guelph, ON N1G 5C9, Canada; sidra9518@gmail.com (S.S.); aileen.hawke@canada.ca (A.H.)

2 School of Pharmacy, Faculty of Medical Sciences, The University of the West Indies, St. Augustine, Trinidad and Tobago; shamjeet.singh@sta.uwi.edu

3 Applied Bioscience Graduate Program and Faculty of Science, University of Ontario Institute of Technology, Oshawa, ON L1G 0C5, Canada; sandra.clarke2@canada.ca

* Correspondence: dan.ramdath@canada.ca

Abstract: The mechanism by which high fat-diet induced obesity affects cardiac protein expression is unclear, and the extent to which this is modulated by prebiotic treatment is not known. These outcomes were assessed in rats initially fed a high-fat diet, then the top 40% weight gain group were randomly allocated to control (CON), high-fat (HF) and HF supplemented with fructooligosaccharide (32 g; HF-FOS) treatments for 12 weeks ($n = 10$/group). At sacrifice, left ventricles were either frozen or preserved in formalin. Serum was stored for glucose and insulin measurements. Protein spectra was obtained using an Orbitrap analyzer, processed with Sequest and fold changes assessed with Scaffold Q +. Treatment effects for body weights, glucose and insulin were assessed using one-way ANOVA, and the differential protein expression was assessed by a Mann–Whitney U test. The Database for Annotation, Visualization and Integrated Discovery and the Kyoto Encyclopedia of Genes and Genomes identified pathways containing overrepresented proteins. Hematoxylin and eosin sections were graded for hypertrophy and also quantified; differences were identified using Chi-square analyses and Mann-Whitney U tests. HF diet fed rats were significantly ($p < 0.05$) heavier than CON, and 23 proteins involved in mitochondrial function and lipid metabolism were differentially expressed between HF and CON. Between HF-FOS and HF, 117 proteins involved in contractility, lipid and carbohydrate metabolism were differentially expressed. HF cardiomyocytes were significantly ($p < 0.05$) more hypertrophic than CON. We conclude that high-fat feeding and FOS are associated with subcellular deviations in cardiac metabolism and contractility, which may influence myocardial function and alter the risk of cardiovascular disease.

Keywords: cardiac; proteomics; mass spectrometry; DAVID; KEGG; fructooligosaccharides; prebiotic; CVD

---

1. Introduction

Cardiovascular diseases (CVDs) continue to be the leading cause of morbidity and mortality globally [1]. While some genetic markers have been identified, they explain less than 15% of the variance in the risk for these diseases [2]. It is well accepted that external factors, such as poor diets, sedentary lifestyles and obesity are the major contributors to CVD risk [3–5]. In particular, obesity contributes significantly to diminished cardiovascular function and increased CVD risk [6]. Cardiac dysfunction associated with obesity is often accompanied by systemic abnormalities such as chronic inflammation, oxidative stress, dyslipidemia, insulin resistance and endothelial dysfunction [7]. On a high fat diet, obese animals display cardiomyocyte hypertrophy, myocardial interstitial fibrosis [8] and disrupted signal transduction in cardiomyocytes, which decrease the ability of these cells to efficiently utilize glucose and lipids [9]. Furthermore, early stage cardiomyopathy caused by high-fat induced obesity in mice is associated with disturbed calcium homeostasis [5]. In humans, increased intake of saturated fatty acids has been shown to promote a pro-inflammatory state and is associated with insulin resistance in muscle and fat tissues [10].

Collectively, biochemical abnormalities associated with high fat diets can lead to cardiac contractile impairments and adaptive myocardial remodelling, which in turn may result in diminished cardiac contractility and an increased risk of heart failure [4,11]. When a proteomic analytical approach was used, insulin resistant mice fed a high fat diet had decreased expression in proteins involved in heart structure, energy metabolism, fat oxidation and the tricarboxylic acid cycle (TCA) cycle [12]. These findings confirm a direct effect of high fat diet on cardiac function, which can be implicated in an increased cardiovascular disease risk. There is now an emerging field of research that suggests the gut microbiome may modulate the relationship between consumption of a high fat diet and the onset of obesity and cardiovascular disease [13]. It is likely that this modulatory effect is mediated through changes in circulating metabolites, but it is not clear what effect this has on tissue level protein expression.

The human gut microbiota is composed of more than 10^{14} bacteria and archaea as well as viruses, fungi, and protozoa. Its variability is affected by genetics, lifestyle and especially dietary components such as prebiotics and probiotics [14]. Prebiotics, or non-digestible food components such as inulin and, fructooligosaccharides (FOS) are associated with favourable modulation of the gut microbiota, and decreased post-prandial glucose and insulin [15,16]. A recent meta-analysis demonstrated that prebiotic intakes are associated with decreases in body mass index (BMI), body weight and fat mass in humans [17]. Review of current evidence also suggests that consumption of prebiotics is inversely associated with obesity, which may be mediated through decreased inflammation and increased production of short chain fatty acids (SCFAs) [18]. It is possible that changes in concentrations of these metabolites may modulate the expression of proteins, and in the case of cardiac function may be associated with a lowering of CVD risk.

This study was undertaken to investigate the effect of high fat-diet induced obesity on cardiac protein expression using a proteomic approach, and to assess the protective effect of supplemental FOS. We hypothesized that obesity would result in impairments in cardiac proteins involved in contractility, insulin signaling and cellular metabolism, and that FOS supplementation would augment these impairments.

2. Materials and Methods

2.1. Experimental Design and Sample Collection

Weanling male Sprague Dawley rats approximately 28 days old were obtained from Charles River (Saint Constant, QC, Canada). Rats were pair-housed in Sealsafe® PLUS Rat individually ventilated cages (IVC, Techniplast, Via I Maggio, Italy) equipped with wire mesh bottoms, gnawing sticks, covered tunnels, and stainless-steel sheets for environmental enrichment, and health checks were performed daily. Room temperature was maintained at 22 °C with 12-hour light/dark cycles, and rats were provided chow and water *ad libitum*.

After an acclimation period of seven days, all rats were initially placed on a high-fat modified AIN-93G diet for two weeks to identify rats that were resistant or susceptible to an obesogenic diet. Rats in the top 40% weight-gain category were categorized as the diet-induced obesity (DIO) phenotype. Following two weeks of high-fat diet consumption and distinction of the obese phenotype, DIO rats ($n = 10$ per group) were further separated into new diet categories, either receiving the base AIN-93G chow as a control diet (CON), a high-fat modified AIN-93G diet (HF), or a high-fat modified AIN-93G diet containing 32.2 g of fructooligosaccharide/1 kg diet (HF-FOS). The amount of FOS included in the test diet (3%) can be reasonably achieved within the human population [19]. The control diet contained 70 g total fat/kg diet and the HF-modified diets each contained 165 g total fat/kg diet. Detailed composition of the different diets is shown in Table 1.

Table 1. Composition of the experimental diets (per 1000 g).

COMPOSITION	CON	HF	HF-FOS
	Ingredient (g)		
Casein (protein)	200	190	190
L-Cystine	3	3	3
Corn Starch	387.5	173.5	172.6
Maltodextrin 10	122	68.3	67.6
Sucrose	100	283.3	282.6
Cellulose, BW200	70	70	40
Fructooligosaccharide	0	0	32.2
Soybean Oil	70	120.3	120.3
Milk Fat, Anhydrous	0	44.2	44.2
tBHQ	0.014	0.014	0.014
Mineral Mix S10022G	35	35	35
	Nutrient (g)		
Protein	179.0	170.2	170.2
Carbohydrate (digestible)	609.5	524.9	522.8
Fat	70.0	164.5	164.5
Fibre	70.0	70.0	72.2
	Nutrient (kcal)		
Protein	716	681	681
Carbohydrate	2438	2100	2091
Fat	630	1481	1481
Total	3784	4261	4253

CON, control diet (AIN-93G); HF, high fat diet (AIN-93G + high fat content); HF-FOS, high-fat diet supplemented with fructooligosaccharides.

Following 12 weeks of experimental diet feeding, necropsies were conducted. Rats were humanely euthanized under isoflurane anesthesia by terminal cardiac bleeds. Non-fasted blood samples were distributed in BD Vacutainer® SST™ Tubes (BD, Franklin Lakes, NJ, USA) and processed according to the manufacturer's directions. Serum was used immediately for glucose measurements or stored at −80 °C for future analyses. Fasted samples (beyond 3 hours) were not possible for this experiment as it would have impacted other critical measures of the major study. Following blood draws, the heart was excised, and the left ventricular tissue was collected, washed in cold PBS and a portion was immediately cryopreserved in liquid nitrogen for protein analysis by mass spectrometry at the SPARC BioCentre (SickKids Hospital, Toronto, ON, Canada). The other portion of the heart was fixed in 10% neutral-buffered formalin at ambient temperature for histological analysis at the Department of Preclinical Sciences, the University of the West Indies, Trinidad. All animal care procedures were approved by the animal care committees at Health Canada and at the University of Ontario Institute of Technology.

2.2. *Serum Insulin and Glucose Measurements*

Serum glucose concentrations were measured on the day of necropsy using a glucose test kit (Ortho-Clinical Diagnostics, Markham, ON, Canada) on a VITROS® 5,1 FS automated clinical chemistry analyser. Circulating insulin concentrations were determined from previously frozen serum samples using a Rat Metabolic Bead Panel Milliplex Map Kit (EMD Millipore Corp. Billerica MA, USA) on a Luminex 200 analyser (Luminex, Austin, TX, USA). There were two levels of commercial quality controls on each Luminex assay plate, and insulin concentrations were found to be within the expected range.

2.3. Histology

Formalin preserved tissue was oriented and embedded in paraffin wax. Sections (7 μm) were cut cross-sectionally and stained with haematoxylin and eosin (Sigma-Aldrich, MO, USA) to visualise tissue morphology. Micrographs were taken at a magnification of 40 × and assessed qualitatively for hypertrophy (cardiomyocyte size) and evidence of interstitial (collagen) deposition/extracellular matrix depositions using four categories: no-evidence, mild, moderate or severe. Chi-squared analyses were used to detect significant associations between cardiac hypertrophy and interstitial deposition and the treatment groups. Micrographs were also quantified using ImageJ2. Briefly, images were converted to 16 bit, and thresholds were used to estimate the percentage of the micrograph occupied by the cardiomyocyte. Mann–Whitney U tests were used to detect any significant differences in cardiomyocyte area between CON and HF and HF and HF-FOS. A p-value of < 0.05 was considered significant.

2.4. Mass Spectrometry

Mass spectrometry analysis was performed at the SPARC BioCentre at the Hospital for Sick Children in Toronto, ON Canada. Cryopreserved cardiac tissue was sliced, incubated with 1 mL cold RIPA (1% Triton X-100, 1% sodium deoxycholate, 0.1% sodium dodecyl sulfate, 150 mM NaCl, 50 mM Tris pH = 7.5, 1 mM EDTA buffer) and homogenised using a TissueLyser LT (Qiagen, Inc., MD, USA). The homogenate was centrifuged at 23,000 × g for 15 minutes, and protein concentrations estimated (Pierce™ BCA Protein Assay Kit, ThermoFisher Scientific, MD, USA) using bovine serum albumin as a standard. Homogenate (100 μg) was mixed with 100 mM triethylammonium bicarbonate (TEAB) to make a final volume of 100 μL. Each protein digest (50 μg) was then labelled with TMT tags and placed into one of three groups of 10; groups were divided to include at least three random samples from each dietary group (CON, HF, HF-FOS) per 10-plex. Samples were cleaned using Strong Cation Exchange clean up tips. Peptides were bound to strong cation exchange material, washed, and eluted off in two stages/TMT group. Each elution was then lyophilised and individually analyzed by LC-MS/MS.

Samples were analyzed on an Orbitrap mass spectrometer (Q-Exactive, ThermoFisher, San Jose, CA, USA) using the method outlined by Ayoub et al. with some modifications [20]. Peptides were eluted over 180 min at a rate of 250 nL/min using a gradient set up as 0%–40% of buffer A (0.1% formic acid) and buffer B (0.1% formic acid in 80% acetonitrile). The method included one MS full scan (525–1600 m/z) followed by 15 data-dependent MS/MS scans with a resolution of 35,000. Fragmentation occurred in the higher energy collisional dissociation (HCD) trap with normalized collision energy set to 27V.

2.5. Protein Identification and Quantitation

All MS/MS samples were analyzed using Sequest (Thermo Fisher Scientific, San Jose, CA, USA; version 1.4.1.14) and X! Tandem (version CYCLONE (2010.12.01.1)). Peptide probabilities from Sequest were assigned by the Scaffold Local FDR (false discovery rate) algorithm [21]. Peptide Probabilities from X! Tandem were assigned by the Peptide Prophet algorithm [22] with Scaffold delta-mass correction. Scaffold Q + (Proteome Software Inc., Portland, OR; version Scaffold_4.7.3) was used to quantitate peptide and protein identifications. Protein identification was accepted if it could be established at greater than 95.0% probability and contained at least two identified peptides. Normalisation was performed as described previously [23].

2.6. Statistical Analyses

This work represents secondary analyses of tissues provided from a larger animal study and characterizes heart muscle collected from a subset of 10 obese rats per diet group. Analyses sought to detect significant differences between (i) HF vs. CON and (ii) HF-FOS vs. HF experimental groups. Glucose, insulin and body weights were normally distributed and analyzed by one-way ANOVA followed by a post-hoc Tukey test. For insulin measures only, there was a sample number of 5 due to constraints on analyzing serum metabolic hormones for the larger study. Fold changes between these groups were calculated by Scaffold Q +. Differentially expressed proteins were determined by using Mann–Whitney U tests, with unadjusted significance level $p < 0.05$ corrected by Benjamini–Hochberg.

2.7. In-Silico Functional Analyses

In silico methods were used to establish the possible functional relationships between differentially expressed proteins in HF vs. CON hearts and HF-FOS vs. HF hearts. The official gene names were utilised in the Database for Annotation, Visualization and Integrated Discovery (DAVID) [24] to perform functional enrichment analyses and elucidate the biological processes where differentially expressed proteins were overrepresented. The enriched Kyoto Encyclopedia of Genes and Genomes (KEGG) pathways and gene ontology (GO) terms for biological processes in the list of the differentially expressed proteins were identified. The p-values of these enrichment analyses were adjusted using Benjamini–Hochberg ($p < 0.05$).

3. Results and Discussions

3.1. Obesity

At the end of this 12-week study, HF diet-fed rats were significantly heavier ($p < 0.05$; 549.4 ± 17.1 g) than CON rats (513.6 ± 14.8 g; Figure 1A), and FOS supplementation (554.3 ± 28.4 g) did not attenuate the obesity phenotype. HF diet-fed rats with or without FOS supplementation gained more weight during this period than CON rats ($p < 0.01$; Figure 1B). This finding is in contrast to results of a recent meta-analysis of human trials that concluded prebiotic consumption was associated with significant decreases in BMI and body weight. It has been suggested that products of FOS fermentation (e.g., SCFA) can modulate glucagon-like peptide-1 (GLP-1) secretion [25], and therefore, influence satiety and weight gain [26]. However, it is possible that the dose of FOS used in this study may not have been sufficiently high; anti-obesogenic effects of FOS have been demonstrated at 5% to 20% [18]. The dose used in our current study was not based on the efficacy of FOS to prevent obesity; rather it is based on a previous human study that examined changes in gut microbiota [19].

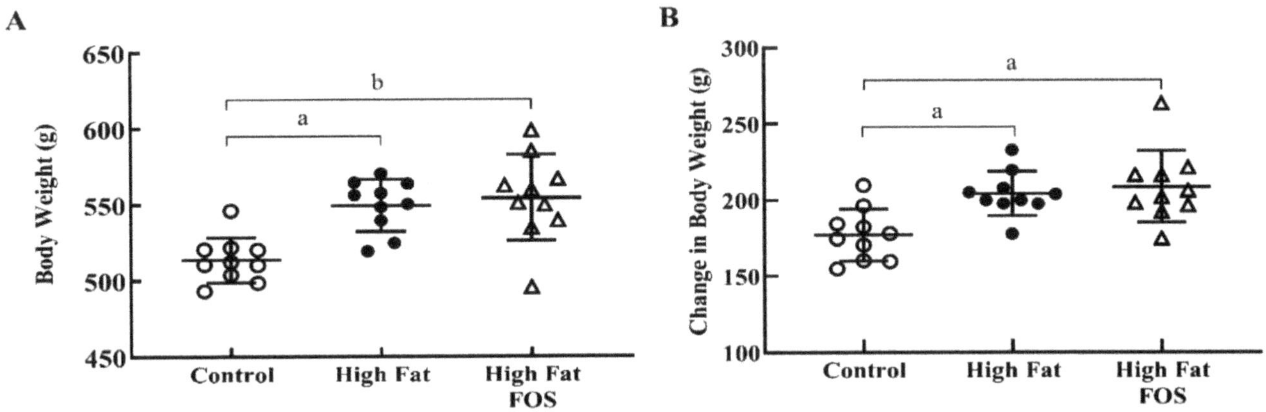

Figure 1. Body weights (mean ± standard deviation) for control, high-fat, and high fat-fructooligosaccharide (FOS) ($n = 10$ each group). (**A**) Total body weight after 12 weeks on experimental diets. (**B**) Change in total body weight after 12 weeks on experimental diets. (a) Tukey-adjusted p-value < 0.01; (b) Tukey-adjusted p-value < 0.001.

3.2. Glucose and Insulin

Serum glucose (Figure 2) and insulin (Figure 3) concentrations between experimental groups were not significantly different. This may be attributed to the blood samples not being obtained in the fasting state. Additionally, the dose of FOS used in the diet may have been too low to produce significant changes in these measures.

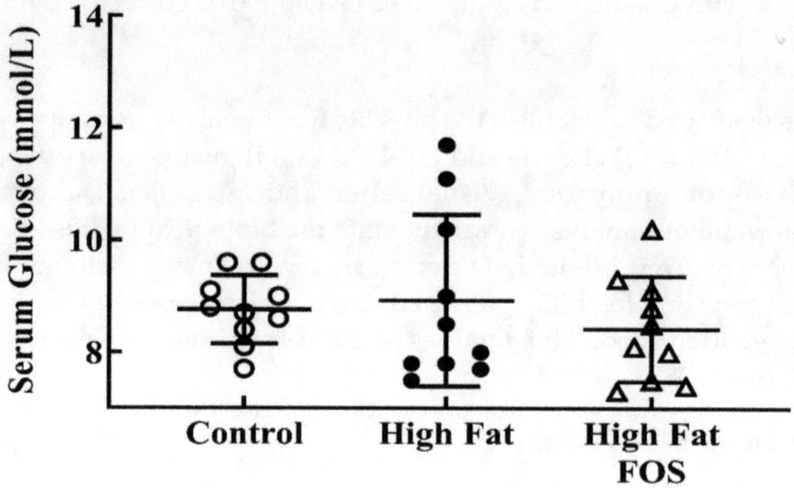

Figure 2. Non-fasting serum glucose (mmol/L) (mean ± standard deviation) for control, high-fat, and high fat-FOS (n = 10 each group) after 12 weeks were not significant by ANOVA.

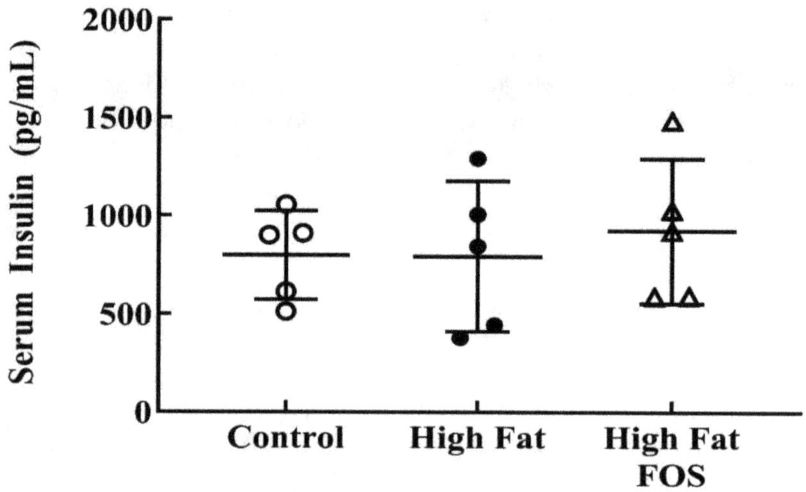

Figure 3. Non-fasting serum insulin (mean ± standard deviation) for control, high-fat, and high fat-FOS (n = 5 each group) after 12 weeks were not significant by ANOVA. Glucose and insulin were not measured for all animals in a group.

3.3. Histology

Figure 4 shows representative micrographs, with representative cardiomyocytes identified in cardiac tissue from rats on CON, HF and HF-FOS diets after 12 weeks of feeding. As shown in Figure 5, qualitative assessment revealed that HF diet was associated with hypertrophic cardiomyocytes ($p < 0.001$), but not increased interstitial fibrotic depositions, and hypertrophy was not attenuated by prebiotic treatment. This qualitative assessment was confirmed by quantification of cardiomyocyte area using Image J2 ($p < 0.05$). Cardiomyocyte area (mean percentage ± SD) was significantly increased ($p < 0.05$) in HF heart (84.69 ± 2.15) when compared to CON hearts (71.60 ± 2.75); this was not reversed by prebiotic treatment. Cardiomyocyte hypertrophy is a noted consequence of obesity [27], but increased cardiac fibrosis following HF has mainly been reported in long-term studies ranging over 7–16 months [28,29]. Although not measured directly in this study, it is likely that cardiac dysfunction would have resulted from HF feeding over a longer period of time [4].

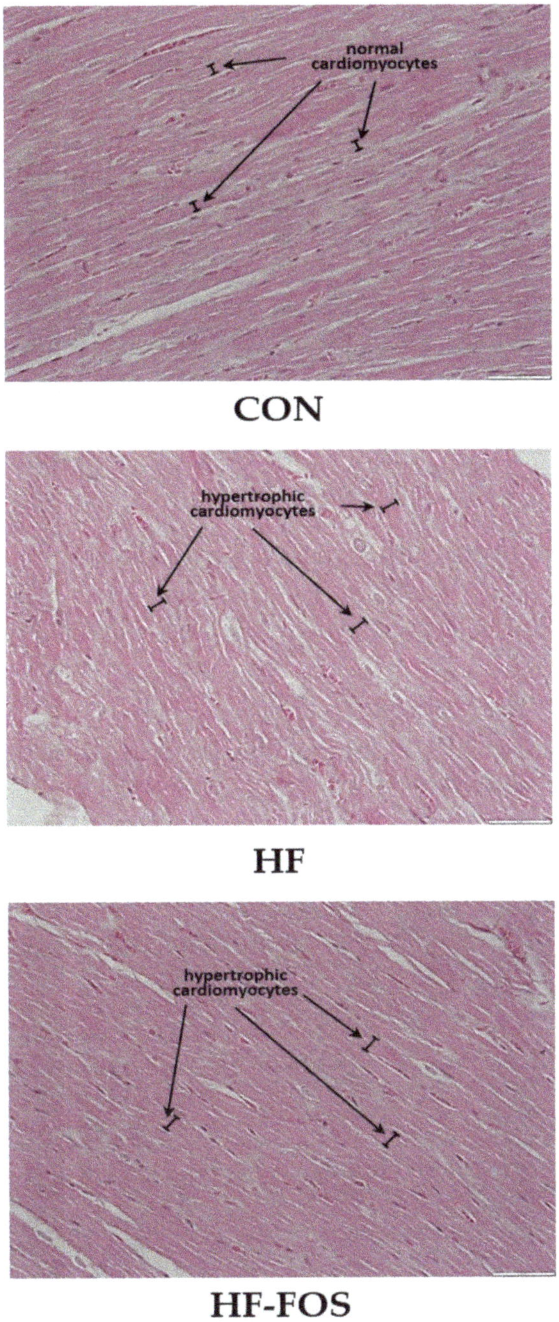

Figure 4. Sample micrographs (40 ×) of left ventricular tissue from CON, HF and HF-FOS groups with representative cardiomyocytes identified. CON, control diet; HF, high-fat diet; HF-FOS, high-fat diet supplemented with fructooligosacchride.

3.4. Cardiac Tissue Protein Expression

Of the 52,664 spectra obtained via mass spectrometry, 45,730 (87%) were quantitated at the thresholds used for this study, and 1501 proteins were identified and quantified (Supplemental Table S1). Compared to CON, HF treatment resulted in significant changes in protein expression: 10 were upregulated and 13 were downregulated (Supplemental Table S2). Five KEGG pathways and 11 GO biological processes were identified by DAVID (Table 2). Between the HF and HF-FOS groups, 117 proteins were significantly different with 96 downregulated and 21 upregulated (Table 3). DAVID identified 6 different GO biological processes that were significantly enriched (Table 4).

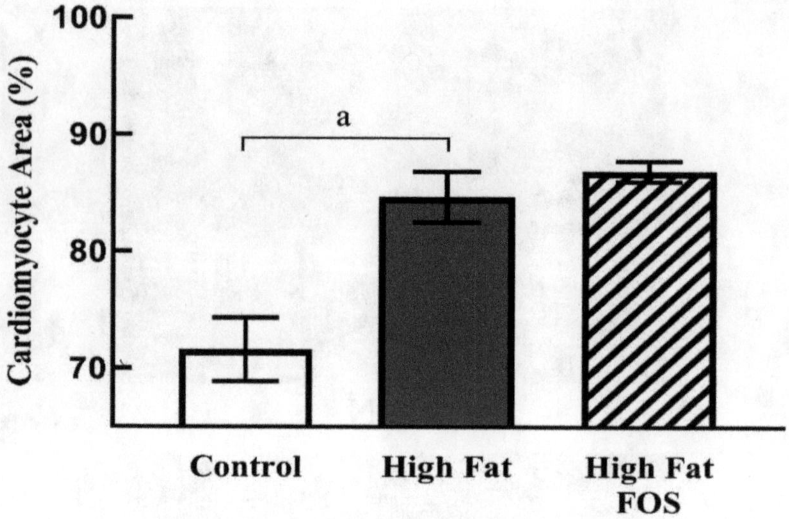

Figure 5. Cardiomyocyte area (mean ± SD) as a percentage of total area from left ventricular tissue in CON, HF and HF-FOS groups. Quantitation was done using ImageJ2. CON, control diet; HF, high-fat diet; HF-FOS, high-fat diet supplemented with fructooligosacchride; **a**: significantly different at $p < 0.05$; $n = 7$.

Table 2. Enriched gene ontology (GO) terms and KEGG pathways in the list of differentially expressed proteins in HF hearts compared to CON.

Biological Theme *	Gene Names ‡	GO and KEGG Pathways †	*p*-Value §
Metabolism (cholesterol)	**apolipoprotein A1 (*Apoa1*)** **apolipoprotein A4 (*Apoa4*)** apolipoprotein E (*Apoe*) **catalase (*Cat*)** **hydroxysteroid (17-beta) dehydrogenase 4 (*Hsd17b4*)**	Cholesterol metabolic process	3.3×10^{-4}
		KEGG:	
		Fat digestion and absorption	3.7×10^{-1}
		Peroxisome	1.6×10^{-1}
		Vitamin digestion and absorption	3.6×10^{-1}
Metabolism (lipid)	**apolipoprotein A1 (*Apoa1*)** **apolipoprotein A4 (*Apoa4*)** apolipoprotein E (Apoe)	VLDL remodelling	3.5×10^{-3}
		Positive regulation of cholesterol esterification	3.5×10^{-3}
		HDL particle assembly	3.5×10^{-3}
		Peripheral nervous system axon regeneration	6.5×10^{-3}
		Reverse cholesterol transport	6.5×10^{-3}
		Phospholipid efflux	7.5×10^{-3}
		Triglyceride catabolic process	2.1×10^{-2}
		Triglyceride homeostasis	2.0×10^{-2}
		Cholesterol Efflux	1.9×10^{-2}
		Lipoprotein metabolic process	1.9×10^{-2}
		KEGG:	
		Fat digestion and absorption	3.7×10^{-1}
		Vitamin digestion and absorption	3.6×10^{-1}

CON, control diet; HF, high fat diet. * The Functional Annotation Clustering general theme as indicated by DAVID. † GO (BP) is gene ontology (GO) biological process component (BP) and KEGG pathway is Kyoto Encyclopedia of Genes and Genomes biological pathway. ‡ **Gene names in bold** indicate that the protein respective to that gene was upregulated between groups; un-bolded gene names indicate downregulation of the respective protein between groups. § *p*-value of the enrichment analyses is significant at Benjamini–Hochberg $p < 0.05$.

Table 3. Differentially expressed proteins in heart tissue following high-fat with fructooligosaccharide vs. high-fat treatments.

Differentially Expressed Protein	Protein Accession No.	Log_2Fold Change (HF-FOS/HF) *	*p*-Value †	Gene Name
apolipoprotein A-IV (APOA4)	EDL95397.1	−0.16	<0.0001	*Apoa4*
catalase, isoform CRA_b (CAT)	EDL79667.1	−0.07	0.0011	*Cat*
creatine kinase, brain, isoform CRA_b (CKB)	EDL97457.1	−0.14	<0.0001	*Ckb*
electron transferring flavoprotein, alpha polypeptide (ETFA)	EDL95569.1	0.06	0.0010	*Etfa*
filamin, alpha (predicted), isoform CRA_b (FLNA)	EDL84990.1 (+1)	−0.12	<0.0001	*Flna*
four and a half LIM domains 1, isoform CRA_b (FHL1)	EDL75140.1	−0.13	0.0003	*Fhl1*
PREDICTED: annexin A6 isoform X1 (ANXA6)	XP_017453031.1	0.09	<0.0001	*Anxa6*
preproapolipoprotein A-I (APOA1)	CAA25224.1	−0.16	<0.0001	*Apoa1*
stress-70 protein, mitochondrial (HSPA9)	NP_001094128.2	−0.06	<0.0001	*Hspa9*
myosin regulatory light chain 2, ventricular/cardiac muscle isoform (MLY2)	NP_001030329.2	0.16	0.0001	*Myl2*
PREDICTED: guanylate-binding protein 1 (GBP1)	XP_006224340.1 (+1)	0.21	0.0002	*Gbp1*
tropomyosin 4 (TPM4)	EDL90830.1	−0.16	0.0002	*Tpm4*
glycerol-3-phosphate dehydrogenase 1-like protein (GPD11)	NP_001178814.1	−0.12	<0.0001	*Gpd1l*
heat shock protein, alpha-crystallin-related, B6/ Hsp20 (HSPB6)	EDM07749.1	−0.11	0.0026	*Hspb6*
LIM and cysteine-rich domains protein 1 (LMCD1)	NP_001008562.1	−0.13	<0.0001	*Lmcd1*
myomesin-1 (MYOM1)	NP_001178513.1	0.09	<0.0001	*Myom1*
nebulette (NEB1)	NP_001178623.1	−0.09	<0.0001	*Nebl*
nexilin, isoform CRA_c (NEXN)	EDL82495.1 (+1)	−0.09	0.0004	*Nexn*
PREDICTED: cAMP-dependent protein kinase type I-alpha regulatory subunit isoform X1 (PRKAR1a)	XP_017452536.1	−0.07	0.0015	*Prkar1a*
PREDICTED: cysteine and glycine-rich protein 3 isoform X1/ cardiac LIM protein (CSRP3)	XP_006229299.1	−0.11	0.0005	*Csrp3*
PREDICTED: heat shock protein HSP 90-alpha (LOC103692716)	XP_008763191.1	−0.07	0.0013	*LOC103692716*
PREDICTED: myomesin-2 isoform X1 (MYOM2)	XP_017455650.1	0.06	<0.0001	*Myom2*
actinin alpha 2 (ACTN2)	EDM06982.1	0.1	<0.0001	*Actn2*
ROK-alpha (Rho-associated protein expression kinase) (ROCK2)	AAB37540.1 (+1)	−0.1	0.0029	*Rock2*
sarcoplasmic/endoplasmic reticulum calcium ATPase 2 isoform a (ATP2A2)	NP_001103609.1	0.04	<0.0001	*Atp2a2*
vinculin (predicted), isoform CRA_a (VCL)	EDL86257.1	−0.05	0.0002	*Vcl*
acetyl-Coenzyme A dehydrogenase, short chain, isoform CRA_a (ACADS)	EDM13909.1	0.06	0.0003	*Acads*
aldehyde dehydrogenase (ALDH1A1)	AAA96657.1	0.25	0.0004	*Aldh1a1*
kynurenine—oxoglutarate transaminase 1, mitochondrial (KYAT1)	NP_001013182.3	−0.24	< 0.0001	*Kyat1*
PREDICTED: mimitin, mitochondrial (NDUFAF2)	XP_001073799.1	−0.18	0.0014	*Ndufaf2*
prolyl endopeptidase (PREP)	EDL99674.1 (+1)	−0.16	0.0005	*Prep*

Table 3. *Cont.*

Differentially Expressed Protein	Protein Accession No.	Log_2Fold Change (HF-FOS/HF) *	*p*-Value †	Gene Name
pyridine nucleotide-disulfide oxidoreductase domain-containing protein 2 (PYRDOXD2)	NP_001004261.1 (+3)	−0.27	<0.0001	*Pyroxd2*
cytochrome c-1 (predicted), isoform CRA_c (CYC1)	EDM15989.1	0.13	<0.0001	*Cyc1*
glutathione S-transferase omega 1 (GSTO1)	ACI32122.1	−0.12	0.0036	*Gsto1*
heat shock 70kDa protein 5 (glucose-regulated protein), isoform CRA_a (HSPA5)	EDL93170.1	−0.08	<0.0001	*Hspa5*
inter alpha-trypsin inhibitor, heavy chain 4, isoform CRA_a (LTIH4)	EDL88978.1	−0.12	<0.0001	*Ltih4*
kynurenine—oxoglutarate transaminase 3 (KYAT3)	NP_001015037.1	−0.13	0.0006	*Kyat3*
leucine-rich PPR motif-containing protein, mitochondrial precursor (LRPPRC)	NP_001008519.1	−0.06	<0.0001	*Lrpprc*
methylcrotonoyl-CoA carboxylase beta chain, mitochondrial (MCCC2)	NP_001012177.1	−0.07	<0.0001	*Mccc2*
methylcrotonoyl-CoA carboxylase subunit alpha, mitochondrial (MCCC1)	NP_001009653.1	−0.09	<0.0001	*Mccc1*
muscle glycogen phosphorylase (PYGM)	EDM12601.1	0.07	<0.0001	*Pygm*
Pgm1 protein, partial (PGM1)	AAI28704.1	−0.05	0.0003	*Pgm1*
PREDICTED: isobutyryl-CoA dehydrogenase, mitochondrial isoform X2 (ACAD8)	XP_003754442.1	−0.07	0.0025	*Acad8*
PREDICTED: triosephosphate isomerase (LOC100911515)	XP_003750702.2	−0.06	<0.0001	*LOC100911515*
rCG20653 (ACOT2)	EDL81468.1	0.07	0.0002	*Acot2*
rCG45082 (C3)	EDL83571.1	−0.05	<0.0001	*C3*
Tu translation elongation factor, mitochondrial (predicted), isoform CRA_c (TUFM)	EDM17456.1	−0.05	0.0001	*Tufm*
ubiquinol cytochrome c reductase core protein 2, isoform CRA_c (UQCRC2)	EDM17618.1	0.05	0.0005	*Uqcrc2*
glutathione peroxidase 1 (GPX1)	NP_110453.3	−0.1	0.0003	*Gpx1*
arginine-tRNA-protein transferase 1 (predicted), isoform CRA_a (ATE1)	EDM17146.1	−0.21	0.0026	*Ate1*
DnaJ (Hsp40) homolog, subfamily A, member 2, isoform CRA_b (DNAJ)	EDL87492.1	−0.15	<0.0001	*DnaJ*
rCG22471, isoform CRA_b (EEF1B2)	EDL98899.1	−0.21	<0.0001	*Eef1b2*
chaperonin subunit 8 (theta) (predicted), isoform CRA_a (CCT8)	EDM10642.1	−0.06	0.0026	*Cct8*
crystallin, alpha B, isoform CRA_a (CRYAB)	EDL95479.1	−0.12	<0.0001	*Cryab*
guanosine diphosphate dissociation inhibitor 1, isoform CRA_a (GDI1)	EDL84976.1	−0.08	0.0011	*Gdi1*
heat shock protein 27 (HSPB1)	AAA41353.1	−0.12	<0.0001	*Hspb1*
peptidylprolyl isomerase F (cyclophilin F), isoform CRA_a (PPIF)	EDL75095.1	−0.07	0.0026	*Ppif*
proteasomal ATPase (rat TBP1) (PSMC3)	BAA11939.1	−0.11	0.0003	*Psmc3*
proteasome (prosome, macropain) subunit, alpha type 1, isoform CRA_d (PSMA1)	EDM17781.1	−0.09	0.0037	*Psma1*
rCG38543, isoform CRA_a (PSMA7)	EDL88834.1	−0.07	0.0013	*Psma7*

Table 3. *Cont.*

Differentially Expressed Protein	Protein Accession No.	Log_2 Fold Change (HF-FOS/HF) *	*p*-Value †	Gene Name
drebrin-like, isoform CRA_b (DBN1)	EDM00307.1	−0.17	0.0011	*Dbnl*
oxidative-stress responsive 1 (predicted) (OXSR1)	EDL76918.1	−0.16	0.0019	*Oxsr1*
Ehd1 protein, partial (EHD1)	AAI60908.1	−0.08	<0.0001	*Ehd1*
EH-domain containing 4 (EHD4)	EDL79933.1	−0.1	<0.0001	*Ehd4*
heat shock 27kD protein family, member 7 (cardiovascular) (HSPB7)	EDL80988.1	−0.12	0.0038	*Hspb7*
nonmuscle myosin heavy chain-A (MYH9)	AAA74950.1	−0.12	<0.0001	*Myh9*
PDZ and LIM domain 1 (elfin), isoform CRA_a (PDLIM1)	EDL94180.1	−0.1	0.0017	*Pdlim1*
PREDICTED: adenylyl cyclase-associated protein 2 isoform X1 (CAP2)	XP_006253816.1	−0.12	< 0.0001	*Cap2*
PREDICTED: beta-1-syntrophin isoform X1 (SNTB1)	XP_017450243.1	−0.11	< 0.0001	*Sntb1*
PREDICTED: spectrin alpha chain, non-erythrocytic 1 isoform X1 (SPTAN1)	XP_008759895.1	0.06	0.0004	*Sptan1*
PREDICTED: tubulin-folding cofactor B (LOC103690005)	XP_017444696.1	−0.2	0.0011	*LOC103690005*
rCG27764, isoform CRA_a (DYNC1H1)	EDL97508.1	−0.08	<0.0001	
acyl-CoA synthetase family member 2, mitochondrial precursor (ACSF2)	NP_001030123.1	0.04	0.0012	*Acsf2*
acyl-Coenzyme A dehydrogenase, very long chain, isoform CRA_c (ACADVL)	EDM04964.1	0.06	<0.0001	*Acadvl*
arginine–tRNA ligase, cytoplasmic (RARS)	NP_001099247.2	−0.11	0.0002	*Rars*
catenin beta-1 (CTNNB1)	NP_445809.2 (+1)	−0.08	0.0026	*Ctnnb1*
calsequestrin 2, isoform CRA_a (CASQ2)	EDL85514.1	−0.05	0.0037	*Casq2*
cellular nucleic acid binding protein 1, isoform CRA_b (CNBP)	EDL91294.1	−0.12	0.0036	*Cnbp*
enoyl coenzyme A hydratase 1, peroxisomal (ECH1)	EDM07870.1	−0.1	<0.0001	*Ech1*
glutamate dehydrogenase 1, isoform CRA_a (GLUD1)	EDL88881.1	−0.05	0.0019	*Glud1*
GrpE-like 1, mitochondrial (GRPEL1)	EDM00047.1	−0.1	0.0007	*Grpel1*
Hagh protein, partial (HAGH)	AAH97301.1	−0.1	0.0025	*Hagh*
Keratin 5 (KRT5)	AAH62086.1	−0.56	0.0018	*Krt5*
L-3-hydroxyacyl-Coenzyme A dehydrogenase, short chain, isoform CRA_a (HADH)	EDL82212.1	0.09	0.0002	*Hadh*
PREDICTED: glycogen phosphorylase, brain form isoform X1 (PYGB)	XP_017446988.1	0.05	0.0026	*Pygb*
PREDICTED: microtubule-associated protein 4 isoform X1 (MAP4)	XP_006243875.1	−0.1	0.001	*Map4*
PREDICTED: myosin-binding protein C, cardiac-type isoform X1 (MYBPC3)	XP_006234566.1	0.07	<0.0001	*Mybpc3*
thioredoxin 2, isoform CRA_b (TXN2)	EDM15902.1	−0.27	0.0034	*Txn2*
TPA_exp: type II keratin Kb1 (KRT1)	DAA02055.1	−0.43	0.0038	*Krt1*
transcription factor A, mitochondrial, isoform CRA_a (TFAM)	EDL97257.1	−0.1	0.0023	*Tfam*
glutamate oxaloacetate transaminase 1, isoform CRA_a (GOT1)	EDL94253.	−0.07	<0.0001	*Got1*
Gpc1 protein (GPC1)	AAH61572.1	−0.08	0.0005	*Gpc1*

Table 3. *Cont.*

Differentially Expressed Protein	Protein Accession No.	Log_2Fold Change (HF-FOS/HF) *	*p*-Value †	Gene Name
isocitrate dehydrogenase 3 (NAD+) alpha, isoform CRA_a (IDH3a)	EDL95540.1	−0.06	0.0038	*Idh3a*
PREDICTED: myosin-7 isoform X2 (MYH7)	XP_006252013.1	−0.17	<0.0001	*Myh7*
ATPase family, AAA domain containing 3A (ATAD3A)	EDL81320.1	−0.17	0.0009	*Atad3a*
glyoxylase 1 (GLO1)	EDL96989.1	−0.14	0.0007	*Glo1*
PREDICTED: pre-B-cell leukemia transcription factor-interacting protein 1 isoform X4 (PBXIP1)	XP_017446382.1	−0.14	0.0012	*Pbxip1*
PREDICTED: solute carrier family 12 member 7 isoform X2 (SLC12A7)	XP_006227851.1	−0.19	<0.0001	*Slc12a7*
PREDICTED: transportin-1 isoform X1 (TNPO1)	XP_008758890.1	−0.25	0.0029	*Tnpo1*
AFG3-like protein 2 (AFG312)	NP_001128336.1	−0.08	0.0002	*Afg3l2*
annexin A5 (ANXA5)	NP_037264.1 (+ 4)	−0.12	<0.0001	*Anxa5*
clathrin heavy chain 1 (CLTC)	NP_062172.1	−0.06	<0.0001	*Cltc*
complement inhibitory factor H (CFH)	CAC67513.1	−0.09	<0.0001	*Cfh*
elongation factor 1-delta (EEFLD)	NP_001013122.1	−0.09	<0.0001	*Eef1d*
fibrinogen B beta chain (FGB)	AAA64866.1	−0.1	<0.0001	*Fgb*
inter-alpha-trypsin inhibitor heavy chain H3 precursor (ITIH3)	NP_059047.1 (+ 4)	−0.13	0.0033	*Itih3*
lumican (LUM)	EDM16832.1	0.06	0.0029	*Lum*
PREDICTED: dynamin-like 120 kDa protein, mitochondrial isoform X1 (OPA1)	XP_006248559.1	−0.07	<0.0001	*Opa1*
PREDICTED: fibrinogen alpha chain isoform X1 (FGA)	XP_006232594.1	−0.13	<0.0001	*Fga*
rat ribosomal protein L13a (RPL13A)	CAA48343.1	−0.11	0.0010	*Rpl13a*
rCG27551, isoform CRA_b (DSTN)	EDL95182.1	−0.1	0.0017	*Dstn*
rCG35863 (LAP3)	EDL99928.1	−0.11	<0.0001	*Lap3*
selenium-binding protein 1 (LOC103689947)	NP_001316822.1	−0.06	0.0023	*LOC103689947*
PREDICTED: similar to RIKEN cDNA 2310039E09 (CAVIN4)	EDL78187.1	−0.13	0.0023	*Cavin4*
Sucla2 protein, partial; succinate-coA ligase subunit beta (SUCLA2)	AAI66998.1	−0.06	0.0003	*Sucla2*
thioredoxin-like 5 (predicted), isoform CRA_b (TXNDC17)	EDM05095.1	−0.09	0.0014	*Txndc17*

HF-FOS, high-fat diet supplemented with fructooligosaccharide; HF, high fat diet. * Log_2Fold change of each protein (HF-FOS/HF). $-^{ve}$ values indicate downregulation and $+^{ve}$ values indicate upregulation of the protein in the HF-FOS group compared to HF. † *p*-value of the Mann–Whitney test with Benjamini–Hochberg multiple corrections test. Significant if $p < 0.0040$.

Table 4. Enriched GO terms and KEGG pathways of differentially expressed proteins between HF-FOS and HF diet groups in heart tissue according to biological theme.

Biological Theme *	Gene Names ‡	GO Terms and KEGG Pathways †	p-Value §
Fatty acid homeostasis	acyl-CoA dehydrogenase family, member 8 (*Acad8*) **acyl-CoA dehydrogenase, C-2 to C-3 short chain (*Acads*)** **acyl-CoA dehydrogenase, very long chain (*Acadvl*)** apolipoprotein A4 (*Apoa4*) **electron transfer flavoprotein alpha subunit (*Etfa*)**	GO-lipid homeostasis	3.0×10^{-2}
	acyl-CoA dehydrogenase family, member 8 (*Acad8*) **acyl-CoA dehydrogenase, C-2 to C-3 short chain (*Acads*)** **acyl-CoA dehydrogenase, very long chain (*Acadvl*)** **electron transfer flavoprotein alpha subunit (*Etfa*)**	GO-fatty acid beta-oxidation using acyl-CoA dehydrogenase	3.8×10^{-2}
Cardiac muscle regulation	calsequestrin 2 (*Casq2*) cysteine and glycine rich protein 3 (*Csrp3*) **myosin binding protein C, cardiac (*Mybpc3*)** myosin heavy chain 7 (*Myh7*) **myosin light chain 2 (*Myl2*)**	GO-cardiac muscle contraction	3.6×10^{-2}
	actinin alpha 2 (*Actn2*) **myomesin 1 (*Myom1*)** **myomesin 2 (*Myom2*)** **myosin binding protein C, cardiac (*Mybpc3*)** myosin heavy chain 7 (*Myh7*) tropomyosin 4 (*Tpm4*)	GO-muscle contraction	6.6×10^{-3}
Carbohydrate metabolism	**acyl-CoA dehydrogenase, C-2 to C-3 short chain (*Acads*)** catalase (*Cat*) glutamate dehydrogenase 1 (*Glud1*) glutamic-oxaloacetic transaminase 1 (*Got1*) isocitrate dehydrogenase 3 (NAD+) alpha (*Idh3a*) succinate-CoA ligase ADP-forming beta subunit t (*Sucla2*) triosephosphate isomerase-like (*LOC100911515*)	KEGG-carbon metabolism	7.3×10^{-2}
	glycerol-3-phosphate dehydrogenase 1-like (*Gpd1l*) glyoxalase 1(*Glo1*) hydroxyacyl glutathione hydrolase (*Hagh*) phosphoglucomutase 1 (*Pgm1*) **phosphorylase, glycogen, muscle (*Pygm*)** **phosphorylase, glycogen; brain (*Pygb*)**	GO-carbohydrate metabolic process	8.8×10^{-2}
Protein processes	GrpE-like 1, mitochondrial (*Grpel1*) chaperonin containing TCP1 subunit 8 (*Cct8*) crystallin, alpha B (*Cryab*) heat shock protein HSP 90-alpha (*LOC103692716*) heat shock protein family A member 9 (*Hspa9*) peptidylprolyl isomerase F (*Ppif*) thioredoxin 2 (*Txn2*)	KEGG-Protein folding	2.1×10^{-2}
Adhesion and cytoskeletal regulation	PDZ and LIM domain 1 (*Pdlim1*) arginyl-tRNA synthetase (*Rars*) chaperonin containing TCP1 subunit 8 (*Cct8*) drebrin-like protein (*Dbnl*) eukaryotic translation elongation factor 1 delta (*Eef1d*) heat shock protein family A member 5 (*Hspa5*) **spectrin, alpha, non-erythrocytic 1 (*Sptan1*)**	GO-cell-cell adhesion	4.5×10^{-2}

HF-FOS, high-fat diet with fructooligosaccharides; HF, high-fat diet. * The functional annotation clustering general theme as indicated by Database for Annotation, Visualization and Integrated Discovery (DAVID). † GO is gene ontology biological process component and KEGG is Kyoto Encyclopedia of Gene and Genomes biological pathway. ‡ **Gene names in bold** indicate that the protein respective to that gene was upregulated between groups; un-bolded gene names indicate downregulation of the respective protein between groups. § *p*-value of the enrichment analyses is significant at Benjamini–Hochberg $p < 0.05$.

3.4.1. Lipid Metabolism (HF vs. CON Diet): Supplemental Table S2 and Table 2

The expression of several proteins involved in lipid metabolism were affected by HF treatment apolipoprotein A-IV (APOA4) and preproapolipoprotein A-I (apolipoprotein A-I; APOA1) proteins were upregulated. In both animal and human experiments, increased APOA4 was associated with decreased atherogenicity [30,31] and increased apolipoprotein B to APOA1 ratio correlated with congestive heart failure in overweight and obese patients [32]. Therefore, an upregulation of these apolipoproteins may reflect a protective response following HF treatment.

Acyl-CoA synthetase family member 2, mitochondrial precursor (ACSF2) is involved in fatty acid synthesis [33] and was downregulated following HF treatment. In contrast, enoyl coenzyme A hydratase 1 (peroxisomal) (ECH1), which is involved in the beta-oxidation of fatty acids, was upregulated on HF presumably due to increased substrate flux. An upregulation of this enzyme has been shown to be protective in rodent models of obesity [34]. In addition to the aforementioned changes, the upregulation of hydroxysteroid (17-beta) dehydrogenase 4, isoform CRA b, partial (HSD17B4) (Supplemental Table S2 and Table 2), which is involved in the formation of 3-ketoacyl-CoA intermediates, suggests that more acetyl-CoA units were produced by fatty acid catabolism following HF treatment, but not utilised for ATP production.

In cardiac tissue, increased beta-oxidation has been suggested to be both adaptive and pathological. This is because lipid uptake can become toxic for the heart when excess fatty acids are converted to diacylglycerols or ceramides, both of which have roles in cardiac dysfunction and insulin resistance [35]. We have shown that HF feeding by obese rats over 12 weeks results in decreased expression of proteins associated with fatty acid synthesis and an increase in those involved in beta-oxidation. Pellieux et al. demonstrated that healthy mice had increased fatty acid oxidation proteins after HF feeding [36]. However, whether HF induced cardiomyopathy occurs because of increased fatty acid oxidation or lipid accumulation remains to be clarified [37].

Several proteins involved in ubiquinone metabolism were decreased by HF feeding; these included coenzyme Q9 partial (COQ9), ADCK3, mitochondrial isoform X1 (COQ8A) and electron transferring flavoprotein, alpha polypeptide (ETFA). Increased dietary COQ9 was shown to improve left ventricular performance, reduce myocardial infarct size and reduce cardiomyocyte apoptosis [38]. The observed reductions in these three proteins could reflect compromised cardiac function via disruption of oxidative phosphorylation, potentially leading to a reduction in ATP synthesis. Similarly, creatine kinase, brain isoform CRA_b (CKB), which catalyzes the transfer of phosphate between ATP and creatine, was downregulated (Table 2). This may be a protective adaptation since excessive myocardial creatine is associated with cardiac hypertrophy, dilatation, impaired contractile function [39] and impaired energy generating pathways including reduced glycolytic function [40].

3.4.2. Protein Metabolism (HF vs. CON Diet): Supplemental Table S2 and Table 2

Isovaleryl coenzyme A dehydrogenase, isoform CRA_a (IVD), RCG20683, isoform CRA_b, (maleylacetoacetate isomerase) (GSTZ1), Aldh4a1 protein, partial (ALDH4A1) and adenylosuccinate synthetase isozyme 1 (ADSSL1) proteins were all downregulated in the HF diet group (Table 2 and Supplemental Table S2). These proteins are all involved in various aspects of amino acid metabolism [41] with the exception of *Adssl1*, which encodes for a muscle-specific enzyme that catalyzes the first step in the conversion of IMP to AMP. As such, decreased production of these proteins suggest that HF treatment might have diminished amino acid catabolism and compromised energy production, likely in favour of fatty acid catabolism.

3.4.3. Oxidative Stress (HF vs. CON Diet): Supplemental Table S2 and Table 2

In terms of the regulation of ROS, catalase isoform CRA_b (CAT) was upregulated while tripartite motif protein 50 (predicted) (TRIM72) was downregulated in the HF group. The change in CAT expression is consistent with other studies that employed HF feeding. Increased fatty acid oxidation leads to more mitochondrial H_2O_2 production, and subsequently larger amounts of catalase is needed [42]. The decreased production of TRIM72 is contrary to this finding, since it is a membrane repair protein that is activated by the type of membrane damage that occurs during ischemic reperfusion injury or with exposure to oxidants such as H_2O_2 [43]. In hearts of a transgenic type I diabetes mellitus model, increased expression of CAT preserved normal cardiac morphology, prevented contractile defects, and reduced malondialdehyde-modified proteins. These authors also demonstrated that the source of the ROS and oxidative damage was the functioning mitochondria [44]. The NAD(P) transhydrogenase, mitochondrial isoform X1 (NNNT) protein regenerates NADPH that is utilised by glutathione peroxidase (GPX) and the thioredoxin/peroxiredoxin systems to convert H_2O_2 to H_2O and optimise ROS balance during cellular respiration [45]. Its downregulation in this experiment matches the trend seen with TRIM72, where ROS regulatory proteins were downregulated.

3.4.4. Cellular Growth and Proliferation (HF vs. CON Diet): Supplemental Table S2 and Table 2

Expression of several proteins involved in cellular growth and proliferation was affected by HF treatment: Annexin A6 isoform X1 (ANXA6), a calcium dependent protein involved in cardiac contractility, was decreased, while there were increases in Filamin, alpha (predicted), isoform CRA_b (FLNA), RCG49564, isoform CRA_a (Cadherin-2) (CDH2) and Stress-70 protein, (heat shock protein-70) mitochondrial (HSPA9). These all have different roles in cell membrane structure, proliferation and aging [46]. FLNA links actin to membrane glycoprotein and is therefore involved in cytoskeletal effects such as changes in cell shape, cell migration and adhesion. Altered expression of *AnxA6* might impair cardiac contraction and relaxation cycles [47]. CDH2 comes from a superfamily of adhesion molecules that mediate Ca^{2+}- dependent cell-to-cell adhesion in tissues [48]. In a model of myocardial hypertrophy, CDH2 was postulated as one of the mechanisms that enables the heart to maintain its physical structure and mechanical function by enhancing cell-to-cell contact and membrane connections [49]. Mitochondrial HSPA9 is a chaperone protein in the biogenesis and refolding of mitochondrial iron-sulfur proteins; it may also have a role in cell proliferation and cellular aging [46]. While the biochemistry of myocardial remodeling remains a mystery, these changes may reflect initial adaptations in cell growth, proliferation and migration consistent with the hypertrophy observed in hematoxylin and eosin stained tissues, and may eventually threaten cardiac compliance.

3.4.5. Lipid Metabolism (HF-FOS vs. HF Diet): Tables 3 and 4

Several proteins involved in the fatty acid homeostasis cluster were upregulated in the HF-FOS group compared to the HF group, with the exception of isobutyryl-CoA dehydrogenase (ACAD8) and apolipoprotein A4 (APOA4). HF rats had greater APOA4 levels compared to CON whereas FOS supplementation downregulated APOA4, which may have resulted in decreased intestinal lipid absorption [50] and/or altered fatty acid oxidation. Further, it was shown that SCFA infusion results in reduced APOA4 synthesis compared to long chain fatty acids [51]. Therefore, increased bacterial SCFA production following FOS supplementation may have downregulated APOA4, but it is unclear what impact this would have on cardiac function. HF-FOS also altered several acyl-coA dehydrogenases. While ACAD8 was downregulated, the upregulation of other dehydrogenases such as acyl-coenzyme A dehydrogenase, very long chain, isoform CRA_c (ACADVL) and acyl-CoA dehydrogenase short chain (ACADS) in the HF-FOS group indicates increased rates of beta-oxidation [52]. The upregulation of acyl-coA dehydrogenases, which require electron transfer flavoprotein alpha subunit (ETFA) as an electron acceptor [53], was associated with increased ETFA observed in HF-FOS hearts. Collectively, these changes point to increased oxidation of fatty acids, presumably as a result of high substrate availability from HF diets, and this was potentiated by FOS supplementation and the action of the gut microbiota.

Fermentation of FOS by the gut microbiota, specifically bifidobacteria [54], produces acetate and lactate which can then be interconverted to butyrate [55]. Butyrate that is leftover from colonocyte metabolism is transported to the liver and peripheral tissues, where it reduces lipid synthesis and increases beta-oxidation [56]. This is similar to the results seen with HF feeding in our study; however, FOS supplementation is expected to have an additive effect via the production of SCFAs, which would likely further reduce the synthesis of diacylglycerols or ceramides and protect against cardiac dysfunction and insulin resistance [35].

3.4.6. Protein Folding (HF-FOS vs. HF Diet): Tables 3 and 4

FOS-treatment downregulated all proteins in the protein folding cluster. Specifically, FOS supplementation decreased the expression of antioxidant and chaperone-like proteins, which tend to increase with obesity or diabetes. This reduction may be due to lower cellular stress in FOS-treated animals [57,58].

3.4.7. Adhesion and Cytoskeletal Regulation (HF-FOS vs. HF Diet): Tables 3 and 4

Most adhesion and cytoskeletal proteins also decreased with FOS. Specifically, eukaryotic translation elongation factor 1 delta (EEF1D) and drebrin-like protein (DBNL) were decreased with FOS treatment, whereas spectrin, alpha, non-erythrocytic 1 (SPTAN1) was increased. By upregulating SPTAN1, FOS treatment may have enhanced cardiomyocyte cell adhesion, and the transmittance of force between contractile proteins and the extracellular matrix [59], thereby promoting cardiac contractility.

3.4.8. Cardiac Muscle Regulation (HF-FOS vs. HF Diet): Tables 3 and 4

The HF-FOS group showed changes in several contractile proteins compared to the HF group. Calsequestrin 2 (CASQ2), which interacts with ryanodine receptors and modulate the duration of calcium efflux from the sarcoplasmic reticulum [60,61], decreased with FOS supplementation. While calcium handling and ryanodine receptor dysregulation are characteristics of cardiac pathologies, including heart failure [60], the specific role of CASQ2 in these diseases remains unclear. HF treatment alone did not result in a change in CASQ2 after 15 weeks [62], therefore the decrease found in our study is likely attributed to FOS and may protect against cardiac hypertrophy and failure [63]. However, further research into CASQ2 and its role in regulating sarcoplasmic calcium handling is needed to clarify whether the CASQ2 reduction seen in the HF-FOS group is advantageous.

Sarcomeric and cytoskeletal proteins were also altered in the HF-FOS group. Myosin binding protein C, cardiac (MYBPC3) was higher in the HF-FOS group compared to HF. MYBPC3 determines the number of myosin heads that can interact with actin [64,65] and during diastole, it decreases myosin-actin interaction to ensure complete relaxation [66]. Myosin light chain 2 (MYL2) is another protein associated with the myosin complex [67], and was upregulated in the HF-FOS group relative to HF. While FOS upregulated MYL2 levels, it is a reduction in MYL2 phosphorylation that is implicated in cardiac diseases [67]. The present study did not assess MYL2 phosphorylation, but increased levels may contribute to stability of the myosin complex. Hearts from FOS-supplemented rats also had lower expression of myosin heavy chain 7 (MYH7), also known as myosin heavy chain (MHC)-β. This protein has been shown to be elevated in diabetes due to a switch in the myosin isozyme from MHC-α to the less-efficient MHC-β [67,68]. Heightened levels of MHC-β hinder actin-myosin kinetics and increase the chance of cardiac dysfunction [67]. Therefore, the reduction in MHC-β seen in the HF-FOS group may be beneficial to cardiac function. The expression of myomesin1 and myomesin-2 isoform X1 (MYOM1 and MYOM2, respectively), found in the M-band of the sarcomere, were increased with FOS supplementation and likely improve myosin stability [69–71].

Expression of cysteine and glycine rich protein 3 (CSRP3) and actinin alpha 2 (ACTN2) were both changed with HF-FOS treatment. Both proteins are found in the Z-band, the protein complex that separates adjacent sarcomere units and anchors the sarcomere to the sarcolemma. A decrease in the ratio of cytoplasmic to nuclear CSRP3 correlates with impaired mechanosensing seen in heart failure [72]. Since ACTN2 is associated with thin filament stability, its upregulation could result in improved cardiac contractility [73].

3.4.9. Carbohydrate Metabolism (HF-FOS vs. HF Diet): Tables 3 and 4

FOS supplementation was associated with decreases in almost all proteins in the carbon metabolism cluster. In the mitochondria, glutamate dehydrogenase 1 (GLUD1) forms a tri-enzyme complex with glutamic-oxaloacetic transaminase 1 (GOT1) and malate dehydrogenase [74]; GOT1 and GLUD1 levels both decreased with HF-FOS feeding in the present study. IDH3A, a subunit of isocitrate dehydrogenase 3 associated with NADH production in the TCA cycle [75], was slightly decreased with FOS supplementation. Given our consistent finding of increased fatty acid oxidation associated with the HF diet, it is reasonable to expect that NADH production via the TCA cycle, and therefore GOT1,

GLUD1 and IDH3A would decrease. Succinate-CoA ligase ADP-forming beta subunit (SUCLA2) also functions in the TCA cycle. FOS was shown to increase intestinal succinate production in mice fed a HF/high-sucrose diet [76], and while the authors suggested that most of the succinate was metabolized in the cecum, our data indicates that FOS may also increase succinate within the heart. This increase in succinate supply could reduce TCA-production of succinate, causing the observed downregulation in SUCLA2 and other upstream TCA enzymes. Collectively, our data suggests that FOS affects metabolism by reducing TCA enzymes during HF feeding.

Glyoxalase 1, hydroxyacyl glutathione hydrolase (GLO1 and HAGH, respectively) and glutathione form the glyoxalase system that degrades methylglyoxal. Methylglyoxal is a by-product of glycolysis that leads to apoptosis and the production of advanced glycation end products (AGE) and ROS, and increases in diabetes [77,78] along with GLO1 activity and expression [79]. The decrease in GLO1 with FOS supplementation indicates that FOS could reduce inflammation and oxidative stress, resulting in less AGE production. A clinical trial is currently underway to determine whether inulin/FOS will decrease AGE formation in pre-diabetic adults [80]. Phosphoglucomutase 1 (PGM1) and glycogen phosphorylase, muscle (PYGM) are both involved in glycogen metabolism. PYGM breaks down glycogen into glycogen-1-phosphate while PGM1 carries out the reversible conversion of glucose-1-phosphate to glucose-6-phosphate. It is difficult to ascertain whether glycogen metabolism was up or downregulated with FOS, given that HF-FOS fed rats had greater levels of PYGM, but lower levels of PGM1. PGM1 was upregulated in skeletal muscle from diabetic patients [81], and glycogen accumulation is common in diabetic cardiomyocytes [82]. However, the role of glycogen in cardiac metabolism has yet to be fully understood [82] and thus we cannot discern whether the FOS-induced changes in PGM1 and PYGM would improve cardiac function.

4. Conclusions

We have attempted to reconcile the numerous changes in cardiac protein expression detected in the obese state with and without dietary FOS supplementation. Cardiomyocyte hypertrophy may be one of the earliest morphological changes. HF dietary treatment consistently resulted in increased fatty acid oxidation and reduction of energy production pathways; these were potentiated by FOS consumption. It is evident that obesity alters cardiac protein expression, including those associated with contractility, and some of these changes are modulated by FOS treatment. Importantly, these changes were not associated with significant differences in non-fasting blood insulin or glucose among experimental groups. Further research may elucidate the proteins and biochemical mechanisms that mediate these changes and predispose the heart to contractile failure. While a 12-week duration is longer than average prebiotic studies [83], extending the study period may help determine whether the observed fold changes translate to functional improvements at the organ level. Furthermore, a longer study duration may be more representative of the chronic nature of obesity and thus provide a clearer understanding of whether FOS mediates obesity-induced cardiac changes. Future research could also evaluate post-translational modifications, such as phosphorylation, which may be more indicative of cardiac function compared to protein abundance. Additionally, an assessment of the microbiome could support the proteomic findings, though studies have found an increase in *Bifidobacterium* with FOS supplementation in healthy adults [83]. To our knowledge, this is one of the first studies to describe the effects of HF feeding and FOS supplementation on the cardiac proteome and can therefore serve as a foundation for future work.

Author Contributions: Conceptualization, methodology, D.D.R., A.H. and S.T.C.; data analysis and manuscript writing, A.H., S.S. (Sidra Sarfaraz) and S.S. (Shamjeet Singh); writing—reviewing and editing, D.D.R., A.H. and S.T.C. All authors have read and approved of the manuscript. All authors have read and agreed to the published version of the manuscript.

Acknowledgments: We thank Stephen P.J. Brooks from the Bureau of Nutrition, Health Canada, for sharing tissues collected during the animal study and for valuable discussions; Judy Green, also from Health Canada, for excellent technical assistance; Jonathan Krieger from SPARC BioCentre, the Hospital for Sick Children, for performing the proteomic analysis.

References

1. Benjamin, E.J.; Muntner, P.; Alonso, A.; Bittencourt, M.S.; Callaway, C.W.; Carson, A.P.; Chamberlain, A.M.; Chang, A.R.; Cheng, S.; Das, S.R.; et al. Heart Disease and Stroke Statistics-2019 Update: A Report From the American Heart Association. *Circulation* **2019**, *139*, e56–e528. [CrossRef] [PubMed]
2. Peden, J.F.; Farrall, M. Thirty-five common variants for coronary artery disease: The fruits of much collaborative labour. *Hum. Mol. Genet.* **2011**, *20*, R198–R205. [CrossRef] [PubMed]
3. Piche, M.E.; Poirier, P.; Lemieux, I.; Despres, J.P. Overview of Epidemiology and Contribution of Obesity and Body Fat Distribution to Cardiovascular Disease: An Update. *Prog. Cardiovasc. Dis.* **2018**, *61*, 103–113. [CrossRef]
4. Travers, J.G.; Kamal, F.A.; Robbins, J.; Yutzey, K.E.; Blaxall, B.C. Cardiac Fibrosis: The Fibroblast Awakens. *Circ. Res.* **2016**, *118*, 1021–1040. [CrossRef]
5. Zhai, A.B.; Haddad, H. The impact of obesity on heart failure. *Curr. Opin. Cardiol.* **2017**, *32*, 196–202. [CrossRef]
6. Dixon, J.B. The effect of obesity on health outcomes. *Mol. Cell Endocrinol.* **2010**, *316*, 104–108. [CrossRef]
7. Akiyama, T.; Tachibana, I.; Shirohara, H.; Watanabe, N.; Otsuki, M. High-fat hypercaloric diet induces obesity, glucose intolerance and hyperlipidemia in normal adult male Wistar rat. *Diabetes Res. Clin. Pract.* **1996**, *31*, 27–35. [CrossRef]
8. Martins, F.; Campos, D.H.; Pagan, L.U.; Martinez, P.F.; Okoshi, K.; Okoshi, M.P.; Padovani, C.R.; Souza, A.S.; Cicogna, A.C.; Oliveira, S.A., Jr. High-fat Diet Promotes Cardiac Remodeling in an Experimental Model of Obesity. *Arq. Bras. Cardiol.* **2015**, *105*, 479–486. [CrossRef] [PubMed]
9. Abel, E.D.; O'Shea, K.M.; Ramasamy, R. Insulin resistance: Metabolic mechanisms and consequences in the heart. *Arter. Thromb. Vasc. Biol.* **2012**, *32*, 2068–2076. [CrossRef] [PubMed]
10. Silva Figueiredo, P.; Carla Inada, A.; Marcelino, G.; Maiara Lopes Cardozo, C.; De Cássia Freitas, K.; De Cássia Avellaneda Guimarães, R.; Pereira de Castro, A.; Aragão do Nascimento, V.; Aiko Hiane, P. Fatty Acids Consumption: The Role Metabolic Aspects Involved in Obesity and Its Associated Disorders. *Nutrients* **2017**, *9*, 1158. [CrossRef] [PubMed]
11. Wang, Z.V.; Li, D.L.; Hill, J.A. Heart failure and loss of metabolic control. *J. Cardiovasc. Pharmacol.* **2014**, *63*, 302–313. [CrossRef] [PubMed]
12. Cruz-Topete, D.; List, E.O.; Okada, S.; Kelder, B.; Kopchick, J.J. Proteomic changes in the heart of diet-induced pre-diabetic mice. *J. Proteom.* **2011**, *74*, 716–727. [CrossRef]
13. Miele, L.; Giorgio, V.; Alberelli, M.A.; De Candia, E.; Gasbarrini, A.; Grieco, A. Impact of Gut Microbiota on Obesity, Diabetes, and Cardiovascular Disease Risk. *Curr. Cardiol. Rep.* **2015**, *17*, 120. [CrossRef]
14. David, L.A.; Materna, A.C.; Friedman, J.; Campos-Baptista, M.I.; Blackburn, M.C.; Perrotta, A.; Erdman, S.E.; Alm, E.J. Host lifestyle affects human microbiota on daily timescales. *Genome Biol.* **2014**, *15*, R89. [CrossRef]
15. Kim, Y.A.; Keogh, J.B.; Clifton, P.M. Probiotics, prebiotics, synbiotics and insulin sensitivity. *Nutr. Res. Rev.* **2018**, *31*, 35–51. [CrossRef]
16. Le Bourgot, C.; Apper, E.; Blat, S.; Respondek, F. Fructo-oligosaccharides and glucose homeostasis: A systematic review and meta-analysis in animal models. *Nutr. Metab.* **2018**, *15*, 9. [CrossRef]
17. John, G.K.; Wang, L.; Nanavati, J.; Twose, C.; Singh, R.; Mullin, G. Dietary Alteration of the Gut Microbiome and Its Impact on Weight and Fat Mass: A Systematic Review and Meta-Analysis. *Genes* **2018**, *9*, 167. [CrossRef]
18. Choque Delgado, G.T.; Tamashiro, W. Role of prebiotics in regulation of microbiota and prevention of obesity. *Food Res. Int.* **2018**, *113*, 183–188. [CrossRef]
19. Clarke, S.T.; Green-Johnson, J.M.; Brooks, S.P.; Ramdath, D.D.; Bercik, P.; Avila, C.; Inglis, G.D.; Green, J.; Yanke, L.J.; Selinger, L.B.; et al. beta2-1 Fructan supplementation alters host immune responses in a manner consistent with increased exposure to microbial components: Results from a double-blinded, randomised, cross-over study in healthy adults. *Br. J. Nutr.* **2016**, *115*, 1748–1759. [CrossRef]
20. Ayoub, H.M.; McDonald, M.R.; Sullivan, J.A.; Tsao, R.; Meckling, K.A. Proteomic Profiles of Adipose and Liver Tissues from an Animal Model of Metabolic Syndrome Fed Purple Vegetables. *Nutrients* **2018**, *10*, 456. [CrossRef]
21. Nesvizhskii, A.I.; Keller, A.; Kolker, E.; Aebersold, R. A statistical model for identifying proteins by tandem mass spectrometry. *Anal. Chem.* **2003**, *75*, 4646–4658. [CrossRef] [PubMed]
22. Keller, A.; Nesvizhskii, A.I.; Kolker, E.; Aebersold, R. Empirical statistical model to estimate the accuracy of peptide identifications made by MS/MS and database search. *Anal. Chem.* **2002**, *74*, 5383–5392. [CrossRef]

23. Oberg, A.L.; Mahoney, D.W.; Eckel-Passow, J.E.; Malone, C.J.; Wolfinger, R.D.; Hill, E.G.; Cooper, L.T.; Onuma, O.K.; Spiro, C.; Therneau, T.M.; et al. Statistical analysis of relative labeled mass spectrometry data from complex samples using ANOVA. *J. Proteome Res.* **2008**, *7*, 225–233. [CrossRef]
24. Da Huang, W.; Sherman, B.T.; Lempicki, R.A. Systematic and integrative analysis of large gene lists using DAVID bioinformatics resources. *Nat. Protoc.* **2009**, *4*, 44–57. [CrossRef]
25. Canfora, E.E.; Jocken, J.W.; Blaak, E.E. Short-chain fatty acids in control of body weight and insulin sensitivity. *Nat. Rev. Endocrinol.* **2015**, *11*, 577–591. [CrossRef] [PubMed]
26. MacDonald, P.E.; Salapatek, A.M.; Wheeler, M.B. Glucagon-like peptide-1 receptor activation antagonizes voltage-dependent repolarizing K(+) currents in beta-cells: A possible glucose-dependent insulinotropic mechanism. *Diabetes* **2002**, *51* (Suppl. 3), S443–S447. [CrossRef]
27. Brady, T.M. The Role of Obesity in the Development of Left Ventricular Hypertrophy Among Children and Adolescents. *Curr. Hypertens. Rep.* **2016**, *18*, 3. [CrossRef]
28. Calligaris, S.D.; Lecanda, M.; Solis, F.; Ezquer, M.; Gutierrez, J.; Brandan, E.; Leiva, A.; Sobrevia, L.; Conget, P. Mice long-term high-fat diet feeding recapitulates human cardiovascular alterations: An animal model to study the early phases of diabetic cardiomyopathy. *PLoS ONE* **2013**, *8*, e60931. [CrossRef]
29. Oliveira, S.A., Jr.; Martinez, P.F.; Guizoni, D.M.; Campos, D.H.; Fernandes, T.; Oliveira, E.M.; Okoshi, M.P.; Okoshi, K.; Padovani, C.R.; Cicogna, A.C. AT1 receptor blockade attenuates insulin resistance and myocardial remodeling in rats with diet-induced obesity. *PLoS ONE* **2014**, *9*, e86447. [CrossRef]
30. Kronenberg, F.; Stuhlinger, M.; Trenkwalder, E.; Geethanjali, F.S.; Pachinger, O.; von Eckardstein, A.; Dieplinger, H. Low apolipoprotein A-IV plasma concentrations in men with coronary artery disease. *J. Am. Coll. Cardiol.* **2000**, *36*, 751–757. [CrossRef]
31. Wang, F.; Kohan, A.B.; Lo, C.M.; Liu, M.; Howles, P.; Tso, P. Apolipoprotein A-IV: A protein intimately involved in metabolism. *J. Lipid Res.* **2015**, *56*, 1403–1418. [CrossRef]
32. Lu, M.; Lu, Q.; Zhang, Y.; Tian, G. ApoB/apoA1 is an effective predictor of coronary heart disease risk in overweight and obesity. *J. Biomed. Res.* **2011**, *25*, 266–273. [CrossRef]
33. Black, P.N.; DiRusso, C.C. Transmembrane movement of exogenous long-chain fatty acids: Proteins, enzymes, and vectorial esterification. *Microbiol. Mol. Biol. Rev.* **2003**, *67*, 454–472. [CrossRef]
34. Xie, W.D.; Wang, H.; Zhang, J.F.; Li, J.N.; Can, Y.; Qing, L.; Kung, H.F.; Zhang, Y.O. Enhanced peroxisomal beta-oxidation metabolism in visceral adipose tissues of high-fat diet-fed obesity-resistant C57BL/6 mice. *Exp. Ther. Med.* **2011**, *2*, 309–315. [CrossRef]
35. Zhang, L.; Ussher, J.R.; Oka, T.; Cadete, V.J.; Wagg, C.; Lopaschuk, G.D. Cardiac diacylglycerol accumulation in high fat-fed mice is associated with impaired insulin-stimulated glucose oxidation. *Cardiovasc. Res.* **2011**, *89*, 148–156. [CrossRef]
36. Pellieux, C.; Montessuit, C.; Papageorgiou, I.; Pedrazzini, T.; Lerch, R. Differential effects of high-fat diet on myocardial lipid metabolism in failing and nonfailing hearts with angiotensin II-mediated cardiac remodeling in mice. *Am. J. Physiol. Heart Circ. Physiol.* **2012**, *302*, H1795–H1805. [CrossRef]
37. Drosatos, K.; Schulze, P.C. Cardiac lipotoxicity: Molecular pathways and therapeutic implications. *Curr. Heart Fail. Rep.* **2013**, *10*, 109–121. [CrossRef]
38. Lekli, I.; Das, S.; Das, S.; Mukherjee, S.; Bak, I.; Juhasz, B.; Bagchi, D.; Trimurtulu, G.; Krishnaraju, A.V.; Sengupta, K.; et al. Coenzyme Q9 provides cardioprotection after converting into coenzyme Q10. *J. Agric. Food Chem.* **2008**, *56*, 5331–5337. [CrossRef]
39. Cao, F.; Zervou, S.; Lygate, C.A. The creatine kinase system as a therapeutic target for myocardial ischaemia-reperfusion injury. *Biochem. Soc. Trans.* **2018**, *46*, 1119–1127. [CrossRef]
40. Zervou, S.; Yin, X.; Nabeebaccus, A.A.; O'Brien, B.A.; Cross, R.L.; McAndrew, D.J.; Atkinson, R.A.; Eykyn, T.R.; Mayr, M.; Neubauer, S.; et al. Proteomic and metabolomic changes driven by elevating myocardial creatine suggest novel metabolic feedback mechanisms. *Amino Acids* **2016**, *48*, 1969–1981. [CrossRef] [PubMed]
41. Fernandez-Canon, J.M.; Baetscher, M.W.; Finegold, M.; Burlingame, T.; Gibson, K.M.; Grompe, M. Maleylacetoacetate isomerase (MAAI/GSTZ)-deficient mice reveal a glutathione-dependent nonenzymatic bypass in tyrosine catabolism. *Mol. Cell Biol.* **2002**, *22*, 4943–4951. [CrossRef]
42. Rindler, P.M.; Plafker, S.M.; Szweda, L.I.; Kinter, M. High dietary fat selectively increases catalase expression within cardiac mitochondria. *J. Biol. Chem.* **2013**, *288*, 1979–1990. [CrossRef] [PubMed]

43. Kohr, M.J.; Evangelista, A.M.; Ferlito, M.; Steenbergen, C.; Murphy, E. S-nitrosylation of TRIM72 at cysteine 144 is critical for protection against oxidation-induced protein degradation and cell death. *J. Mol. Cell Cardiol.* **2014**, *69*, 67–74. [CrossRef]
44. Carlson, E.C.; Ye, G.; Xu, M.; Metreveli, N.S.; Epstein, P.N.; Donthi, R.V.; Xia, S. Catalase protects cardiomyocyte function in models of type 1 and type 2 diabetes. *Diabetes* **2004**, *53*, 1336–1343.
45. Kohlhaas, M.; Nickel, A.G.; Maack, C. Mitochondrial energetics and calcium coupling in the heart. *J. Physiol.* **2017**, *595*, 3753–3763. [CrossRef]
46. Hu, F.; Liu, F. Mitochondrial stress: A bridge between mitochondrial dysfunction and metabolic diseases? *Cell Signal* **2011**, *23*, 1528–1533. [CrossRef]
47. Mishra, S.; Chander, V.; Banerjee, P.; Oh, J.G.; Lifirsu, E.; Park, W.J.; Kim, D.H.; Bandyopadhyay, A. Interaction of annexin A6 with alpha actinin in cardiomyocytes. *BMC Cell Biol.* **2011**, *12*, 7. [CrossRef] [PubMed]
48. Chopra, A.; Tabdanov, E.; Patel, H.; Janmey, P.A.; Kresh, J.Y. Cardiac myocyte remodeling mediated by N-cadherin-dependent mechanosensing. *Am. J. Physiol. Heart Circ. Physiol.* **2011**, *300*, H1252–H1266. [CrossRef]
49. Mu, L.; Jing, C.; Guo, Z. Expression of N-cadherin proteins in myocardial hypertrophy in rats. *Exp. Ther. Med.* **2014**, *7*, 355–359. [CrossRef]
50. Kohan, A.B.; Wang, F.; Lo, C.M.; Liu, M.; Tso, P. ApoA-IV: Current and emerging roles in intestinal lipid metabolism, glucose homeostasis, and satiety. *Am. J. Physiol. Gastrointest. Liver Physiol.* **2015**, *308*, G472–G481. [CrossRef]
51. Kalogeris, T.J.; Monroe, F.; Demichele, S.J.; Tso, P. Intestinal synthesis and lymphatic secretion of apolipoprotein A-IV vary with chain length of intestinally infused fatty acids in rats. *J. Nutr.* **1996**, *126*, 2720–2729. [CrossRef] [PubMed]
52. Marín-García, J.; Goldenthal, M.J.; Moe, G.W. *Post-Genomic Cardiology*; Academic Press: Boston, MA, USA, 2007; p. 680.
53. Ikeda, Y.; Okamura-Ikeda, K.; Tanaka, K. Purification and characterization of short-chain, medium-chain, and long-chain acyl-CoA dehydrogenases from rat liver mitochondria. Isolation of the holo- and apoenzymes and conversion of the apoenzyme to the holoenzyme. *J. Biol. Chem.* **1985**, *260*, 1311–1325. [PubMed]
54. Damian, F.; Van den Mooter, G.; Samyn, C.; Kinget, R. In vitro biodegradation study of acetyl and methyl inulins by Bifidobacteria and inulinase. *Eur. J. Pharm. Biopharm.* **1999**, *47*, 275–282. [CrossRef]
55. Morrison, D.J.; Mackay, W.G.; Edwards, C.A.; Preston, T.; Dodson, B.; Weaver, L.T. Butyrate production from oligofructose fermentation by the human faecal flora: What is the contribution of extracellular acetate and lactate? *Br. J. Nutr.* **2006**, *96*, 570–577. [CrossRef]
56. Den Besten, G.; van Eunen, K.; Groen, A.K.; Venema, K.; Reijngoud, D.J.; Bakker, B.M. The role of short-chain fatty acids in the interplay between diet, gut microbiota, and host energy metabolism. *J. Lipid Res.* **2013**, *54*, 2325–2340. [CrossRef]
57. Cani, P.D.; Possemiers, S.; Van de Wiele, T.; Guiot, Y.; Everard, A.; Rottier, O.; Geurts, L.; Naslain, D.; Neyrinck, A.; Lambert, D.M.; et al. Changes in gut microbiota control inflammation in obese mice through a mechanism involving GLP-2-driven improvement of gut permeability. *Gut* **2009**, *58*, 1091–1103. [CrossRef]
58. Yoo, J.Y.; Kim, S.S. Probiotics and prebiotics: Present status and future perspectives on metabolic disorders. *Nutrients* **2016**, *8*, 173. [CrossRef]
59. Bennett, P.M.; Baines, A.J.; Lecomte, M.C.; Maggs, A.M.; Pinder, J.C. Not just a plasma membrane protein: In cardiac muscle cells alpha-II spectrin also shows a close association with myofibrils. *J. Muscle Res. Cell Motil.* **2004**, *25*, 119–126. [CrossRef]
60. Gyorke, I.; Hester, N.; Jones, L.R.; Gyorke, S. The role of calsequestrin, triadin, and junctin in conferring cardiac ryanodine receptor responsiveness to luminal calcium. *Biophys. J.* **2004**, *86*, 2121–2128. [CrossRef]
61. Terentyev, D.; Viatchenko-Karpinski, S.; Gyorke, I.; Volpe, P.; Williams, S.C.; Gyorke, S. Calsequestrin determines the functional size and stability of cardiac intracellular calcium stores: Mechanism for hereditary arrhythmia. *Proc. Natl. Acad. Sci. USA* **2003**, *100*, 11759–11764. [CrossRef]
62. Lima-Leopoldo, A.P.; Leopoldo, A.S.; da Silva, D.C.; do Nascimento, A.F.; de Campos, D.H.; Luvizotto, R.A.; de Deus, A.F.; Freire, P.P.; Medeiros, A.; Okoshi, K.; et al. Long-term obesity promotes alterations in diastolic function induced by reduction of phospholamban phosphorylation at serine-16 without affecting calcium handling. *J. Appl. Physiol.* **2014**, *117*, 669–678. [CrossRef]

63. Sato, Y.; Ferguson, D.G.; Sako, H.; Dorn, G.W., II; Kadambi, V.J.; Yatani, A.; Hoit, B.D.; Walsh, R.A.; Kranias, E.G. Cardiac-specific overexpression of mouse cardiac calsequestrin is associated with depressed cardiovascular function and hypertrophy in transgenic mice. *J. Biol. Chem.* **1998**, *273*, 28470–28477. [CrossRef]
64. Flashman, E.; Redwood, C.; Moolman-Smook, J.; Watkins, H. Cardiac myosin binding protein C: Its role in physiology and disease. *Circ. Res.* **2004**, *94*, 1279–1289. [CrossRef]
65. Winegrad, S. Cardiac myosin binding protein C. *Circ. Res.* **1999**, *84*, 1117–1126. [CrossRef]
66. Pohlmann, L.; Kroger, I.; Vignier, N.; Schlossarek, S.; Kramer, E.; Coirault, C.; Sultan, K.R.; El-Armouche, A.; Winegrad, S.; Eschenhagen, T.; et al. Cardiac myosin-binding protein C is required for complete relaxation in intact myocytes. *Circ. Res.* **2007**, *101*, 928–938. [CrossRef]
67. Waddingham, M.T.; Edgley, A.J.; Tsuchimochi, H.; Kelly, D.J.; Shirai, M.; Pearson, J.T. Contractile apparatus dysfunction early in the pathophysiology of diabetic cardiomyopathy. *World J. Diabetes* **2015**, *6*, 943–960. [CrossRef] [PubMed]
68. Rundell, V.L.; Geenen, D.L.; Buttrick, P.M.; de Tombe, P.P. Depressed cardiac tension cost in experimental diabetes is due to altered myosin heavy chain isoform expression. *Am. J. Physiol. Heart Circ. Physiol.* **2004**, *287*, H408–H413. [CrossRef]
69. Agarkova, I.; Perriard, J.C. The M-band: An elastic web that crosslinks thick filaments in the center of the sarcomere. *Trends Cell Biol.* **2005**, *15*, 477–485. [CrossRef]
70. Pask, H.T.; Jones, K.L.; Luther, P.K.; Squire, J.M. M-band structure, M-bridge interactions and contraction speed in vertebrate cardiac muscles. *J. Muscle Res. Cell Motil.* **1994**, *15*, 633–645. [CrossRef]
71. Rozanski, A.; Takano, A.P.; Kato, P.N.; Soares, A.G.; Lellis-Santos, C.; Campos, J.C.; Ferreira, J.C.; Barreto-Chaves, M.L.; Moriscot, A.S. M-protein is down-regulated in cardiac hypertrophy driven by thyroid hormone in rats. *Mol. Endocrinol.* **2013**, *27*, 2055–2065. [CrossRef] [PubMed]
72. Paudyal, A.; Dewan, S.; Ikie, C.; Whalley, B.J.; de Tombe, P.P.; Boateng, S.Y. Nuclear accumulation of myocyte muscle LIM protein is regulated by heme oxygenase 1 and correlates with cardiac function in the transition to failure. *J. Physiol.* **2016**, *594*, 3287–3305. [CrossRef]
73. Communal, C.; Sumandea, M.; de Tombe, P.; Narula, J.; Solaro, R.J.; Hajjar, R.J. Functional consequences of caspase activation in cardiac myocytes. *Proc. Natl. Acad. Sci. USA* **2002**, *99*, 6252–6256. [CrossRef]
74. Fahien, L.A.; Macdonald, M.J. The complex mechanism of glutamate dehydrogenase in insulin secretion. *Diabetes* **2011**, *60*, 2450–2454. [CrossRef]
75. Kim, H.K.; Thu, V.T.; Heo, H.J.; Kim, N.; Han, J. Cardiac proteomic responses to ischemia-reperfusion injury and ischemic preconditioning. *Expert Rev. Proteom.* **2011**, *8*, 241–261. [CrossRef]
76. De Vadder, F.; Kovatcheva-Datchary, P.; Zitoun, C.; Duchampt, A.; Backhed, F.; Mithieux, G. Microbiota-Produced Succinate Improves Glucose Homeostasis via Intestinal Gluconeogenesis. *Cell Metab.* **2016**, *24*, 151–157. [CrossRef]
77. Brownlee, M. Biochemistry and molecular cell biology of diabetic complications. *Nature* **2001**, *414*, 813–820. [CrossRef] [PubMed]
78. Rabbani, N.; Thornalley, P.J. Glyoxalase in diabetes, obesity and related disorders. *Semin. Cell Dev. Biol.* **2011**, *22*, 309–317. [CrossRef]
79. Brouwers, O.; de Vos-Houben, J.M.; Niessen, P.M.; Miyata, T.; van Nieuwenhoven, F.; Janssen, B.J.; Hageman, G.; Stehouwer, C.D.; Schalkwijk, C.G. Mild oxidative damage in the diabetic rat heart is attenuated by glyoxalase-1 overexpression. *Int. J. Mol. Sci.* **2013**, *14*, 15724–15739. [CrossRef]
80. Kellow, N.J.; Coughlan, M.T.; Savige, G.S.; Reid, C.M. Effect of dietary prebiotic supplementation on advanced glycation, insulin resistance and inflammatory biomarkers in adults with pre-diabetes: A study protocol for a double-blind placebo-controlled randomised crossover clinical trial. *BMC Endocr. Disord.* **2014**, *14*, 55. [CrossRef] [PubMed]
81. Hojlund, K.; Wrzesinski, K.; Larsen, P.M.; Fey, S.J.; Roepstorff, P.; Handberg, A.; Dela, F.; Vinten, J.; McCormack, J.G.; Reynet, C.; et al. Proteome analysis reveals phosphorylation of ATP synthase beta -subunit in human skeletal muscle and proteins with potential roles in type 2 diabetes. *J. Biol. Chem.* **2003**, *278*, 10436–10442. [CrossRef] [PubMed]
82. Varma, U.; Koutsifeli, P.; Benson, V.L.; Mellor, K.M.; Delbridge, L.M.D. Molecular mechanisms of cardiac pathology in diabetes—Experimental insights. *Biochim. Biophys. Acta Mol. Basis. Dis.* **2018**, *1864*, 1949–1959. [CrossRef]

2

Low Urinary Iodine Concentrations Associated with Dyslipidemia in US Adults

Kyung Won Lee, Dayeon Shin and Won O. Song *

Department of Food Science and Human Nutrition, Michigan State University, 469 Wilson Road, Trout FSHN Building, East Lansing, MI 48824, USA; kyungwon@msu.edu (K.W.L.); shinda@msu.edu (D.S.)
* Correspondence: song@msu.edu

Abstract: Iodine is an essential component of the thyroid hormone which plays crucial roles in healthy thyroid function and lipid metabolism. However, the association between iodine status and dyslipidemia has not been well established at a population level. We aimed to test the hypothesis that the odds of dyslipidemia including elevated total cholesterol, triglycerides, low-density lipoprotein (LDL) cholesterol and apolipoprotein B, and lowered high-density lipoprotein (HDL) cholesterol and HDL/LDL ratio are associated with urinary iodine concentration (UIC) in a population perspective. Data of 2495 US adults (⩾20 years) in the National Health and Nutrition Examination Survey 2007–2012 were used in this study. Two subgroups (*i.e.*, UIC below *vs.* above the 10th percentile) were compared of dyslipidemia as defined based on NCEP ATP III guidelines. The differences between the groups were tested statistically by chi-square test, simple linear regressions, and multiple logistic regressions. Serum lipid concentrations differed significantly between two iodine status groups when sociodemographic and lifestyle covariates were controlled (all, $p < 0.05$). Those with the lowest decile of UIC were more likely to be at risk for elevated total cholesterol (>200 mg/dL) (adjusted odds ratio (AOR) = 1.51, 95% confidence interval (CI): 1.03–2.23) and elevated LDL cholesterol (>130 mg/dL) (AOR = 1.58, 95% CI: 1.11–2.23) and lowered HDL/LDL ratio (<0.4) (AOR = 1.66, 95% CI: 1.18–2.33), compared to those with UIC above the 10th percentile. In US adults, low UIC was associated with increased odds for dyslipidemia. Findings of the present cross-sectional study with spot urine samples highlight the significant association between UIC and serum lipids at population level, but do not substantiate a causal relationship. Further investigations are warranted to elucidate the causal relationship among iodine intakes, iodine status, and serum lipid profiles.

Keywords: iodine; serum lipids; cholesterol; dyslipidemia; NHANES

---

1. Introduction

Iodine is an indispensable component of thyroid hormone biosynthesis and normal thyroid function [1]. Thyroid hormone plays a key role in the regulation of multiple mechanisms, particularly lipid synthesis and absorption [2]. Since every cell in the body is affected by thyroid hormone, iodine status is associated with various health outcomes including goiter, hypothyroidism, mental retardation, and dyslipidemia [3]. Impaired lipid metabolism may be resulted from inadequate thyroid hormone production due to insufficient iodine [4]. In an iodine deficient population, serum thyroid stimulating hormone (TSH) levels is elevated to prompt an uptake of circulating iodine by the thyroid [5]. It has been reported that elevated TSH has a positive association with risk for dyslipidemia [6]. Additionally, abnormal thyroid hormone due to iodine deficiency may lead to adverse aftereffects such as hypothyroidism throughout various life stages [7]. It is well-known that hypothyroidism is a major risk factor for the development of dyslipidemia, hypercholesterolemia and cardiovascular disease (CVD) [8,9]. Hypothyroidism accelerates elevations in serum total cholesterol and low-density lipoprotein (LDL) cholesterol by increasing cholesterol absorption in the intestines and lowering LDL cholesterol clearance from the serum. Moreover, hypothyroidism may increase serum triglycerides by decreasing lipoprotein lipase activity [10,11].

Dyslipidemia broadly describes abnormalities associated with serum lipid metabolism. Its clinical consequences are elevated levels of total cholesterol, triglycerides, and LDL cholesterol, and decreased high-density lipoprotein (HDL) cholesterol levels [12]. Dyslipidemia is one of the risk factors of CVD and a main component of metabolic syndrome. Increased social burdens resulting from CVD and metabolic syndrome have led to extensive investigations to prevent them in the field of nutrition [13,14]. Dyslipidemia consisting of elevated total cholesterol and LDL cholesterol has been observed in patients with hypothyroidism [15,16]. The majority of previous studies noted that abnormalities in total cholesterol and LDL cholesterol were normalized after the successful treatment of hypothyroidism [17,18]. Although many studies examined the association between thyroid dysfunction and lipid levels, we still have no adequate information regarding the relationship between iodine status and serum lipid levels. Only a very few studies have investigated the development of dyslipidemia in relation to iodine status. Uncontrolled and small scale studies have been conducted on the effects of iodine treatments in goitrous subjects with CVD and lipid abnormalities. Previous studies reported that iodine treatments for subjects with goiter resulting from iodine deficiency improved serum lipid profiles by lowering previously elevated total cholesterol and LDL cholesterol [19,20]. In a recent study with mice, hypothyroidic function due to insufficient iodine intake changed lipid profiles, while excessive iodine intake had a beneficial effect on lipid metabolism [21].

Considering that the prevalence of both iodine deficiency and dyslipidemia still remain high among some subgroups in the US [22,23], further research is appropriate to elucidate the association between iodine status and lipids. It takes a long time to develop dyslipidemia from hypothyroidism [11,24] and hypothyroidism from iodine deficiency [25]. If dyslipidemia is associated with inadequate iodine status, the correction for iodine status may have considerable benefits for prevention and treatment of dyslipidemia. Therefore, we hypothesized that urinary iodine concentration (UIC) is associated with the odds of dyslipidemia in the US population. The specific aims of our study were to identify sociodemographic and lifestyle variables affecting UIC and serum lipids, to determine the association of UIC with serum lipid levels, and to estimate risks for dyslipidemia by UIC using recently available National Health and Nutrition Examination Survey (NHANES) data collected from 2007 to 2012. UIC from a spot urine sample is the only indicator of iodine status that is currently available in the NHANES. UIC is a reliable indicator for the iodine status assessment, because more than 90% of dietary iodine appears in urine [26]. UIC from ten repeat collections from spot urine samples or 24-h urine samples can be applied to as a measurement for individual's iodine status, whereas single spot urine samples should be used to assess iodine status only at a population level [22,27]. Although it is hard to conclude anything at the individual level due to limitation of indicators for iodine status in the NHANES, we can describe an association between below *vs.* above the 10th percentile of UIC subgroups with serum lipid concentrations based on large population-based analyses.

2. Methods

2.1. Data Source and Study Sample

The NHANES, a cross-sectional examination survey, is conducted by the National Center for Health Statistics (NCHS) of the Centers for Disease Control and Prevention (CDC). Each NHANES survey is based on a complex, stratified, multistage, and probability cluster designed to obtain nationally representative samples of civilian, noninstitutionalized residents in the US [28]. The NHANES consists of interviews, laboratory tests, and physical examinations administered by highly trained staff [29]. NHANES protocols were approved by the NCHS Research Ethics Review Board and all subjects aged ⩾18 years participated voluntarily after giving their informed consent [30].

Detailed descriptions of survey plan and design have been previously provided in the NHANES analytic guidelines [28] and thus will not be explained here.

In 1999, the NHANES became a continuous survey with collecting data in every two-year cycles. In this study, we merged three continuous NHANES cycles (2007–2008, 2009–2010, and 2011–2012) and focused on 9164 US adults (⩾20 years) who participated in the NHANES 2007–2012 and have urinary iodine information. We excluded those who were pregnant and lactating women (n = 267), not eligible for data analyses because of missing information on serum lipids (n = 4871), those who were taking any medications for thyroid dysfunction or dyslipidemia (n = 824), and those with missing information on key sociodemographic and lifestyle characteristics (n = 707). The final analytic sample consisted of 2495 adults.

2.2. Definition of Dyslipidemia

We utilized NHANES serum laboratory information on total cholesterol, triglycerides, HDL cholesterol, LDL cholesterol, and apolipoprotein B levels to assess dyslipidemia. For this study, dyslipidemia was defined based on the guidelines provided in the third report of the US National Cholesterol Education Programme Adult Treatment Panel III (NCEP ATP III) [31]: total cholesterol >200 mg/dL for elevated total cholesterol; triglycerides >150 mg/dL for elevated triglycerides; HDL cholesterol <40 mg/dL in men and <50 mg/dL in women for lowered HDL cholesterol; LDL cholesterol >130 mg/dL for elevated LDL cholesterol; HDL/LDL ratio <0.4 for lowered HDL/LDL ratio; apolipoprotein B >130 mg/dL for elevated apolipoprotein B.

2.3. Iodine Status

The NHANES has included measured UIC to monitor the iodine status among US population aged 6 years and older since 1971. Information on UIC has been collected through spot urine samples by the Elemental Analysis Laboratory of the CDC's Division of Laboratory Sciences. UIC was measured by inductively coupled plasma mass spectroscopy (ICP-MS) based on the method by Caldwell *et al.* [32,33] using the same equipment at the same laboratories [34,35]. To examine the association of UIC and serum lipid levels, the participants included in this study were divided into deciles according to UIC distribution and the lowest decile of them was defined as having low UIC (9.0–47.2 μg/L). Then, serum lipid levels were compared between two subgroups (below *vs.* above the 10th percentile of UIC) [36].

2.4. Covariates

The NHANES included information collected on the sociodemographic and lifestyle characteristics through interviews administered by trained interviewers. In this study, variables included in the statistical analytic models were sex (men and women); age (20–39, 40–59, and ⩾60 years); race/ethnicity (non-Hispanic whites, non-Hispanic blacks, all Hispanics, and others); education (less than high school, high school, and more than high school); family poverty income ratio (PIR) (low, ⩽1.85; medium, 1.85 to ⩽3.5; and high >3.5) [28]; supplement use (reported use of a dietary supplement in the last 30 days; yes and no) [37]; smoking (serum cotinine level; low, <0.015 mg/L; medium, 0.015 to <10 mg/L; high, ⩾10 mg/L) [38]; alcohol consumption (average number of drinks/day; no drink, >0 to <1, 1 to <2, and ⩾2 drinks/day) [37]; BMI (underweight, <18.5 kg/m^2; normal, 18.5 to <25 kg/m^2; overweight, 25 to <30 kg/m^2; and obese, ⩾30 kg/m^2) [39]; physical activity (Metabolic Equivalent Task (MET)-minutes/week) from leisure-time physical activity: no activity, 0 to <500, 500 to <1000, and ⩾1000 MET-minutes/week [40].

2.5. Statistical Analyses

We analyzed all data with SAS (version 9.3, SAS Institute Inc, Cary, NC, USA). To account for complex survey design, survey nonresponse, and planned oversampling, we used SURVEY procedure including sample weight, stratum (SDMVSTRA), and primary sampling unit (SDMVPSU) recommended by NCHS for the NHANES analysis [29].

The chi-square test was performed to investigate the distributions (%) and the association between UIC and sociodemographic and lifestyle variables (categorical variables) (Table S1). We used bivariate methods based on simple linear regressions to test the differences in serum lipid profiles by sociodemographic and lifestyle variables (Tables 1 and 2). The variables that were significantly associated were considered as covariates in subsequent analyses. Serum lipid levels including total cholesterol, triglycerides, HDL cholesterol, LDL cholesterol, HDL/LDL ratio and apolipoprotein B (continuous variables) were compared between two subgroups (*i.e.*, below *vs.* above the 10th percentile of UIC) using linear regression (Table 3 and Table S2). Multiple logistic regression analyses were used to determine risks for abnormal lipid levels according to UIC (Table 4). Odds ratios (ORs) with 95% confidence intervals (CIs) were calculated after controlling for covariates in two models: unadjusted (model 1) and adjusted for sex, age, race/ethnicity, education, income, supplement use, smoking, alcohol consumption, BMI, and physical activity (model 2). Two-sided p values were considered to be statistically significant if $p < 0.05$.

Table 1. Unadjusted serum lipid status biomarker levels by sociodemographic variable categories for US adults, NHANES 2007–2012 [1].

Sociodemographic Variable		TC	TG	HDL-C	LDL-C	Apo B
		mg/dL	mg/dL	mg/dL	mg/dL	mg/dL
Sex	Men	196.8 ± 1.3 [2,*]	130.5 ± 2.3 **	48.9 ± 0.5 **	121.8 ± 1.2	95.1 ± 0.9 *
	Women	201.6 ± 1.5	112.0 ± 2.6	59.8 ± 0.7	119.4 ± 1.3	91.4 ± 1.0
	r^2, % [3]	<1	2.12	11.31	<1	<1
Age	20–39 years	184.8 ± 1.4 **	112.8 ± 2.8 **	51.6 ± 0.7 **	110.6 ± 1.3 **	85.9 ± 0.9 **
	40–59 years	208.3 ± 1.7	129.0 ± 2.1	54.7 ± 0.8	127.8 ± 1.6	98.7 ± 1.1
	⩾60 years	212.6 ± 2.7	123.8 ± 3.1	59.9 ± 1.2	127.9 ± 2.3	98.3 ± 1.3
	r^2, %	9.80	1.41	3.06	6.20	6.85
Race/ Ethnicity	NHW	200.5 ± 1.3 *	122.0 ± 2.2 **	54.7 + 0.7 **	121.4 ± 1.1	93.4 ± 0.9 *
	NHB	193.5 ± 2.1	97.1 ± 3.9	58.1 ± 1.1	116.0 ± 1.9	90.1 ± 1.7
	All Hispanics	197.1 ± 1.6	133.6 ± 2.4	49.8 ± 0.6	120.5 ± 1.3	95.6 ± 1.1
	Other	197.5 ± 4.1	128.2 ± 9.8	52.8 ± 1.5	119.1 ± 3.2	92.3 ± 3.0
	r^2, %	<1	2.12	1.75	<1	<1
Education	Less than high school	199.0 ± 1.9	127.9 ± 2.5 **	50.5 ± 0.8 **	122.9 ± 1.5	96.7 ± 1.2 **
	High school	200.7 ± 2.1	129.5 ± 3.4	52.0 ± 1.0	122.8 ± 1.8	96.4 ± 1.4
	More than high school	198.6 ± 1.6	116.5 ± 2.3	56.1 ± 0.5	119.2 ± 1.3	91.2 ± 0.9
	r^2, %	<1	<1	2.16	<1	1.20
PIR	Low	198.1 ± 1.6	124.9 ± 2.2	52.8 ± 0.7 *	120.3 ± 1.4	93.8 ± 0.9
	Medium	198.0 ± 2.3	118.1 ± 3.5	53.7 ± 1.0	120.7 ± 2.0	93.5 ± 1.6
	High	200.6 ± 1.7	120.5 ± 2.6	55.7 ± 0.8	120.9 ± 1.4	92.9 ± 0.9
	r^2, %	<1	<1	<1	<1	<1

[1] Data are from the National Health and Nutrition Examination Surveys. All data except for sample size are weighted accounting for the complex study design according to the directions of the National Center for Health Statistics. Biomarker levels represent mean ± SEM. The total n size was 2495. TC, total cholesterol; TG, triglyceride; HDL-C, HDL cholesterol; LDL-C, LDL cholesterol; Apo B, apolipoprotein B; NHW, non-Hispanic white; NHB, non-Hispanic black; PIR, family poverty-income ratio (low: 0–1.85; medium: 1.85 < to 3.5; high: >3.5); [2] p values were based on Wald F test, which tests whether at least 1 of the means across the sociodemographic variable categories is significantly different (* $p < 0.05$, ** $p < 0.01$); [3] values for r^2 are based on model 1, simple linear regression, by categories as shown.

Table 2. Unadjusted serum lipid status biomarker levels by lifestyle variable categories for US adults, NHANES 2007–2012 [1].

Lifestyle Variable		TC	TG	HDL-C	LDL-C	Apo B
		mg/dL	mg/dL	mg/dL	mg/dL	mg/dL
Supplement use [2]	Yes	203.2 ± 1.8 [3],**	117.7 ± 2.7	58.1 ± 0.9 **	121.5 ± 1.6	93.7 ± 1.1
	No	197.0 ± 1.1	123.4 ± 1.7	52.2 ± 0.5	120.1 ± 1.0	93.1 ± 0.8
	r^2, % [4]	<1	<1	3.09	<1	<1
Smoking [5]	Low	203.1 ± 2.3	110.9 ± 3.2 **	59.2 ± 0.8 **	121.7 ± 2.2	92.3 ± 1.4
	Medium	197.8 ± 1.3	122.9 ± 2.6	53.6 ± 0.7	119.6 ± 1.1	92.9 ± 0.9
	High	198.5 ± 2.0	126.8 ± 2.5	51.7 ± 1.0	121.5 ± 1.8	94.7 ± 1.3
	r^2, %	<1	<1	2.84	<1	<1
Alcohol consumption [6]	None	202.9 ± 2.1 *	128.7 ± 3.3 *	51.7 ± 1.0 *	125.5 ± 1.6 **	97.0 ± 1.2 *
	>0 to <1 drink/day	197.2 ± 1.3	119.1 ± 1.7	54.0 ± 0.6	119.4 ± 1.1	92.1 ± 0.8
	1 to <2 drinks/day	202.8 ± 3.0	119.5 ± 5.8	57.1 ± 1.6	121.8 ± 2.2	93.9 ± 1.8
	⩾2 drinks/day	202.8 ± 3.7	128.5 ± 6.4	57.5 ± 1.8	119.6 ± 3.8	94.9 ± 2.6
	r^2, %	<1	<1	1.08	<1	<1
BMI [7]	Underweight	189.4 ± 5.2 **	95.2 ± 7.5 **	62.6 ± 3.1 **	107.8 ± 4.7 **	82.5 ± 2.7 **
	Normal weight	193.9 ± 2.0	99.2 ± 1.7	61.3 ± 1.0	112.8 ± 1.5	85.4 ± 1.0
	Overweight	203.1 ± 1.5	128.0 ± 2.9	52.8 ± 0.8	124.8 ± 1.4	96.3 ± 1.0
	Obese	200.9 ± 1.9	139.4 ± 3.1	47.8 ± 0.6	125.2 ± 1.6	99.1 ± 1.1
	r^2, %	1.15	7.22	11.92	3.09	6.40
Physical activity [8]	No activity	200.5 ± 1.2	127.1 ± 2.0 **	52.7 ± 0.6 **	122.4 ± 1.1	95.4 ± 0.7 **
	0 to <500 MET-min/week.	199.9 ± 3.5	121.7 ± 3.2	54.0 ± 1.0	121.7 ± 2.7	93.3 ± 1.6
	500 to <1000 MET-min/week.	199.2 ± 3.6	117.2 ± 5.3	56.7 ± 1.1	119.0 ± 2.6	92.0 ± 2.0
	⩾1000 MET-min/week.	196.5 ± 1.9	114.4 ± 2.6	55.7 ± 1.1	117.9 ± 2.0	90.6 ± 1.2
	r^2, %	<1	<1	<1	<1	<1

[1] Data are from the National Health and Nutrition Examination Surveys. All data except for sample size are weighted accounting for the complex study design according to the directions of the National Center for Health Statistics. Biomarker levels represent mean ± SEM. The total n size was 2495. TC, total cholesterol; TG, triglyceride; HDL-C, HDL cholesterol; LDL-C, LDL cholesterol; Apo B, apolipoprotein B; [2] reported taking supplement containing iodine within the past 30 days; [3] p values were based on Wald F test, which tests whether at least 1 of the means across the lifestyle variable categories is significantly different (* $p < 0.05$, ** $p < 0.01$); [4] values for r^2 are based on model 1, simple linear regression, by categories as shown; [5] smoking status defined by a serum cotinine concentration (low: <0.015 mg/L; medium: 0.015 to <10 mg/L; high: ⩾10 mg/L); [6] calculated as average daily number of drinks/day [(frequency × quantity)/365.25]; 1 drink ≈ 15 g ethanol; [7] underweight: <18.5 kg/m^2; normal weight: 18.5 to >25 kg/m^2; overweight: 25 to <30 kg/m^2; and obese: ⩾30 kg/m^2; [8] calculated as total MET (metabolic equivalent task minutes)-min/week from self-reported leisure-time physical activities.

Table 3. Serum lipid profiles by urinary iodine concentration in US women, NHANES 2007–2012 [1].

Serum Lipids	Women	Low UIC, <10th Percentile (n = 148)	UIC ⩾10th Percentile (n = 1008)	p Value
	Age (years)	mean ± SEM [2]	mean ± SEM	
TC	20–39	188.6 ± 6.1	193.2 ± 4.6	0.2699
	40–59	205.6 ± 6.6	207.7 ± 4.5	0.7754
	⩾60	231.6 ± 7.3	215.4 ± 4.3	0.0052 **
TG	20–39	101.1 ± 13.9	90.7 ± 8.1	0.2493
	40–59	110.3 ± 11.2	118.0 ± 10.2	0.3686
	⩾60	82.39 ± 18.3	99.9 ± 10.3	0.2041
HDL-C	20–39	62.5 ± 2.5	62.5 ± 2.2	0.9948
	40–59	65.1 ± 2.8	67.7 ± 1.9	0.2380
	⩾60	67.3 ± 3.8	67.4 ± 2.8	0.9801
LDL-C	20–39	106.2 ± 5.0	102.0 ± 4.3	0.3677
	40–59	118.9 ± 5.4	117.9 ± 4.0	0.8635
	⩾60	151.8 ± 5.6	132.2 ± 3.2	0.0011 **
Apo B	20–39	81.9 ± 5.1	78.9 ± 4.1	0.3305
	40–59	92.4 ± 4.9	95.1 ± 3.8	0.4881
	⩾60	107.8 ± 5.6	96.2 ± 2.9	0.0103 *

[1] Data are from the National Health and Nutrition Examination Surveys. All data except for sample size are weighted accounting for the complex study design according to the directions of the National Center for Health Statistics. The total n size was 2495. UIC, urinary iodine concentration; TC, total cholesterol; TG, triglyceride; HDL-C, HDL cholesterol; LDL-C, LDL cholesterol; Apo B, apolipoprotein B; [2] weighted mean ± SEM. * $p < 0.05$, ** $p < 0.01$.

Table 4. Prevalence of dyslipidemia of adults in relation to urinary iodine concentration in US adults, NHANES 2007–2012 [1].

Dyslipidemia	Model	Low UIC, <10th Percentile (n = 249)	UIC ⩾10th Percentile (n = 2246)	p Value [2]
		AOR (95% CI)	Referent	
Elevated TC (>200 mg/dL)	1	1.35 (0.96–1.89)	1.00	0.0834
	2	1.42 (0.98–2.08)	1.00	0.0666
Elevated TG (>150 mg/dL)	1	0.76 (0.51–1.13)	1.00	0.1652
	2	0.93 (0.63–1.37)	1.00	0.7098
Lowered HDL-C (<40 mg/dL in men, <50 mg/dL in women)	1	0.64 (0.47–0.86)	1.00	0.0040 **
	2	0.92 (0.65–1.30)	1.00	0.6329
Elevated LDL-C (>130 mg/dL)	1	1.41 (1.04–1.92)	1.00	0.0283 *
	2	1.63 (1.16–2.28)	1.00	0.0054 **
Lowered HDL/LDL ratio (<0.4)	1	0.88 (0.65–1.19)	1.00	0.3991
	2	1.71 (1.09–2.67)	1.00	0.0199 *
Elevated Apo B (>130 mg/dL)	1	0.98 (0.50–1.91)	1.00	0.9567
	2	0.98 (0.46–2.08)	1.00	0.9505

[1] Data are from the National Health and Nutrition Examination Surveys. All data except for sample size are weighted accounting for the complex study design according to the directions of the National Center for Health Statistics. Multiple logistic regression analysis was performed to estimate odds ratio for dyslipidemia for subjects from the NHANES 2007–2012 in two models: unadjusted (model 1) and adjusted for sex, age, race/ethnicity, education, income, supplement use, smoking, alcohol consumption, BMI, physical activity (model 2). UIC, urinary iodine concentration; AOR, adjusted odds ratio; 95% CI, 95% confidence interval. TC, total cholesterol; TG, triglyceride; HDL-C, HDL cholesterol; LDL-C, LDL cholesterol; Apo B, apolipoprotein B; [2] p value obtained from multiple logistic regression model with diagnosis of dyslipidemia as the outcome variables (* $p < 0.05$, ** $p < 0.01$).

3. Results

The sociodemographic and lifestyle characteristics of the study population categorized by UIC are presented in Table S1. Compared to those with UIC above the 10th percentile, those with UIC below the 10th percentile were more likely to be women, have a poorer level of education, and less likely to take iodine-containing supplements and to be obese.

Unadjusted biomarker concentrations of serum lipid according to sociodemographic and lifestyle characteristics are shown in Tables 1 and 2. Among the sociodemographic variables, sex, age, race/ethnicity, and education (except for total cholesterol) were significantly associated with the majority of serum lipid biomarkers, except for LDL cholesterol which was associated only with age (Table 1). Unlike other sociodemographic variables, PIR was associated only with HDL cholesterol levels. Almost all of the lifestyle variables also had a significant relation with serum lipid status biomarkers (Table 2). Particularly, alcohol consumption and BMI were significantly associated with all five serum lipid biomarkers. The lifestyle variables, supplement use and smoking (except for LDL cholesterol and apolipoprotein B), and physical activity (except for total cholesterol and LDL cholesterol) were also significantly associated with most lipid biomarker concentrations. In our bivariate model, sex, age, and BMI explained the largest portion of the variability in the majority of serum lipid biomarkers; and other sociodemographic and lifestyle variables accounted for little variance in most serum lipid biomarkers.

Serum lipid levels by UIC are shown in Table 3 and Table S2. In men, serum lipid levels did not differ according to UIC, whereas in women, two serum lipid biomarkers differed significantly by UIC. Particularly in older women ($\geqslant$60 years), serum lipid levels such as total cholesterol, LDL cholesterol, and apolipoprotein B were significantly different according to UIC (all, $p < 0.05$). Older women with low UIC had a higher level of total cholesterol, LDL cholesterol and apolipoprotein B levels (231.6 ± 7.3 mg/dL, 151.8 ± 5.6 mg/dL and 107.8 ± 5.6 mg/dL, respectively) than those with UIC above the 10th percentile (215.4 ± 4.3 mg/dL, 132.2 ± 3.2 mg/dL and 96.2 ± 2.9 mg/dL, respectively).

The adjusted ORs and 95% CIs for risk factors of dyslipidemia after adjustment for covariates by UIC are described in Table 4. In comparison to adults with UIC above the 10th percentile, adults with the lowest decile of UIC were more likely to have dyslipidemia. The adjusted ORs of dyslipidemia risk factors among adults with low UIC *vs.* UIC at or above the 10th percentile were 1.63 (95% CI, 1.16–2.28) for elevated LDL cholesterol (>130 mg/dL) and 1.71 (95% CI, 1.09–2.67) for lowered HDL/LDL ratio (<0.4). Adults with low UIC had increased risk of elevated total cholesterol (>200 mg/dL) at marginally significant levels ($p = 0.0666$).

4. Discussion

In this study, significant differences were found in multiple lipid measures according to UIC. Majority of adults with UIC above the 10th percentile had desirable serum lipid range, whereas, those with UIC below the 10th percentile had elevated total cholesterol, LDL cholesterol, and apolipoprotein B. Our findings are consistent with previous researches regarding lipid profiles related to iodine status and iodine treatments in European [19,41] and African countries [42]. The research on 136 adolescents with endemic goitrous in Germany demonstrated that those with iodine deficiency-induced goiter had abnormally higher average total cholesterol and LDL cholesterol levels compared to non-goitrous control subjects [19]. In another study conducted by the same research group, the effects of iodine treatment for six months improved serum lipid levels [41]. Iodine supplement treatment for euthyroid goiter on children resulted significant decrease in total cholesterol and LDL cholesterol to their normal level [43]. A recent randomized controlled intervention study also reported that 6-month intervention with iodine supplementation significantly decreased risks for hypercholesterolemia in overweight and obese Moroccan women [44]. Additionally, a rural African population-based study reported that pregnant women and their offspring in an iodine deficient area are more likely to have a risk of coronary complications and hyperlipidemia compared to non-iodine deficient region [42]. Empirical evidence from clinical studies has demonstrated that iodine treatment was successful for those with CVD and high blood pressure [45]. There have also been many studies on thyroid dysfunction as a risk factor of lipid abnormalities and CVD. In adolescents with type 1 diabetes, subclinical hypothyroidism was positively correlated with mild dyslipidemia and increased the risk of CVD [46]. In 40 Spanish children aged 2–9 years, mean HDL cholesterol level was significantly lower in children with hypothyroidism compared to healthy children [47]. As thyroid failure has become one of determinants for dyslipidemia, an assertion has been raised that biochemical screening for thyroid disorders is needed for every dyslipidemia patient [48]. These existing studies suggest that long-term inadequate iodine intake may increase risks for dyslipidemia and CVD even though no clinical sign of thyroid dysfunction are present. We significantly expanded the scope of prior study using data from the representative US population and found that this association is still significant among US adults.

No association was found between TSH and UIC except for the case of excessive iodine intake where TSH levels were elevated by inhibiting thyroid hormone synthesis, which is known as the Wolff-Chaikoff effect [32,49]. It is hard to find UIC associated with TSH, particularly in the case of low UIC. Low UIC stimulates thyroid auto-regulation and an offsetting increase in serum triiodothyronine (T3), which normalize thyroid function [50]. Therefore, thyroid function test measuring TSH and thyroxine (T4) levels cannot be a good indicator for reflecting iodine status. Even though insufficient iodine intakes assessed by a single spot urine sample is not necessarily consistent with chronic iodine deficiency or subclinical hypothyroidism, persistent iodine deficiency leads to decreased thyroid hormone synthesis and elevated TSH easily with low-normal serum T4 concentration and high-normal serum T3 range [6]. As mentioned earlier, thyroid hormone is closely link to many metabolic pathways. Thus, the decrease in thyroid hormone synthesis induced by inadequate iodine intake raises the possibility of abnormal lipid metabolism [4]. In addition to classic pathway of lipid metabolism related to thyroid hormone, thyroid hormone-independent effect of TSH on lipid abnormalities was observed [51,52]. Lowered activity of hepatic lipase, which plays an important role in modulation of lipid levels and promoting cholesterol uptake by the liver, due to elevated TSH levels directly affect serum lipid levels [53]. In accordance with this mechanism, biochemical responses iodine deficiency may produce a more atherogenic lipid and higher risk for CVD [54]. Although iodine is also an essential component of the thyroid hormone and healthy thyroid function, iodine itself may play an important role in the cardiovascular health such as cancer-fighting properties and anti-inflammation [55]. However, only limited data support the proposition that iodine status was inversely associated with risk for CVD and iodine intakes were the largest contributor to mortalities due to CVD [20]. The underlying mechanism influencing serum lipid abnormalities by iodine status still remains partially unclear. A perspective and population-based study is required to elucidate a mechanism connected to iodine deficiency, thyroid function, and serum lipid. Therefore, continual monitoring of the independent role of iodine status in dyslipidemia allows us to put a new perspective on the treatment and possible prevention of CVD as well as dyslipidemia.

This study has several limitations. An important limitation of the study is that our findings are based on the cross-sectionally designed survey data. Such a fact makes it difficult to determine a causal relationship between UIC and dyslipidemia. However, this study highlighted that those with low UIC had increased risk of lipid abnormalities. In an animal study conducted by Zhao *et al.* [21], they confirmed the decreasing effect of high iodine intake on hyperlipidemia in mice, but did not investigate that kind of effect in humans. Therefore, adding to our results, it will be necessary to make further efforts to identify a casual effect of high iodine exposure on lipid concentration among those with iodine excess. Investigating potential mechanism between a wide range of iodine intake and lipid levels can provide us with a better understanding of the role of iodine status in pathogenesis of lipid metabolism. Another limitation is the lack of key information on iodine intake. Spot urine sample UIC is the only indicator for iodine status measurement in the NHANES. It has been well-documented that UIC obtained from spot urine sample is a suitable indicator for assessment of population's iodine status, but not for individual's [27]. Moreover, assessing iodine status based on UIC could not determine the actual amount of iodine intake from dietary sources. To overcome recognized limitations, we used the decile approach. Using this approach, we could have significant findings regarding the association between UIC and serum lipids. However, findings from decile grouping of study samples' UIC distribution still have the limitation that inconsistent results can be found with the different populations. Therefore, their association should be interpreted with circumspection. Understanding the impact of actual dietary iodine intakes and individual's iodine status on serum lipids is worth further investigation as well. Lastly, the study using mice reported that the effect of iodine intake on lipid metabolism may vary depending on the sex of the mice, mentioning needs of considering interaction between iodine status and the sex hormone in the lipid metabolism [21]. Further investigation is needed to explore the effect of these interactions. Adding the strengths of the present study mentioned above, this is a recent and unique study investigating the association between UIC and serum lipid profiles based on larger samples of the US adult population. We confirmed that sociodemographic and lifestyle factors affect UIC and serum lipids, the significant association between low UIC and lipid profiles persisted even after controlling for those confounding factors in our analysis models.

5. Conclusions

In summary, according to the NHANES 2007–2012, we found a cross-sectional association between low UIC measured by a spot urine sample and serum lipid profiles, particularly among total cholesterol, LDL cholesterol, and apolipoprotein B. Thus, efforts for maintaining adequate level of urinary iodine are recommended to prevent risk factors for dyslipidemia among US adults. However, there is a limitation in that, even though UIC used in this study as a biomarker might capture iodine status at the population level, but not at the individual level. Therefore, there is a need for further study investigating the relationship between biomarkers for iodine status that can reflect the iodine status of individuals and serum lipid levels. Additionally, further prospective research regarding the effect of iodine status on lipid metabolism and vice versa will establish epidemiological evidence for a causal relationship between them and help develop effective educational and clinical interventions in this area.

Acknowledgments: The manuscript was prepared using the NHANES 2007–2012 data obtained from the CDC. All authors would like to appreciate the CDC for the availability of the NHANES survey data.

Author Contributions: Kyung Won Lee conceptualized the study, conducted the analyses and wrote the draft of manuscript. Dayeon Shin provided inputs for the data analyses and critically contributed to the manuscript development and revision. Won O. Song guided the manuscript development and substantially revised the paper. All authors have reviewed the submitted manuscript and approved its current form for submission in the journal.

References

1. Zimmermann, M.B.; Jooste, P.L.; Pandav, C.S. Iodine-deficiency disorders. *Lancet* **2008**, *372*, 1251–1262. [CrossRef]
2. Feingold, K.R. The regulation and role of epidermal lipid synthesis. *Adv. Lipid Res.* **2014**, *24*, 57–82.
3. Mullur, R.; Liu, Y.-Y.; Brent, G.A. Thyroid hormone regulation of metabolism. *Physiol. Rev.* **2014**, *94*, 355–382. [CrossRef] [PubMed]
4. Pearce, E.N. Update in lipid alterations in subclinical hypothyroidism. *J. Clin. Endocrinol. Metab.* **2011**, *97*, 326–333. [CrossRef] [PubMed]
5. De Jesus Garduño-Garcia, J.; Alvirde-Garcia, U.; López-Carrasco, G.; Mendoza, M.E.P.; Mehta, R.; Arellano-Campos, O.; Choza, R.; Sauque, L.; Garay-Sevilla, M.E.; Malacara, J.M. TSH and free thyroxine concentrations are associated with differing metabolic markers in euthyroid subjects. *Eur. J. Endocrinol.* **2010**, *163*, 273–278. [CrossRef] [PubMed]
6. Åsvold, B.O.; Vatten, L.J.; Nilsen, T.I.; Bjøro, T. The association between TSH within the reference range and serum lipid concentrations in a population-based study. The HUNT study. *Eur. J. Endocrinol.* **2007**, *156*, 181–186. [CrossRef] [PubMed]
7. Zimmermann, M.B.; Boelaert, K. Iodine deficiency and thyroid disorders. *Lancet Diabetes Endocrinol.* **2015**, *3*, 286–295. [CrossRef]

8. Duntas, L.H. Thyroid disease and lipids. *Thyroid* **2002**, *12*, 287–293. [CrossRef] [PubMed]
9. Nyirenda, M.J.; Clark, D.N.; Finlayson, A.R.; Read, J.; Elders, A.; Bain, M.; Fox, K.A.; Toft, A.D. Thyroid disease and increased cardiovascular risk. *Thyroid* **2005**, *15*, 718–724. [CrossRef] [PubMed]
10. Shin, D.J.; Osborne, T.F. Thyroid hormone regulation and cholesterol metabolism are connected through sterol regulatory element-binding protein-2 (SREBP-2). *J. Biol. Chem.* **2003**, *278*, 34114–34118. [CrossRef] [PubMed]
11. Rizos, C.; Elisaf, M.; Liberopoulos, E. Effects of thyroid dysfunction on lipid profile. *Open Cardiovasc. Med. J.* **2011**, *5*, 76–84. [CrossRef] [PubMed]
12. Tomeleri, C.M.; Ronque, E.R.; Silva, D.R.; Júnior, C.G.C.; Fernandes, R.A.; Teixeira, D.C.; Barbosa, D.S.; Venturini, D.; Okino, A.M.; Oliveira, J.A. Prevalence of dyslipidemia in adolescents: Comparison between definitions. *Rev. Port. Cardiol.* **2015**, *34*, 103–109. [PubMed]
13. Saydah, S.; Bullard, K.M.; Cheng, Y.; Ali, M.K.; Gregg, E.W.; Geiss, L.; Imperatore, G. Trends in cardiovascular disease risk factors by obesity level in adults in the United States, NHANES 1999–2010. *Obesity* **2014**, *22*, 1888–1895. [CrossRef] [PubMed]
14. Peeters, A.; Backholer, K. Is the health burden associated with obesity changing? *Am. J. Epidemiol.* **2012**, *176*, 840–845. [CrossRef] [PubMed]
15. Zhu, X.; Cheng, S. New insights into regulation of lipid metabolism by thyroid hormone. *Curr. Opin. Endocrinol. Diabetes Obes.* **2010**, *17*, 408–413. [CrossRef] [PubMed]
16. Tzotzas, T.; Krassas, G.E.; Konstantinidis, T.; Bougoulia, M. Changes in lipoprotein (a) levels in overt and subclinical hypothyroidism before and during treatment. *Thyroid* **2000**, *10*, 803–808. [CrossRef] [PubMed]
17. Teixeira, P.D.F.D.S.; Reuters, V.S.; Ferreira, M.M.; Almeida, C.P.; Reis, F.A.A.; Buescu, A.; Costa, A.J.L.; Vaisman, M. Lipid profile in different degrees of hypothyroidism and effects of levothyroxine replacement in mild thyroid failure. *Transl. Res.* **2008**, *151*, 224–231. [CrossRef] [PubMed]
18. Adrees, M.; Gibney, J.; El-Saeity, N.; Boran, G. Effects of 18 months of L-T4 replacement in women with subclinical hypothyroidism. *Clin. Endocrinol.* **2009**, *71*, 298–303. [CrossRef] [PubMed]
19. Rönnefarth, G.; Kauf, E.; Deschner, F.; Forberger, M. Therapy of iodine deficiency goiter in adolescents with iodine or a combination of iodine and levothyroxine with special reference to lipid parameters. *Klin. Padiatr.* **1996**, *208*, 123–128. [CrossRef] [PubMed]
20. Keys, A.; Karvonen, M.; Fidanza, F. Serum-cholesterol studies in Finland. *Lancet* **1958**, *272*, 175–178. [CrossRef]
21. Zhao, S.J.; Ye, Y.; Sun, F.J.; Tian, E.J.; Chen, Z.P. The impact of dietary iodine intake on lipid metabolism in mice. *Biol. Trace Elem. Res.* **2011**, *142*, 581–588. [CrossRef] [PubMed]
22. Sullivan, K.M.; Perrine, C.G.; Pearce, E.N.; Caldwell, K.L. Monitoring the iodine status of pregnant women in the United States. *Thyroid* **2013**, *23*, 520–521. [CrossRef] [PubMed]
23. Christian, J.B.; Bourgeois, N.E.; Lowe, K.A. Cholesterol screening in US adults and awareness of high cholesterol among individuals with severe hypertriglyceridemia: National Health and Nutrition Examination Surveys 2001–2008. *J. Cardiovasc. Nurs.* **2015**, *30*, 26–34. [CrossRef] [PubMed]
24. Melse-Boonstra, A.; Mackenzie, I. Iodine deficiency, thyroid function and hearing deficit: A review. *Nutr. Res.* **2013**, *26*, 110–117. [CrossRef] [PubMed]
25. Papi, G.; degli Uberti, E.; Betterle, C.; Carani, C.; Pearce, E.N.; Braverman, L.E.; Roti, E. Subclinical hypothyroidism. *Curr. Opin. Endocrinol. Diabetes Obes.* **2007**, *14*, 197–208. [CrossRef] [PubMed]
26. Hurrell, R. Bioavailability of iodine. *Eur. J. Clin. Nutr.* **1997**, *51*, S9–S12. [PubMed]
27. König, F.; Andersson, M.; Hotz, K.; Aeberli, I.; Zimmermann, M.B. Ten repeat collections for urinary iodine from spot samples or 24-h samples are needed to reliably estimate individual iodine status in women. *J. Nutr.* **2011**, *141*, 2049–2054. [CrossRef] [PubMed]
28. National Center for Health Statistics. National Health and Nutrition Examination Survey: Analytic Guidelines, 1999–2010. Available online: http://www.cdc.gov/nchs/data/series/sr_02/sr02_161.pdf (accessed on 8 January 2015).
29. Centers for Disease Control and Prevention. About the National Health and Nutrition Examination Survey. Available online: http://www.cdc.gov/nchs/nhanes.htm (accessed on 8 January 2015).
30. Centers for Disease Control and Prevention; National Center for Health Statistics. NCHS Research Ethics Review Board (ERB) Approval. Available online: http://www.cdc.gov/nchs/nhanes/irba98.htm (accessed on 1 August 2015).

31. National Institutes of Health. *The Third Report of the National Cholesterol Education Program. Expert Panel on Detection, Evaluation, and Treatment of High. Blood Cholesterol in Adults (Adult Treatment Panel III)*; NIH Publication 01-3670. National Institutes of Health: Bethesda, MD, USA, 2001.
32. Caldwell, K.L.; Jones, R.; Hollowell, J.G. Urinary iodine concentration: United States National Health and Nutrition Examination Survey 2001–2002. *Thyroid* **2005**, *15*, 692–699. [CrossRef] [PubMed]
33. Caldwell, K.L.; Maxwell, C.B.; Makhmudov, A.; Pino, S.; Braverman, L.E.; Jones, R.L.; Hollowell, J.G. Use of inductively coupled plasma mass spectrometry to measure urinary iodine in NHANES 2000: Comparison with previous method. *Clin. Chem.* **2003**, *49*, 1019–1021. [CrossRef] [PubMed]
34. National Health and Nutrition Examination Survey. 2009–2010 Data Documentation, Codebook, and Frequencies. Available online: http://wwwn.cdc.gov/nchs/nhanes/2009-2010/uio_f.htm (accessed on 13 October 2014).
35. National Health and Nutrition Examination Survey. 2011–2012 Data Documentation, Codebook, and Frequencies. Available online: http://wwwn.cdc.gov/nchs/nhanes/2011-2012/uio_g.htm (accessed on 12 October 2014).
36. Van Mil, N.H.; Tiemeier, H.; Bongers-Schokking, J.J.; Ghassabian, A.; Hofman, A.; Hooijkaas, H.; Jaddoe, V.W.; de Muinck Keizer-Schrama, S.M.; Steegers, E.A.; Visser, T.J. Low urinary iodine excretion during early pregnancy is associated with alterations in executive functioning in children. *J. Nutr.* **2012**, *142*, 2167–2174. [CrossRef] [PubMed]
37. Pfeiffer, C.M.; Sternberg, M.R.; Caldwell, K.L.; Pan, Y. Race-ethnicity is related to biomarkers of iron and iodine status after adjusting for sociodemographic and lifestyle variables in NHANES 2003–2006. *J. Nutr.* **2013**, *143*, 977S–985S. [CrossRef] [PubMed]
38. Steinmaus, C.; Miller, M.D.; Howd, R. Impact of smoking and thiocyanate on perchlorate and thyroid hormone associations in the 2001–2002 National Health and Nutrition Examination Survey. *Environ. Health Perspect.* **2007**, *115*, 1333–1338. [CrossRef] [PubMed]
39. World Health Organization. *Obesity: Preventing and Managing the Global Epidemic, Report of a WHO Consultation*; WHO Technical Report Series no. 894; World Health Organization: Geneva, Switzerland, 2000.
40. Wang, C.Y.; Haskell, W.L.; Farrell, S.W.; LaMonte, M.J.; Blair, S.N.; Curtin, L.R.; Hughes, J.P.; Burt, V.L. Cardiorespiratory fitness levels among US adults 20–49 years of age: Findings from the 1999–2004 National Health and Nutrition Examination Survey. *Am. J. Epidemiol.* **2010**, *171*, 426–435. [CrossRef] [PubMed]
41. Rönnefarth, G.; Kauf, E.; Deschner, F.; Forberger, M. Euthyroid goiter in puberty—A harmless illness? *Klin. Padiatr.* **1995**, *208*, 77–82. [CrossRef] [PubMed]
42. Das, S.C.; Mohammed, A.Z.; Al-Hassan, S.U.; Otokwula, A.A.; Isichei, U.P. The triad-iodine deficiency, hyperlipidaemia, high coronary risk—In a "maternal-neonate" population of rural Africa. *Indian J. Clin. Biochem.* **2007**, *22*, 79–83. [CrossRef] [PubMed]
43. Zimmermann, M.B.; Aeberli, I.; Melse-Boonstra, A.; Grimci, L.; Bridson, J.; Chaouki, N.; Mbhenyane, X.; Jooste, P.L. Iodine treatment in children with subclinical hypothyroidism due to chronic iodine deficiency decreases thyrotropin and C-peptide concentrations and improves the lipid profile. *Thyroid* **2009**, *19*, 1099–1104. [CrossRef] [PubMed]
44. Herter-Aeberli, I.; Cherkaoui, M.; el Ansari, N.; Rohner, R.; Stinca, S.; Chabaa, L.; von Eckardstein, A.; Aboussad, A.; Zimmermann, M.B. Iodine supplementation decreases hypercholesterolemia in iodine-deficient, overweight women: A randomized controlled trial. *J. Nutr.* **2015**, *145*, 2067–2075. [CrossRef] [PubMed]
45. Cann, S.A.H. Hypothesis: Dietary iodine intake in the etiology of cardiovascular disease. *J. Am. Coll. Nutr.* **2006**, *25*, 1–11. [CrossRef]
46. Denzer, C.; Karges, B.; Näke, A.; Rosenbauer, J.; Schober, E.; Schwab, K.O.; Holl, R.W. Subclinical hypothyroidism and dyslipidemia in children and adolescents with type 1 diabetes mellitus. *Eur. J. Endocrinol.* **2013**, *168*, 601–608. [CrossRef] [PubMed]
47. Paoli-Valeri, M.; Guzman, M.; Jimenez-Lopez, V.; Arias-Ferreira, A.; Briceno-Fernandez, M.; Arata-Bellabarba, G. Atherogenic lipid profile in children with subclinical hypothyroidism. *An. Pediatr.* **2005**, *62*, 128–134. [CrossRef]
48. Liberopoulos, E.N.; Elisaf, M.S. Dyslipidemia in patients with thyroid disorders. *Hormones (Athens)* **2002**, *1*, 218–223. [CrossRef] [PubMed]

49. Haddow, J.E.; McClain, M.R.; Palomaki, G.E.; Hollowell, J.G. Urine iodine measurements, creatinine adjustment, and thyroid deficiency in an adult United States population. *J. Clin. Endocrinol. Metab.* **2007**, *92*, 1019–1022. [CrossRef] [PubMed]
50. Soldin, O.P.; Tractenberg, R.E.; Pezzullo, J.C. Do thyroxine and thyroid-stimulating hormone levels reflect urinary iodine concentrations? *Ther. Drug Monit.* **2005**, *27*, 178–185. [CrossRef] [PubMed]
51. Brenta, G.; Berg, G.; Arias, P.; Zago, V.; Schnitman, M.; Muzzio, M.L.; Sinay, I.; Schreier, L. Lipoprotein alterations, hepatic lipase activity, and insulin sensitivity in subclinical hypothyroidism: Response to L-T4 treatment. *Thyroid* **2007**, *17*, 453–460. [CrossRef] [PubMed]
52. Zhang, W.; Tian, L.M.; Han, Y.; Ma, H.Y.; Wang, L.C.; Guo, J.; Gao, L.; Zhao, J.J. Presence of thyrotropin receptor in hepatocytes: Not a case of illegitimate transcription. *J. Cell. Mol. Med.* **2009**, *13*, 4636–4642. [CrossRef] [PubMed]
53. Wang, F.; Tan, Y.; Wang, C.; Zhang, X.; Zhao, Y.; Song, X.; Zhang, B.; Guan, Q.; Xu, J.; Zhang, J. Thyroid-stimulating hormone levels within the reference range are associated with serum lipid profiles independent of thyroid hormones. *J. Clin. Endocrinol. Metab.* **2012**, *97*, 2724–2731. [CrossRef] [PubMed]
54. Razvi, S.; Ingoe, L.; Keeka, G.; Oates, C.; McMillan, C.; Weaver, J.U. The beneficial effect of L-thyroxine on cardiovascular risk factors, endothelial function, and quality of life in subclinical hypothyroidism: Randomized, crossover trial. *J. Clin. Endocrinol. Metab.* **2007**, *92*, 1715–1723. [CrossRef] [PubMed]
55. Venturi, S.; Donati, F.M.; Venturi, A.; Venturi, M. Environmental iodine deficiency: A challenge to the evolution of terrestrial life? *Thyroid* **2000**, *10*, 727–729. [CrossRef] [PubMed]

3

Involvement of the Niacin Receptor GPR109a in the Local Control of Glucose Uptake in Small Intestine of Type 2 Diabetic Mice

Tung Po Wong, Leo Ka Yu Chan and Po Sing Leung *

School of Biomedical Sciences, Faculty of Medicine, The Chinese University of Hong Kong, Shatin, Hong Kong, China; wongtp@cuhk.edu.hk (T.P.W.); leokychan@link.cuhk.edu.hk (L.K.Y.C.)

* Correspondence: psleung@cuhk.edu.hk

Abstract: Niacin is a popular nutritional supplement known to reduce the risk of cardiovascular diseases by enhancing high-density lipoprotein levels. Despite such health benefits, niacin impairs fasting blood glucose. In type 2 diabetes (T2DM), an increase in jejunal glucose transport has been well documented; however, this is intriguingly decreased during niacin deficient state. In this regard, the role of the niacin receptor GPR109a in T2DM jejunal glucose transport remains unknown. Therefore, the effects of diabetes and high-glucose conditions on GPR109a expression were studied using jejunal enterocytes of 10-week-old *m+/db* and *db/db* mice, as well as Caco-2 cells cultured in 5.6 or 25.2 mM glucose concentrations. Expression of the target genes and proteins were quantified using real-time polymerase chain reaction (RT-PCR) and Western blotting. Glucose uptake in Caco-2 cells and everted mouse jejunum was measured using liquid scintillation counting. 10-week T2DM increased mRNA and protein expression levels of GPR109a in jejunum by 195.0% and 75.9%, respectively, as compared with the respective *m+/db* control; high-glucose concentrations increased mRNA and protein expression of GPR109a in Caco-2 cells by 130.2% and 69.0%, respectively, which was also confirmed by immunohistochemistry. In conclusion, the enhanced GPR109a expression in jejunal enterocytes of T2DM mice and high-glucose treated Caco-2 cells suggests that GPR109a is involved in elevating intestinal glucose transport observed in diabetes.

Keywords: enterocytes; jejunum; glucose transport; SGLT1; GLUT2; Caco-2; hyperglycemia; hyperlipidemia

---

1. Introduction

Diabetes mellitus is classically one of the most common chronic metabolic disorders, which is characterized by a plethora of clinical complications; they include, but are not limited to, cardiovascular disease, end-stage renal diseases, diabetic foot disorders, and blindness. One of the most notable clinical manifestations of diabetic patients is dyslipidemia, which is the major risk factor for cardiovascular disease in type 2 diabetes mellitus (T2DM). It has been reported that diabetics have significantly higher coronary-event-associated deaths than the non-diabetics [1]. Furthermore, diabetic individuals without known clinical coronary heart disease (CHD) are exposed to comparable risk of mortality compared to those non-diabetics who have experienced a myocardial infarction [2], thus leading to the recognition of diabetes as a CHD-risk-equivalent condition [3].

In order to address this issue, scientists have taken strides to develop novel therapeutic agents that ameliorate cardiovascular disease by specifically targeting dyslipidemia in diabetic patients. In recent years, niacin, also known as nicotinic acid or Vitamin B3, has been a popular nutritional supplement; in fact, it is widely used to treat cardiovascular disease which is associated with dyslipidemia by lowering the level of low-density lipoprotein and triglycerides, while raising the level of high-density lipoprotein simultaneously [4]. Notwithstanding the existence of these health benefits, niacin has been shown to induce glucose intolerance in patients, as evidenced by significant increases in blood glucose levels (5.83 mg/dL) after three years of niacin treatment in euglycemic patients (9.88 mg/dL for niacin *vs.* 4.05 mg/dL for without niacin) [5]. Meanwhile, the incidence rate of impaired fasting blood glucose was increased by 29%. In patients suffering from hyperglycemia, high doses of niacin also increased their level of Hemoglobin A1c by about 0.3% [6]. It is recognized that oral niacin elevated blood glucose levels and thereby deteriorated diabetes in some patients; however, the precise mechanism still remains unknown [7]. In contrast, a lower V_{max} for jejunal glucose uptake *vs.* control group was observed in rats fed with niacin deficient diet [8]. Niacin deficiency also significantly lowers the active electrogenic absorption of glucose across jejunal mucosa [9]. Collectively, these findings have shown that niacin, to a certain extent, might not be beneficial in terms of its adverse effects on glucose homeostasis observed in diabetic patients.

Of interest in this context is our recent data showing that such a niacin-induced hyperglycemia is probably mediated via the activation of niacin receptor GPR109A-mediated ROS-PPARγ-UCP2 (reactive oxygen species-peroxisome proliferator-activated receptor-γ-uncoupling protein 2) signaling pathway in the pancreatic islet β-cells [10]. In addition, previous studies have shown that niacin exerts its effects by binding to its specific G protein-coupled receptors HM74 (GPR109B) and its homologues HM74A (GPR109A) [11–13]. In terms of its potency, niacin activates GPR109A and GPR109B with half maximal effective concentration (EC_{50}) values of 0.1 mM and 100 mM, respectively [14]. Both GPR109A and GPR109B have been expressed in the human colon and localized to the apical membrane of colonocytes [15]. In mice, GPR109A is expressed in both small and large intestines [12,16]. Despite these findings, the role of GPR109A in jejunal glucose uptake is still elusive. Interestingly, jejunal glucose transport via both sodium-dependent glucose transporter (SGLT1) and glucose transporter 2 (GLUT2) is greatly increased in early diabetes [17]. In this respect, SGLT1 is a high-affinity, low-capacity transporter localized at the brush border membrane (BBM) of jejunal enterocytes, which is responsible for active uptake of glucose from the intestinal lumen; however, GLUT2 is a glucose transporter normally situated on the basolateral membrane of the jejunal enterocytes but it is translocated and inserted into the BBM during enhanced SGLT1-mediated glucose uptake [18–20]. In this way, glucose transport capability of GLUT2 can be up to three times greater than that of SGLT1 [21].

Given the fact that dietary glucose is a critical component in determining our blood glucose homeostasis and in light of the above-mentioned findings, the present study was designed to unravel the undiscovered role of niacin in the regulation of intestinal glucose uptake, with particular emphasis on T2DM, and its potential interaction with the intestinal glucose transporters, SGLT1 and GLUT2, thus its consequence on glucose homeostasis.

2. Experimental Section

2.1. Animals

4- to 12-week-old male *m+/db* and *db/db* mice in this study were used and supplied by the Laboratory Animal Services Centre at The Chinese University of Hong Kong. Animals were maintained on a standard chow (Prolab RMH 2500, 5P14; Lab Diet, St. Louis, MO, United States) and water *ad libitum* up to the time of experiment. Only those diabetic mice with blood glucose levels above 10 mM were included in the diabetic group. Anesthesia before experimentation was achieved with pentobarbitone sodium (50 mg/kg) intraperitoneally. All procedures have been approved by the Animal Experimentation Ethics Committee of the Chinese University of Hong Kong (No. 10/064/MIS).

2.2. Isolation of Enterocytes

Enterocytes were prepared from 4 cm long jejunal segments, beginning 4 cm distal to the ligament of Treitz. Intestinal epithelia cells were isolated and harvested by a Ca^{2+}-chelation technique [22]. Briefly, isolated intestinal segments were flushed through with ice-cold saline followed by air. The segment was tied off at one end and filled with Ca^{2+}-free hypertonic isolation buffer (7 mM K_2SO_4,

44 mM K_2HPO_4, 9 mM $NaHCO_3$, 10 mM HEPES, 2 mM L-glutamine, 0.5 mM dithiothreitol, 1 mM Na_2EDTA, and 180 mM glucose, pH 7.4), equilibrated with 95% O_2 and 5% CO_2, where over-distention was avoided. The segment was then tied off to form a closed sac and incubated in 0.9% saline at 37 °C with gentle shaking for 16 min. Cells were dislodged manually, and the resulting suspension was collected and centrifuged for 30 s at 500 g; the pellet was re-suspended in freshly prepared cold buffer and this procedure was repeated twice, as we reported previously [23,24].

2.3. Western Blot Analysis

The procedures of Western blot have been described previously [25]. Proteins from the enterocyte and Caco-2 cells were extracted using the CytoBuster protein extraction reagent (Novagen, Darmstadt, Germany) and quantified using Bio-Rad Bradford assay kit (Bio-Rad, Munich, Germany). Proteins (10 μg/lane) were subjected to electrophoresis on a 10% (weight (wt)/volume (vol)) polyacrylamide gel. Proteins from the polyacrylamide gel were transferred to the polyvinylidene difluoride membrane using a semi-dry transblot unit (Bio-Rad, Munich, Germany). The protein-blotted membrane was saturated by submersion in 5% (wt/vol) nonfat skimmed milk in phosphate buffered saline (PBS) (pH 7.4) with 0.1% (vol/vol) Tween-20 for one hour at room temperature. The membranes were incubated with anti-HM74(M-65) receptor rabbit polyclonal antibodies (SC-134583; Santa Cruz Biotechnology, Dallas, TX, United States)(1:100), anti-NIACR1 (Niacin receptor 1) rabbit polyclonal antibodies (NBP1-92180, Novus Biologicals, Littleton, CO, United States) (1:100), and anti-β-actin mouse polyclonal antibodies (EMD Millipore, Danvers, Massachusetts, United States) (1:5000) overnight at 4 °C. After washing with 0.1% Tween-20 in Phosphate-buffered saline (PBS), membranes were incubated with the following corresponding peroxidase-labeled secondary antibodies for one hour at room temperature: anti-rabbit Immunoglobulin G (IgG) antibody (GE Healthcare Bio-Sciences, Pittsburgh, PA, United States) (1:1300) and anti-mouse IgG antibody (GE Healthcare Bio-Sciences, Pittsburgh, PA, United States) (1:2500). The positive signal was revealed using Enhanced Chemiluminescence-plus (ECL-plus); GE Healthcare Bio-Sciences, Pittsburgh, PA, United States) western blotting detection reagent and Fuji Medical Super RX-N autoradiography film (FUJIFILM, Valhalla, NY, United States). The intensity of the bands was quantified using FluorChem software (ProteinSimple, San Jose, CA, United States). The corresponding expression of β-actin of each sample was used to normalize its expression of the target protein.

2.4. Real-Time PCR Analysis

Quantitative RT-PCR was performed using StepOne™ Real-Time PCR Systems (ThermoFisher Scientific, Grand Island, NY, United States). The procedure has been described previously [26]. Briefly, total RNA was extracted from freshly prepared enterocytes or Caco-2 cells grown in 5.6, 11.2, or 25.2 mM glucose using Trizol reagent (ThermoFisher Scientific, Grand Island, NY, United States) according to the manufacturer's instructions. RNase Out (ThermoFisher Scientific, Grand Island, NY, United States) was added to the RNA solutions to prevent degradation by RNase. Total RNA served as the template for cDNA preparation using iScript™ Select cDNA Synthesis Kit (Bio-Rad Laboratories, Munich, Germany). Primers were designed from mice and human cDNA sequences using Primer Express Software provided by ThermoFisher Scientific. Mice β-actin and Human β-actin were used as reference genes to normalize the relative expression of each target gene. The sequences of primers used are shown in Table 1. Sybergreen reactions were set up in a volume of 25 μL with ABI two-step sybergreen PCR reagents (ThermoFisher Scientific, Grand Island, NY, United States). Each reaction consisted of 12.5 μL PCR master mix, 0.05 to 0.30 μM of each amplification primer, and 1 μL cDNA. Each sample was run in duplicate with an initial 10-min period at 95 °C to enable the reaction, followed by 40 cycles at 95 °C for 15 s and 60 °C for 1 min. The samples were heated to 60 °C for 1 min, then to 95 °C over the next minute, and finally cooled slowly from 95 °C to 60 °C over 20 min to collect data for the analysis of dissociation curve. Amplification data were collected by the detector of the StepOne™ Real-Time PCR Systems and analyzed with Sequence Detection System software

(ThermoFisher Scientific, Grand Island, NY, United States). The threshold cycle (C_T) of each sample was determined from the time point where fluorescence was first detected, with the cycle number being inversely related to cDNA concentration. The fold changes in mRNA expression were calculated using the $2^{-\Delta\Delta CT}$ method [27].

Table 1. Sequences of specific primers used for real-time quantitative RT-PCR.

Gene	Forward Primer	Reverse Primer
Mouse β-actin (NM_007393.4)	TCCTCCTGAGCGCAAGTACTC	GTGGACAGTAGTGAGGCCAGGT
Mouse GPR109a (NM_030701.3)	GGCGTGGTGCAGTGAGCAGT	GGCCCACGGACAGGCTAGGT
Human β-actin (NC_000007.14)	GGCACCCAGCACAATGAAGATC	ATGCTTCTAGGCGGACTATGACTT
Human GPR109a (NM_177551.3)	TGCCGCCCTTCCTGATGGACA	TGTTCAGGGCGTGGTGGGGA

2.5. Immunohistochemistry

Immunofluorescence was carried out as described previously with some modifications to determine the mucosal localization of niacin receptors [23]. Isolated jejunal segments were rinsed with cold saline and then quickly transferred to ice-cold 4% paraformaldehyde (PFA) in 0.1 M PBS (pH 7.4) and incubated at 4 °C overnight. Tissue segments were rinsed with PBS and incubated with 20% sucrose in PBS at 4 °C overnight and later embedded in optimum cutting temperature medium (Tissue-Tek, Sakura Finetek Europe B.V., Zoeterwoude, The Netherlands). Sections (6 μm) were collected on Superforst slides (Gerhard Menzel GmbH, Braunschweig, Germany), and these were boiled in 10 mM citrate buffer for 10 min to retrieve the antigens. Sections were incubated with 1% (wt/vol) bovine serum albumin (BSA) and 6% (wt/vol) normal donkey serum (NDS) (Jackson Immuno Research, West Grove, PA, United States) for one hour at room temperature to block nonspecific antibody binding. The slides were incubated overnight at 4 °C with primary antibody (SC-134583; Santa Cruz Biotechnology, Dallas, TX, United States) (1:100), diluted in PBS with 2% NDS and 0.1% Triton X-100. After three washes with PBS, bound primary antibodies were detected by incubation with their corresponding secondary antibodies labeled with Cyc-3 (Jackson Immuno Research, West Grove, PA, United States) (1:100, diluted with 0.1 M PBS containing 2% NDS) at room temperature for 1 h. Immunoreactivity was captured with a fluorescent microscope equipped with a DC480 digital camera (Leica Microsystems, Buffalo Grove, IL, United States). Human Caco-2 cells were grown on silane-coated cover slips, incubated with ice-cold 4% PFA in 0.1 M PBS (pH 7.4) for 8 min, and washed three times with 0.1 M PBS, followed by the same steps as the immunostaining procedures mentioned above starting from the incubation with 1% BSA and 6% NDS (wt/vol), except that anti-NIACR1 rabbit polyclonal antibodies (NBP1-92180) (1:100) was used as the primary antibody.

2.6. Glucose Uptake by Everted Jejunal Sleeves

Prior to measurements of glucose uptake, long jejunal segments (3 to 4 cm long) were taken 3 cm distal to the ligament of Treitz. Glucose uptake was measured using everted jejunal sleeves [28,29]. In brief, isolated jejunal segments were rinsed with cold saline and everted over a glass rod. The tissue was tied securely to the rod and pre-incubated in gassed carbogen (95% O_2, 5% CO_2) bicarbonate buffer (128 mM NaCl, 4.7 mM KCl, 2.5 mM $CaCl_2$, 1.2 mM KH_2PO_4, 1.2 mM $MgSO_4$, and 20 mM $NaHCO_3$) without glucose for 4 min at 37 °C followed by 15 min using the same buffer, with 0.1 μM to 2 mM of niacin (Sigma-Aldrich, St Louis, MO, United States). Then, concentrated D-glucose was added to the buffer to make up to a final glucose concentration of 50 mM with 0.2 μCi/mL D-[^{14}C]glucose (GE Healthcare Bio-Sciences, Pittsburgh, PA, United States) with trace amounts of 0.1 μCi/mL L-[^{3}H]glucose (Sigma-Aldrich, St Louis, MO, United States) to correct for non-specific uptake. After a 2 min incubation, the segments were washed rapidly with ice-cold saline containing 0.3 mM phlorizin with stirring for 1 min. The tissue was removed from the rod, oven-dried, and weighed. The dried residue was incubated with Soluene-350 (Perkin-Elmer, Waltham, MA, United States) at 60 °C for 4 h. Scintillation fluid (Ultima Gold; Perkin-Elmer, Waltham, MA, United States) was added, and counting of radioactivity was carried out. The rate of glucose uptake was calculated as picomole per milligram dry weight intestine per second.

2.7. *Glucose Uptake by Caco-2 Cells*

Caco-2 cells were purchased from ATCC (catalog no. HTB-37). Cells were grown at 37 °C in minimum essential medium (M2279; Sigma-Aldrich, St Louis, MO, United States) with 20% fetal bovine serum (FBS), 1% nonessential amino acids (#11140; ThermoFisher Scientific, Grand Island, NY, United States), and 1% penicillin-streptomycin and gassed with 95% air–5% CO_2. Cells were subcultured at ~80% confluence, at a cell density of between 8×10^4 and 1×10^5 cells/cm^2. The medium was changed every two days, and cells were used 14 days after confluence, when they expressed characteristics of enterocyte differentiation [30,31]. Caco-2 cells grown in media containing 5.6 and 25.2 mM glucose for 14 days after confluence were harvested by Trizol reagent (Thermo Fisher Scientific, NY, United States) for RNA isolation and real-time PCR reaction, and Cytobuster (EMD Millipore, Danvers, MA, United States) for Western blotting.

Caco-2 cells grown in 5.6 mM glucose were rinsed with 25 °C oxygenated bicarbonate buffer (128 mM NaCl, 4.7 mM KCl, 2.5 mM $CaCl_2$, 1.2 mM KH_2PO_4, 1.2 mM $MgSO_4$, and 20 mM $NaHCO_3$) with 10% FBS, 1% penicillin-streptomycin, and 1% nonessential amino acids. Cells were preincubated in gassed (95% O_2–5% CO_2) bicarbonate buffer containing 50 mM mannitol for 1 h at 37 °C. The buffer was then replaced with fresh bicarbonate buffer containing 50 mM glucose and 0.2 μCi/mL D-[^{14}C]glucose (GE Healthcare Bio-Sciences, Pittsburgh, PA, United States), with or without 0.1 μM to 2 mM niacin. In some experiments, 0.3 mM phlorizin or 0.1 mM phloretin was also present. Cells were washed quickly three times by stirring in ice-cold saline containing 0.3 mM phlorizin. The cells were digested with 0.3 M NaOH, and aliquots were added to scintillation fluid (Ultima Gold; Perkin-Elmer, Waltham, MA, United States). Glucose uptake was measured as disintegrations per min per well of a six-well plate containing a monolayer of Caco-2 cells.

2.8. *siRNA Knockdown of GPR109a in Caco-2 Cells*

Caco-2 cells grown on six wells plates reached 70% confluence at the time of transfection. One day before the transfection, the medium was changed to one containing no antibiotics. Stock Stealth™ RNA (ThermoFisher Scientific, Grand Island, NY, United States) was diluted to 40 nM with 50 μL Opti-MEM® I Reduced Serum Medium without serum. Lipofectamine®2000 (ThermoFisher Scientific, Grand Island, NY, United States) was diluted 50 times with Opti-MEM®I Reduced Serum Medium (ThermoFisher Scientific, Grand Island, NY, United States) and incubated 5 min at room temperature. The diluted Stealth™ RNA and Lipofectamine®2000 was mixed and incubated at room temperature for 10 min. The oligomer-Lipofectamine®2000 complexes were added to each well, followed by incubation of the cells at 37 °C in CO2 incubator for 72 h. The transfected cells were harvested for either protein detection or glucose uptake.

2.9. *Statistical Analysis*

All results were analyzed using Prism 3.0 software. The data were expressed as means ± standard error of the mean (SEM). Student's unpaired two-tailed *t*-test and One-Way Analysis of variance (ANOVA) (Tukey's post-hoc test) were employed to detect significant differences between two groups and among three or more groups, respectively. For all comparisons, $p < 0.05$ was considered statistically significant. For RT-PCR, the C_T value of the target gene of a sample was first corrected for the C_T value of β-actin, before being statistically analyzed [27].

3. Results

3.1. Enterocyte Expression of GPR109a

The real-time PCR analysis of mRNA expression of GPR109a normalized to β-actin revealed the presence of GPR109a mRNA in both *m+/db* and *db/db* mouse jejunal brush border (Figure 1A). Expression of GPR109a mRNA in enterocytes from 10-week-old *db/db* mice was higher than that seen in four-week-old *db/db* mice. At the age of 10 weeks, expression of GPR109a in *db/db* mouse jejunum was 2.96 folds greater than that of the control 10-week-old *m+/db* mouse jejunum. Consistently, Western blotting of enterocyte protein also revealed the presence of GPR109a protein in both *m+/db* and *db/db* mice (Figure 1B). Expression levels of GPR109a protein in enterocytes from 10-week-old diabetic *db/db* mice were 1.76 folds greater than their corresponding control 10-week-old *m+/db* mice.

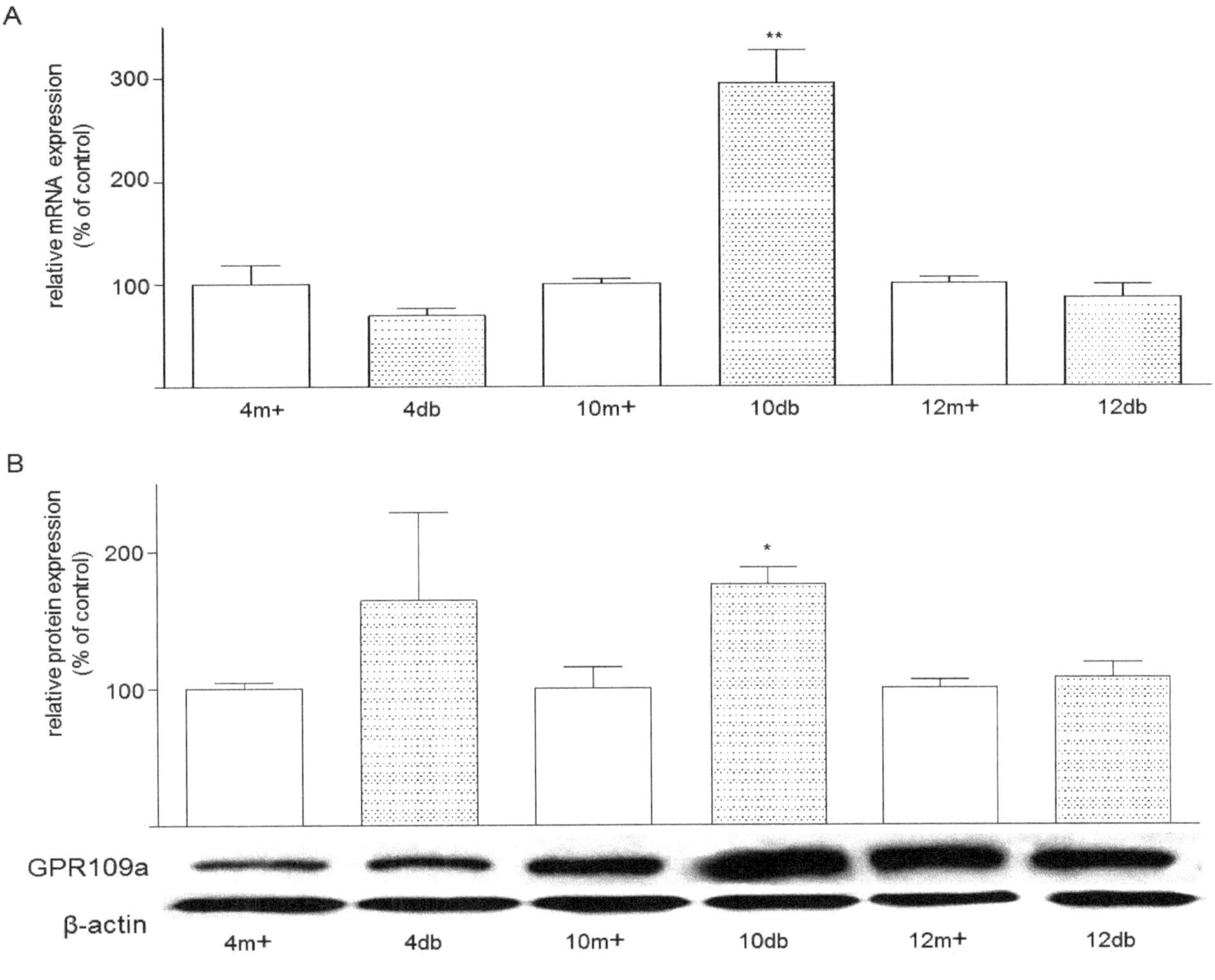

Figure 1. (**A**) Effects of age and Type 2 Diabetes Mellitus (T2DM) on the mRNA expression of GPR109a in jejunal mucosa. Mouse mRNA abundance was determined by real-time PCR using jejunal mucosa and data were calculated as the percentage of their corresponding m+ non-diabetic controls. All results are expressed relative to enterocytes of non-diabetic rats, and are given as mean ± standard error of the mean (SEM), $n = 3$–4; 10 db *vs.* 10 m+, ** $p < 0.01$; (**B**) Effects of age and T2DM on the protein expression of GPR109a in jejunal enterocytes. Western blot analysis showing the relative expression of GPR109a in homogenates of enterocytes prepared from jejuna of *m+/db* and *db/db* mice of 4, 10 or 12 weeks of age. Data were calculated as the percentage change compared to their corresponding *m+* non-diabetic control. Results are expressed as means ± SEM, $n = 3$–5, 10m+ *vs.* 10 db, * $p < 0.05$. 4m+, 8m+, 10m+ and 12m+ represent 4-, 8-, 10- and 12-week-old *m+/db* mice respectively; whereas 4 db, 8 db, 10 db and 12 db represent 4-, 8-, 10- and 12-week-old *db/db* mice, respectively.

3.2. Localization of GPR109a in Jejunal Mucosa of m+/db and db/db Mice, and Caco-2 Cells

Immunohistochemical results showed the localization of GPR109a at the level of the BBM along the entire jejunal villus length in both normal (*m+/db*) (Figure 2A–C) and diabetic (*db/db*) (Figure 2D–F) animals. However, expression of GPR109a was consistently higher in diabetic jejunum and this was particularly apparent at higher magnification (Figure 2H diabetic *vs.* Figure 2G normal). On the other hand, immunocytochemistry also revealed the presence of niacin receptors at the cell membrane of Caco-2 cells from the 14 days after confluence (Figure 2J–O). In examination, expression of niacin receptor was higher in cells grown in 25.2 mM glucose (Figure 2M) compared to those cultured in 5.6 mM glucose (Figure 2J).

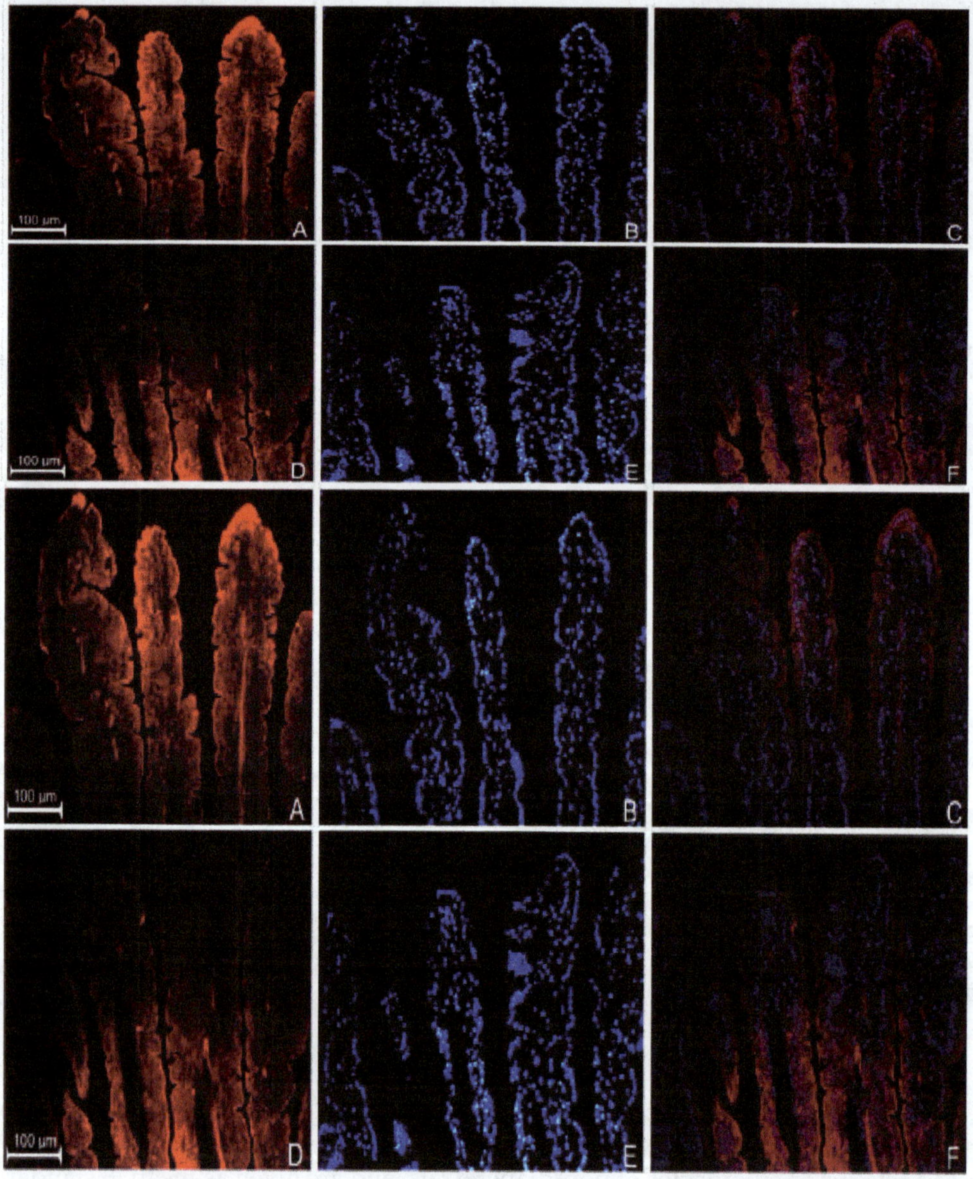

Figure 2. Immunodetection of GPR109a in jejunum of 10-week-old *m+/db* mice (**A**) and 10-week-old *db/db* mice (**D**). (**B,E**) are the nuclear DAPI staining of (**A,D**) respectively; (**C,F**) are their corresponding merged images. Higher magnification of niacin receptor staining of *m+/db* (**G**) and *db/db* (**H**); (**I**) shows jejunal sections prepared in the absence of primary antibodies (negative control). Immunodetection of niacin receptor in Caco-2 cells grown in 5.6 mM (**J**) and 25.2 mM glucose (**M**); (**K,N**) show nuclear 4′,6-diamidino-2-phenylindole (DAPI) staining of (**J**) and (**M**) respectively; (**L,O**) are the corresponding merged images.

3.3. *Effects of Niacin on Jejunal Glucose Uptake*

Next, we attempted to study the role of GPR109a in modulating jejunal glucose uptake. By using the intestine from non-diabetic (*m+/db*) mice, mucosal exposure to niacin for 10 min increased glucose uptake in a dose-dependent fashion (Figure 3). At 1 mM niacin, glucose uptake was increased by 26.8%.

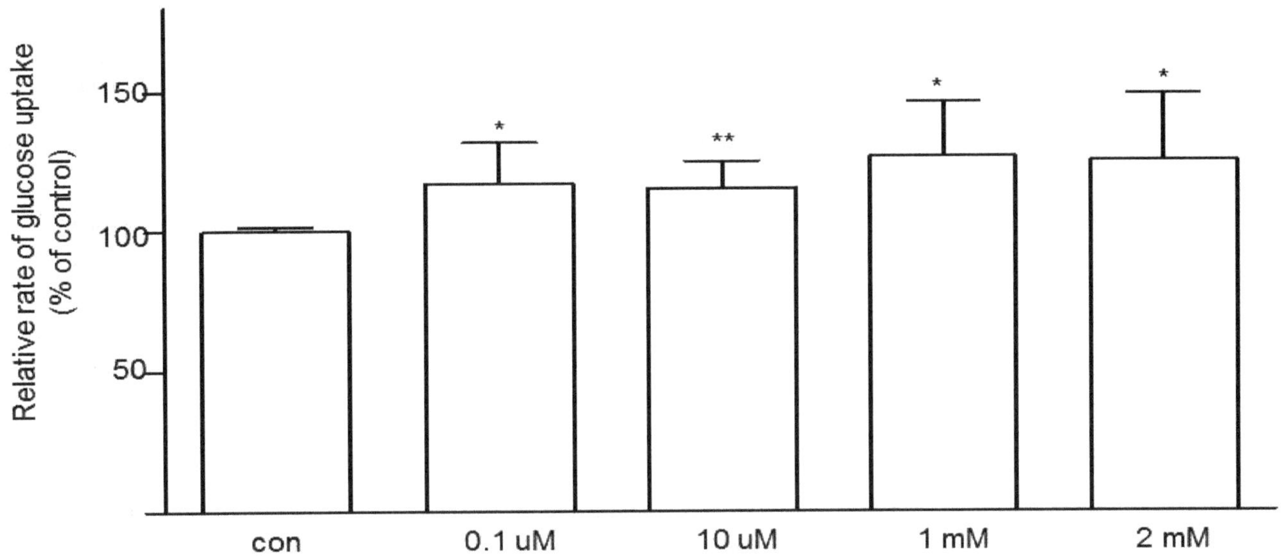

Figure 3. The dose-dependent effect of niacin on jejunal glucose uptake using 10-week-old *m+/db* mice. Data are expressed as relative percentage of glucose uptake relative to the control (con). $n = 6$ for each concentration of niacin. Data are given as means ± standard error of the mean (SEM), * $p < 0.05$ *vs.* control; ** $p < 0.01$ *vs.* control.

3.4. *Effects of Glucose Concentrations on the Expression of GPR109a in Caco-2 Cells*

Caco-2 cells were used to study the effects of glucose concentrations of the growth medium on the gene expression of GPR109a. GPR109a mRNA was expressed in Caco-2 cells grown in both low glucose and high glucose media. In comparison with the low glucose concentration (5.6 mM), it was observed that high glucose concentration (25.2 mM) increased both of the gene and protein levels of niacin receptor expression by 130.2% and 69%, respectively (Figure 4A, B).

3.5. *Effects of Niacin and Glucose Transporter Inhibitors on Glucose Uptake in Caco-2 Cells*

We also sought to study the role of the niacin receptor GPR109a in the modulation of glucose uptake in Caco-2 cells. Caco-2 cells grown on normal glucose (5.6 mM) and exposed to niacin for 10 min increased glucose uptake in a dose-dependent fashion (Figure 5A); at 1 mM niacin, glucose uptake was increased by 20.1%. On the other hand, the effects of the two glucose transporter inhibitors, the SGLT1 blocker phlorizin (0.3 mM) and GLUT2 blocker phloretin (0.1 mM), in the presence or absence, on the glucose uptake of Caco-2 cells grown in normal 5.6 mM glucose were also examined. As shown, 0.3 mM phlorizin and 0.1 mM phloretin inhibited glucose uptake by 23.3% and 62.5%, respectively.In addition, 1 mM niacin further increased glucose uptake when present with 0.3 mM phlorizin and 0.1 mM phloretin (Figure 5B). These data indicate that both SGLT1 and GLUT2 may be involved in the upregulation of niacin-induced glucose uptake.

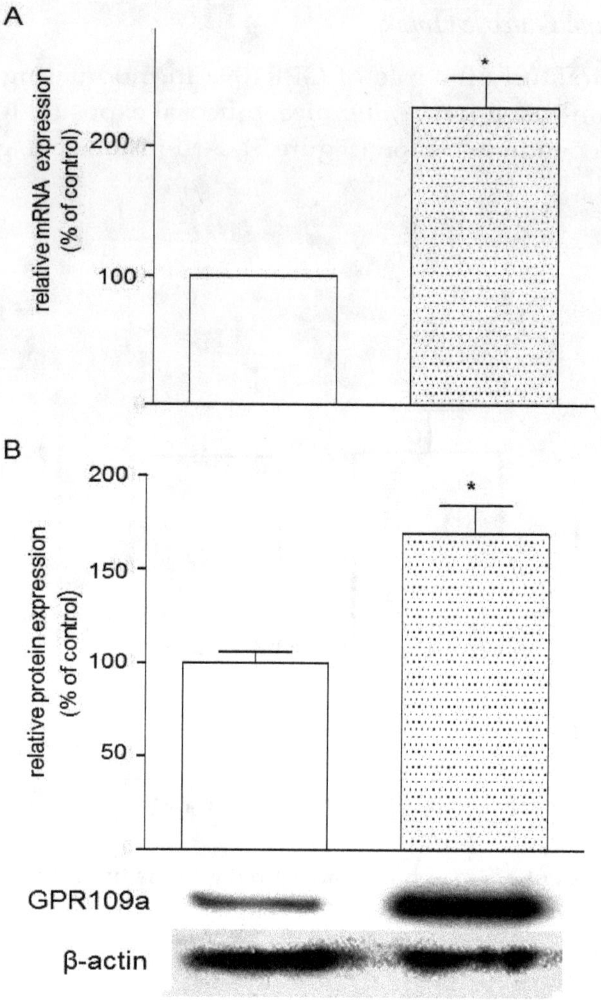

Figure 4. (**A**) Effects of high glucose concentration (25.2 mM) on the mRNA expression of GPR109a in Caco-2 cells *vs.* low glucose concentration (5.6 mM). Results are expressed as means ± standard error of the mean (SEM), $n = 3$, control = 5.6 mM glucose, control *vs.* 25.2 mM glucose, * $p < 0.05$; (**B**) Effects of high glucose (25.2 mM) on GPR109a protein expression in Caco-2 cells *vs.* control 5.6 mM glucose concentrations. Results are expressed as means ± SEM, $n = 6$, control = 5.6 mM *vs.* 25.2 mM, * $p < 0.05$.

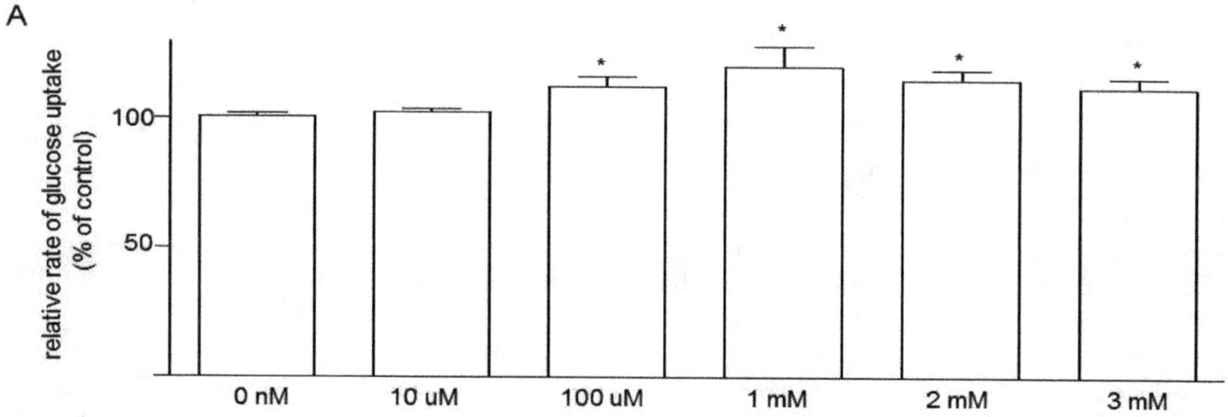

Figure 5. *Cont.*

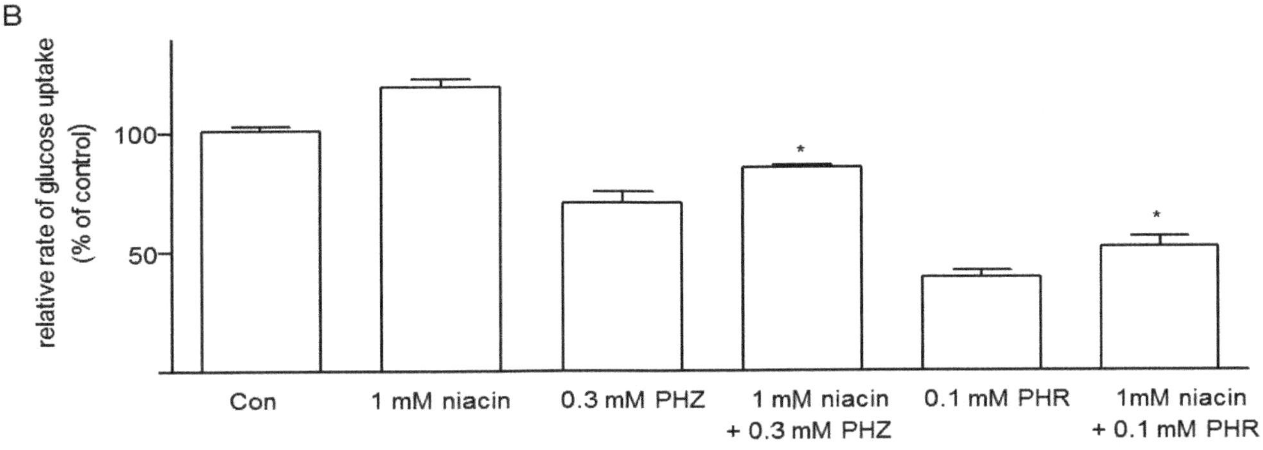

Figure 5. (**A**) Dose dependent effect of niacin on glucose uptake by Caco-2 cells grown in glucose (5.6 mM) (expressed as percentage of glucose uptake relative to their control). n = 6 for each concentration of niacin. Data are given as means ± standard error of the mean (SEM), 0 nM *vs.* treatment groups, * $p < 0.05$; (**B**) Glucose uptake by Caco-2 cells grown in 5.6 mM glucose showing effect of 1 mM niacin, with or without phlorizin (PHZ, 0.3 mM) and phloretin (PHR, 0.1 mM). Results are expressed relative to the respective control value (con). All data are given as means ± SEM, n = 6. 0.3 mM PHZ *vs.* 0.3 mM PHZ + 1 mM niacin and 0.1 mM PHR *vs.* 0.1 mM PHR + 1 mM niacin, * $p < 0.05$.

3.6. *Effects of Knockdown of GPR109a on Glucose Uptake in Caco-2 Cells*

Three different siRNA sequences (HSS155268, HSS155269 and HSS155270) were tried in the study of knockdown of niacin receptor in Caco-2 cells grown in 5.6 mM glucose. Western blot analysis showed that the knockdown experiments with siRNA HSS155269, HSS155270 and HSS155268 decreased protein expression of niacin receptors by 45.0%, 53.7%, and 32.5%, respectively as compared with the negative siRNA control group (Figure 6A). Therefore, we selected the siRNA HSS155270, the most effective knockdown sequence, which decreased the rate of glucose uptake of Caco-2 cells grown in 5.6 mM glucose by 30.2% (Figure 6B).

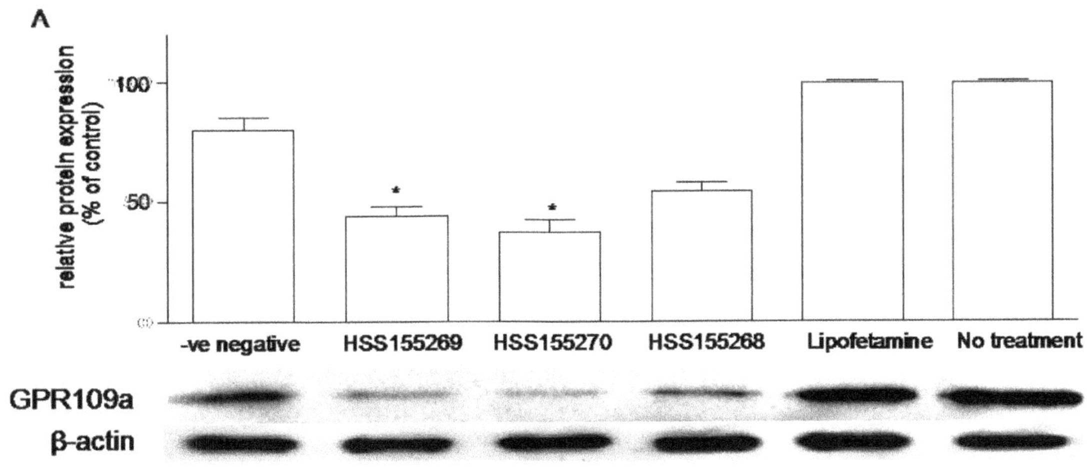

Figure 6. *Cont.*

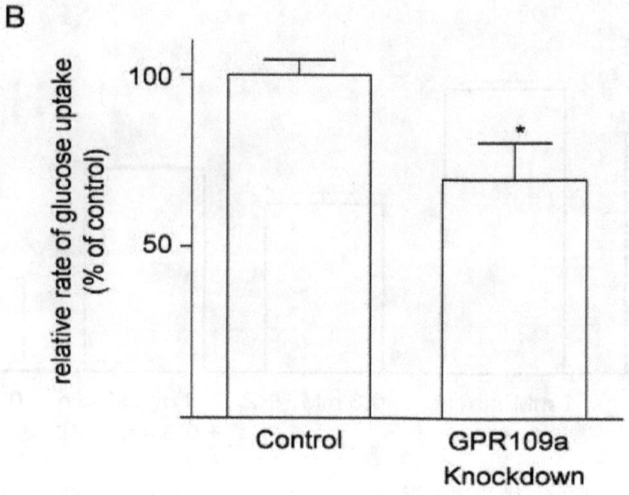

Figure 6. (**A**) Effects of siRNA knockdown of GPR109a on the expression of GPR109a protein in Caco-2 cells grown in 5.6 mM glucose. Western blot analysis showing the relative expression of niacin receptor in homogenates of cells prepared from the -ve negative (negative control siRNA, *Silencer*® Select Negative Control siRNA, non-targeting SiRNA with limited sequence similarity to known genes), and three different sequences of siRNA (HSS155269, HSS155270 and HSS155268). "Lipofetamine" contains only the lipofetamine transfection buffer, without any siRNA. "No treatment" contains neither the transfection buffer nor any siRNA. Results are expressed as means ± standard error of the mean (SEM), $n = 6$. HSS155269 *vs.* negative control, 45% decrease in expression, * $p < 0.05$; HSS155270 *vs.* negative control, 53.8% decrease in expression, * $p < 0.05$; (**B**) Effects of siRNA (HSS155270) knockdown of GPR109a on the glucose uptake of Caco-2 cells grown in 5.6 mM glucose. Knockdown of GPR109a decreased the rate of glucose uptake by 30.2%, $n = 5$, * $p < 0.05$.

4. Discussion

Niacin is a commonly employed anti-hyperlipidemia drug but it is also widely known to induce hyperglycemia during chronic and high-dose therapy [5,6]. Despite this, the mechanistic action of niacin and its receptor GPR109a in the regulation of glucose homeostasis, in particular with intestinal glucose uptake, remains ambiguous. The present study has shown, for the first time, that enterocyte GPR109a is expressed and functional in the local control of intestinal glucose absorption, and that type 2 diabetic and high glucose conditions upregulate the GPR109a expression, thus enhancing niacin-induced intestinal glucose uptake in the mice. Our laboratory has recently reported the novel role of niacin, via its activation of GPR109A, in pancreatic islets [10]. In that study, niacin was found to increase fasting glucose concentrations, reduce glucose-stimulated insulin secretion (GSIS) and insulin secretion, and impair glucose tolerance, thereby inducing pancreatic islet dysfunctions in high-fat diet (HFD) induced obese mice [10]. In this regard, the present study establishes a previously undiscovered role of niacin in local regulation of glucose homeostasis at the level of the small intestine in normal and diabetic states.

In the present study, we have first demonstrated that the mRNA and protein expression levels of the niacin receptor GPR109a were elevated in the diabetic *db/db* mice, as evidenced by real-time qPCR and Western blot, as well as further supported by the immunohistochemical results. Interestingly, an upregulated expression GPR109a was also observed in diabetic mouse and human retina, where GPR109a could serve as an anti-inflammatory receptor in retinal pigement epithelial cells and is closely associated with diabetic retinopathy [32]. It is well recognized that inflammatory process is a key causative factor in the pathogenesis of diabetes and GPR109a has been shown to be a potent anti-inflammatory receptor in various physiologically important organs, including but not limiting to, the colon [33], blood vessels [34], and pancreas [10]. In light of these findings, it prompts us to speculate that such an elevated GPR109a expression may be responsible for acting as a strategic counteractive mechanism against the inflammatory insults, as induced by hyperglycemia in diabetic states.

To address this issue, we sought to examine whether niacin could locally regulate glucose uptake across the small intestinal BBM. In fact, our laboratory has previously shown the functional existence of a local renin-angiotensin system (RAS) in the regulation of intestinal glucose uptake, where binding of the two physiologically active components of this system, angiotensin II, to its angiotensin type 1 receptor and the binding of angiotensin (1–7) to the Mas receptor at the jejunal BBM in enterocytes inhibit SGLT1-mediated glucose transport across this membrane in a dose-dependent fashion [23,35]. Therefore, we explore to investigate whether niacin is also able to regulate glucose uptake locally in the intestine. First of all, it is necessary to address if niacin arriving at the small intestine would be adequate to elicit its physiological function. Studies have shown that niacin is indeed equally absorbed by the stomach and the upper small intestine in human [36]. In fact, up to about four grams of niacin could be almost completely absorbed by adults. Intestinal luminal concentration of niacin under physiological conditions has been reported to lie in the micromolar but not in the millimolar range [37]. As a result, there should be sufficient amount of niacin reaching the jejunum for its physiological actions. Our results showed that niacin increased intestinal glucose uptake in *m+/db* mice significantly and dose-dependently; these data were further substantiated by the observed decrease in glucose uptake after GPR109a knockdown in Caco-2 cells. Our findings are in line with the observation that niacin treatment increases glucose uptake in adipocytes where such an effect of niacin on glucose uptake was antagonized by theophylline and isoprenaline, which are that agents that increase intracellular concentrations of 3′,5′-cyclic adenosine monophosphate (cAMP); in addition, niacin could further increase the maximum rate of glucose transport stimulated by insulin in adipocytes [38]. In adipocytes, niacin treatment significantly lowered the intracellular concentrations of cAMP in adipocytes, and a decrease in cAMP level upregulated glucose uptake [38,39]. However, cAMP has been shown to stimulate SGLT1 and thus mediated intestinal glucose uptake in enterocytes [40], thereby contradicting the findings in adipocytes. Not withstanding these findings, it might be plausible to postulate that cAMP is a downstream signaling molecule of GPR109a for its subsequent mediation of glucose uptake. Despite this, further investigations are warranted in order to confirm the precise role of cAMP in jejunal enterocytes.

Apart from the *in vivo* data, we further investigated the effects of high glucose treatment on the expression profiles of mRNA and protein of GPR109a in human Caco-2 cells. Our data revealed that 25.2 mM glucose concentration raised remarkably the mRNA and protein levels of GPR109a, when compared to those of the Caco-2 cells grown in 5.6 mM glucose. To address which glucose transporters are involved in GPR109a-mediated intestinal glucose uptake, we sought to add phlorizin (SGLT1 blocker) and phloretin (GLUT2 blocker) to examine whether the stimulatory effect of niacin on glucose uptake was mediated via SGLT1 and/or GLUT2. In this regard, we found both SGLT1 and GLUT2 were responsible for this regulatory process. In terms of SGLT1, cAMP has been shown to stimulate SGLT1 function in enterocytes as mentioned above [40] and involved in post-transcriptional stabilization of SGLT1 message [41]. Therefore, it is plausible to propose that cAMP may act as a downstream mediator for the action of niacin on SGLT1-mediated glucose uptake. In term of GLUT2, however, cAMP has been previously reported to prevent glucose-mediated stimulation of GLUT2 in hepatocytes [42], and thus a decrease in cAMP level in hepatocytes is supposed to upregulate GLUT2-mediated glucose uptake; however, this postulate is apparently contradictory with that of SGLT1. In view of this, the signaling molecules rather than GLUT2 might be involved in the regulation of niacin-stimulated GLUT2 activity, which merits intensive investigations in the future.

Besides, we also questioned whether there a crosstalk among GPR109A, SGLT1, and GLUT2 might exist. In this context, niacin binding to GPR109A has been shown to increase the Protein Kinase C (PKC) activity in CHO-K1 cells [43]. Furthermore, GLUT2 can be PKC-dependently translocated apically upon high glucose exposure [44]. In the pancreatic islet, activation of Protein Kinase A (PKA) by adenylyl cyclase inhibited the GLUT2 mediated initial rate of 3-*O*-methyl glucose uptake by 48% [45].

Also, activation of PKC has been shown to activate human SGLT1 [46]. In the apical GLUT2 model, SGLT1-mediated glucose transport promotes insertion of GLUT2 into the apical membrane within minutes, where the capacity of GLUT2 mediated glucose transport can be increased up to more than three fold [21]. On the grounds of the evidence, it might be possible that niacin binding to GPR109a inhibits the PKA activity, and activates PKC activity at the same time. The niacin binding might increase the translocation of GLUT2 to the apical membrane, thus GLUT2-mediated glucose uptake. Another possibility is that GPR109a activation by niacin effects the production of SGLT1. In the uptake experiment, the time of the niacin treatment lasted only few minutes. The time may not be long enough to induce the upregulation of SGLT1 expression. Since an increased SGLT1 activity would upregulate GLUT2 activity [21], the increase in GLUT2 activity by niacin binding to GPR109a might upregulate SGLT1 mediated glucose uptake.

5. Conclusions

In conclusion, the present study is the first to report that niacin is able to bind to the niacin receptor GPR109a to stimulate SGLT1- and GLUT2-mediated jejunal glucose uptake in hyperglycemia observed in diabetes. Given niacin is a crucial nutritional supplement that garners attention over the recent years, our results should provide a clinical implication that the niacin receptor GPR109a may serve as a potential therapeutic target for novel dietary or pharmacological approaches to controlling intestinal sugar delivery, thereby improving glycemic control for diabetes.

Acknowledgments: This work was fully supported by the General Research Fund of the Research Grants Council of the Hong Kong Special Administrative Region, China (Ref. No.: CUHK 14110314), awarded to P.S. Leung.

Author Contributions: Tung Po Wong performed the experiments, analyzed the data, and drafted the manuscript. Leo Ka Yu Chan contributed to the preparation of the manuscript and data analysis. Po Sing Leung conceived and designed the study and experiments, and compiled the manuscript. All authors approved the final version of the manuscript.

References

1. Sprafka, J.M.; Burke, G.L.; Folsom, A.R.; McGovern, P.G.; Hahn, L.P. Trends in prevalence of diabetes mellitus in patients with myocardial infarction and effect of diabetes on survival. The Minnesota Heart Survey. *Diabetes Care* **1991**, *14*, 537–543. [CrossRef]
2. Haffner, S.M.; Lehto, S.; Rönnemaa, T.; Pyörälä, K.; Laakso, M. Mortality from coronary heart disease in subjects with type 2 diabetes and in nondiabetic subjects with and without prior myocardial infarction. *N. Engl. J. Med.* **1998**, *339*, 229–234. [CrossRef]
3. Expert Panel on Detection. Evaluation, and Treatment of High Blood Cholesterol in Adults. Executive summary of the third report of the national cholesterol education program (NCEP) expert panel on detection, evaluation, and treatment of high blood cholesterol in adults (Adult Treatment Panel III). *JAMA* **2001**, *285*, 2486–2497.
4. Guyton, J.R.; Goldberg, A.C.; Kreisberg, R.A.; Sprecher, D.L.; Superko, H.R.; O'Connor, C.M. Effectiveness of once-nightly dosing of extended release niacin alone and in combination for hypercholesterolemia. *Am. J. Cardiol.* **1998**, *82*, 737–743. [CrossRef]
5. Phan, B.A.; Muñoz, L.; Shadzi, P.; Isquith, D.; Triller, M.; Brown, B.G.; Zhao, X.Q. Effects of niacin on glucose levels, coronary stenosis progression, and clinical events in subjects with normal baseline glucose levels (<100 mg/dL): A combined analysis of the Familial Atherosclerosis Treatment Study (FATS), HDL-Atherosclerosis Treatment Study (HATS), Armed Forces Regression Study (AFREGS), and Carotid Plaque Composition by MRI during lipid-lowering (CPC) study. *Am. J. Cardiol.* **2013**, *111*, 352–355.
6. Hochholzer, W.; Berg, D.D.; Giugliano, R.P. The facts behind niacin. *Ther. Adv. Cardiovasc. Dis.* **2011**, *5*, 227–240. [CrossRef]
7. Mcgovern, M.E. Use of nicotinic acid in patients with elevated fasting glucose, diabetes, or metabolic syndrome. *Br. J. Diabetes Vasc. Dis.* **2004**, *4*, 78. [CrossRef]
8. Victoria, C.R.; Meneghelli, U.G. Kinetics of jejunal glucose transport in niacin deficient rats. *Arq. Gastroenterol.* **1990**, *27*, 191–196.

9. Victoria, C.R. Jejunal electrogenic transport of glucose in rats with niacin deficiency. *Arq. Gastroenterol.* **1994**, *31*, 18–23.
10. Chen, L.; So, W.Y.; Li, Y.T.; Cheng, Q.; Boucher, B.J.; Leung, P.S. Niacin-induced hyperglycemia is partially mediated via niacin receptor GPR109a in pancreatic islets. *Mol. Cell. Endocrinol.* **2015**, *404*, 56–66. [CrossRef]
11. Soga, T.; Kamohara, M.; Takasaki, J.; Matsumoto, S.; Saito, T.; Ohishi, T.; Hiyama, H.; Matsuo, A.; Matsushime, H.; Furuichi, K. Molecular identification of nicotinic acid receptor. *Biochem. Biophys. Res. Commun.* **2003**, *303*, 364–369. [CrossRef]
12. Tunaru, S.; Kero, J.; Schaub, A.; Wufka, C.; Blaukat, A.; Pfeffer, K.; Offermanns, S. PUMA-G and HM74 are receptors for nicotinic acid and mediate its anti-lipolytic effect. *Nat. Med.* **2003**, *9*, 352–355. [CrossRef]
13. Wise, A.; Foord, S.M.; Fraser, N.J.; Barnes, A.A.; Elshourbagy, N.; Eilert, M.; Ignar, D.M.; Murdock, P.R.; Steplewski, K.; Green, A.; *et al.* Molecular identification of high and low affinity receptors for nicotinic acid. *J. Biol. Chem.* **2003**, *278*, 9869–9874. [CrossRef]
14. Offermanns, S. The nicotinic acid receptor GPR109A (HM74A or PUMA-G) as a new therapeutic target. *Trends Pharmacol. Sci.* **2006**, *7*, 384–390. [CrossRef]
15. Zellner, C.; Pullinger, C.R.; Aouizerat, B.E.; Frost, P.H.; Kwok, P.Y.; Malloy, M.J.; Kane, J.P. Variations in human HM74 (GPR109B) and HM74A (GPR109A) niacin receptors. *Hum. Mutat.* **2005**, *25*, 18–21. [CrossRef]
16. Cresci, G.A.; Thangaraju, M.; Mellinger, J.D.; Liu, K.; Ganapathy, V. Colonic gene expression in conventional and germ-free mice with a focus on the butyrate receptor GPR109A and the butyrate transporter SLC5A8. *J. Gastrointest. Surg.* **2010**, *14*, 449–461. [CrossRef]
17. Sharp, P.A.; Boyer, S.; Srai, S.K.; Baldwin, S.A.; Debnam, E.S. Early diabetes-induced changes in rat jejunal glucose transport and the response to insulin. *J. Endocrinol.* **1997**, *154*, 19–25. [CrossRef]
18. Kellett, G.L.; Helliwell, P.A. The diffusive component of intestinal glucose absorption is mediated by the glucose-induced recruitment of GLUT2 to the brush-border membrane. *Biochem. J.* **2000**, *350*, 155–162. [CrossRef]
19. Kellett, G.L. The facilitated component of intestinal glucose absorption. *J. Physiol.* **2001**, *531*, 585–595. [CrossRef]
20. Tobin, V.; le Gall, M.; Fioramonti, X.; Stolarczyk, E.; Blazquez, A.G.; Klein, C.; Prigent, M.; Serradas, P.; Cuif, M.H.; Magnan, C.; *et al.* Insulin internalizes GLUT2 in the enterocytes of healthy but not insulin-resistant mice. *Diabetes* **2008**, *57*, 55–62. [CrossRef]
21. Kellett, G.L.; Brot-Laroche, E. Apical GLUT2: A major pathway of intestinal sugar absorption. *Diabetes* **2005**, *54*, 3056–3062. [CrossRef]
22. Del Castillo, J.R. The use of hyperosmolar, intracellular-like solutions for the isolation of epithelial cells from guinea-pig small intestine. *Biochim. Biophys. Acta* **1987**, *901*, 201–208. [CrossRef]
23. Wong, T.P.; Debnam, E.S.; Leung, P.S. Involvement of an enterocyte renin-angiotensin system in the local control of SGLT1-dependent glucose uptake across the rat small intestinal brush border membrane. *J. Physiol.* **2007**, *584*, 613–623. [CrossRef]
24. Wong, T.P.; Debnam, E.S.; Leung, P.S. Diabetes mellitus and expression of the enterocyte renin-angiotensin system: Implications for control of glucose transport across the brush border membrane. *Am. J. Physiol. Cell Physiol.* **2009**, *297*, 601–610. [CrossRef]
25. Ip, S.P.; Wong, T.P.; Tsai, S.J.; Leung, P.S. The recovery of some components of the renin angiotensin system in the rat pancreas after chronic exposure to hypoxic condition. *J. Mol. Endocrinol.* **2003**, *3*, 563–571. [CrossRef]
26. Chu, K.Y.; Leung, P.S. Angiotensin II Type 1 receptor antagonism mediates uncoupling protein 2-driven oxidative stress and ameliorates pancreatic islet β-cell function in young Type 2 diabetic mice. *Antioxid. Redox. Signal.* **2007**, *9*, 869–878. [CrossRef]
27. Lau, T.; Carlsson, P.O.; Leung, P.S. Evidence for a local angiotensin-generating system and dose-dependent inhibition of glucose-stimulated insulin release by angiotensin II in isolated pancreatic islets. *Diabetologia* **2004**, *47*, 240–248. [CrossRef]
28. Debnam, E.S.; Smith, M.W.; Sharp, P.A.; Srai, S.K.; Turvey, A.; Keable, S.J. The effects of streptozotocin diabetes on sodium-glucose transporter (SGLT1) expression and function in rat jejunal and ileal villus-attached enterocytes. *Pflugers* **1995**, *430*, 151–159. [CrossRef]

29. Karasov, W.H.; Pond, R.S.; Solberg, D.H.; Diamond, J.M. Regulation of proline and glucose transport in mouse intestine by dietary substrate levels. *Proc. Natl. Acad. Sci. USA* **1983**, *80*, 7674–7677. [CrossRef]
30. Gilbert, T.; Rodriguez-Boulan, E. Induction of vacuolar apical compartments in the Caco-2 intestinal epithelial cell line. *J. Cell Sci.* **1991**, *100*, 451–458.
31. Jumarie, C.; Malo, C. Caco-2 cells cultured in serum-free medium as a model for the study of enterocytic differentiation *in vitro*. *J. Cell Physiol.* **1991**, *149*, 24–33. [CrossRef]
32. Gambhir, D.; Ananth, S.; Veeranan-Karmegam, R.; Elangovan, S.; Hester, S.; Jennings, E.; Offermanns, S.; Nussbaum, J.J.; Smith, S.B.; Thangaraju, M.; *et al.* GPR109A as an anti-inflammatory receptor in retinal pigment epithelial cells and its relevance to diabetic retinopathy. *Invest. Ophthalmol. Vis. Sci.* **2012**, *53*, 2208–2217. [CrossRef]
33. Singh, N.; Gurav, A.; Sivaprakasam, S.; Brady, E.; Padia, R.; Shi, H.; Thangaraju, M.; Prasad, P.D.; Manicassamy, S.; Munn, D.H.; *et al.* Activation of GPR109a, receptor for niacin and the commensal metabolite butyrate, suppresses colonic inflammation and carcinogenesis. *Immunity* **2014**, *40*, 128–139. [CrossRef]
34. Chai, J.T.; Digby, J.E.; Choudhury, R.P. GPR109A and Vascular inflammation. *Curr. Atheroscler. Rep.* **2013**, *15*, 325. [CrossRef]
35. Wong, T.P.; Ho, K.Y.; Ng, E.K.W.; Debnam, E.S.; Leung, P.S. Upregulation of ACE2-ANG-(1–7)-Mas axis in jejunal enterocytes of type 1 diabetic rats: Implications for glucose transport. *Am. J. Physiol. Endocrinol.* **2012**, *303*, E669–E681. [CrossRef]
36. Bechgaard, H.; Jespersen, S. GI absorption of niacin in humans. *J. Pharm. Sci.* **1977**, *66*, 871–872. [CrossRef]
37. Johnson, R.L.; Ghishan, F.K.; Kaunitz, J.D.; Merchant, J.L.; Said, H.M.; Wood, J.D. *Physiology of the Gastrointestinal Tract*, 5th ed.; Elsevier Inc.: San Diego, CA, USA, 2012; Volume 2.
38. Taylor, W.M.; Mak, M.L.; Halperin, M.L. Effect of 3′,5′-cyclic AMP on glucose transport in rat adipocytes. *Proc. Natl. Acad. Sci. USA* **1976**, *73*, 4359–4363. [CrossRef]
39. Taylor, W.M.; Halperin, M.L. Stimulation of glucose transport in rat adipocytes by insulin, adenosine, nicotinic acid and hydrogen peroxide. Role of adenosine 3′,5′-cyclic monophosphate. *Biochem. J.* **1979**, *178*, 381–389. [CrossRef]
40. Stümpel, F.; Scholtka, B.; Jungermann, K. A new role for enteric glucagon-37: Acute stimulation of glucose absorption in rat small intestine. *FEBS Lett.* **1997**, *410*, 515–519. [CrossRef]
41. Lee, W.Y.; Loflin, P.; Clancey, C.J.; Peng, H.; Lever, J.E. Cyclic nucleotide regulation of Na+/glucose cotransporter (SGLT1) mRNA stability. Interaction of a nucleocytoplasmic protein with a regulatory domain in the 3′-untranslated region critical for stabilization. *J. Biol. Chem.* **2000**, *275*, 33998–34008. [CrossRef]
42. Rencurel, F.; Waeber, G.; Bonny, C.; Antoine, B.; Maulard, P.; Girard, J.; Leturque, A. cAMP prevents the glucose-mediated stimulation of GLUT2 gene transcription in hepatocytes. *Biochem. J.* **1997**, *322*, 441–448. [CrossRef]
43. Li, G.; Deng, X.; Wu, C.; Zhou, Q.; Chen, L.; Shi, Y.; Huang, H.; Zhou, N. Distinct kinetic and spatial patterns of protein kinase C (PKC)- and epidermal growth factor receptor (EGFR)-dependent activation of extracellular signal-regulated kinases 1 and 2 by human nicotinic acid receptor GPR109A. *J. Biol. Chem.* **2011**, *286*, 31199–31212. [CrossRef]
44. Cohen, M.; Kitsberg, D.; Tsytkin, S.; Shulman, M.; Aroeti, B.; Nahmias, Y. Live imaging of GLUT2 glucose dependent trafficking and its inhibition in polarized epithelial cysts. *Open Biol.* **2014**, *4*. [CrossRef]
45. Thorens, B.; Dériaz, N.; Bosco, D.; DeVos, A.; Pipeleers, D.; Schuit, F.; Meda, P.; Porret, A. Protein kinase A-dependent phosphorylation of GLUT2 in pancreatic β cells. *J. Biol. Chem.* **1996**, *271*, 8075–8081.
46. Wright, E.M.; Hirsch, J.R.; Loo, D.D.; Zampighi, G.A. Regulation of Na+/glucose cotransporters. *J. Exp. Biol.* **1997**, *200*, 287–293.

4

Caloric Restriction as a Strategy to Improve Vascular Dysfunction in Metabolic Disorders

Concha F. García-Prieto [1] and María S. Fernández-Alfonso [2,*]

1 The Rolf Luft Research Center for Diabetes and Endocrinology, Karolinska Institutet, Stockholm 17176, Sweden; concepcion.fernandez.garcia-prieto@ki.se
2 Instituto Pluridisciplinar and Facultad de Farmacia, Universidad Complutense, Madrid 28040, Spain
* Correspondence: marisolf@farm.ucm.es

Abstract: Caloric restriction (CR) has proved to be the most effective and reproducible dietary intervention to increase healthy lifespan and aging. A reduction in cardiovascular disease (CVD) risk in obese subjects can be already achieved by a moderate and sustainable weight loss. Since pharmacological approaches for body weight reduction have, at present, a poor long-term efficacy, CR is of great interest in the prevention and/or reduction of CVD associated with obesity. Other dietary strategies changing specific macronutrients, such as altering carbohydrates, protein content or diet glycemic index have been also shown to decrease the progression of CVD in obese patients. In this review, we will focus on the positive effects and possible mechanisms of action of these strategies on vascular dysfunction.

Keywords: caloric restriction; dietary intervention; endothelial dysfunction; cardiovascular disease; obesity

1. Introduction

Obesity is a chronic disease due to an energetic imbalance in which caloric intake is higher than energetic expenditure. It is closely associated with insulin resistance and type 2 diabetes (T2D), leading to several manifestations of cardiovascular disease (CVD), such as hypertension, coronary artery disease, myocardial infarction, heart failure and stroke [1]. CVD is a major health problem worldwide accounting for 30% of all deaths and demands a global approach to prevention and early detection. In obese individuals, the earliest indication of vascular dysfunction preceding the development of prehypertension and hypertension is the impairment of endothelial function [2]. Therefore, endothelial function improvement should become a key approach to prevent and/or treat cardiovascular (CV) complications related to metabolic disorders.

The primary goal to reduce CVD risk in subjects who are overweight and obese is a moderate and sustainable weight loss. An improvement of multiple metabolic and hormonal factors implicated in the pathogenesis of CVD associated with metabolic disorders is already achieved by a weight loss of 5%–10% [3] that needs to be maintained over time. Since pharmacological approaches for body weight (BW) reduction have, at present, a poor long-term efficacy, other strategies such as caloric restriction (CR), exercise programs, or bariatric surgery are of great interest [3,4].

CR is defined as a state in which energy intake is reduced below usual *ad libitum* intake without malnutrition, independently of its duration. It is one of the most common and cost-effective interventions used to induce BW reduction and CV risk factor amelioration. Other dietary strategies changing specific macronutrients have also been shown to decrease progression of CVD. It is important to note that the induction of a negative energy balance is mandatory for achieving the metabolic benefits of weight loss since the sole reduction in fat mass alone by surgical procedures does not improve CV risk factors in obese patients [5,6]. Taking into consideration the complex and vast literature regarding dietary strategies, in this review, we will focus on the positive effects on vascular dysfunction, CV risk factors and CVD exerted by CR and macronutrients intake modification.

2. CR Reduces CV Risk Factors

Benefits on CV risk factors by reducing the daily caloric intake have been widely described in overweight and obese patients [7–19]. CR induces reductions in BW, waist perimeter, total fat, serum triglycerides (TG), or low-density lipoprotein (LDL)-cholesterol concentrations [12,14,20]. It is also associated with a reduction of circulating insulin levels together with an increase in insulin sensitivity [12,14,18,20]. The decrease in adiposity leads to reductions in leptin [14,18], inflammatory cytokines, prostaglandins, and/or oxidative stress [9,10,14,18], as well as to an increase in the anti-inflammatory Il-10 [14] and adiponectin (Figure 1) (see Section 4.4). In obese patients with or without associated hypertension, weight loss enhances flow-mediated vasodilation (FMD, which determines endothelial function *in vivo*) [8,11], and induces a reduction in blood pressure (BP) [7,20].

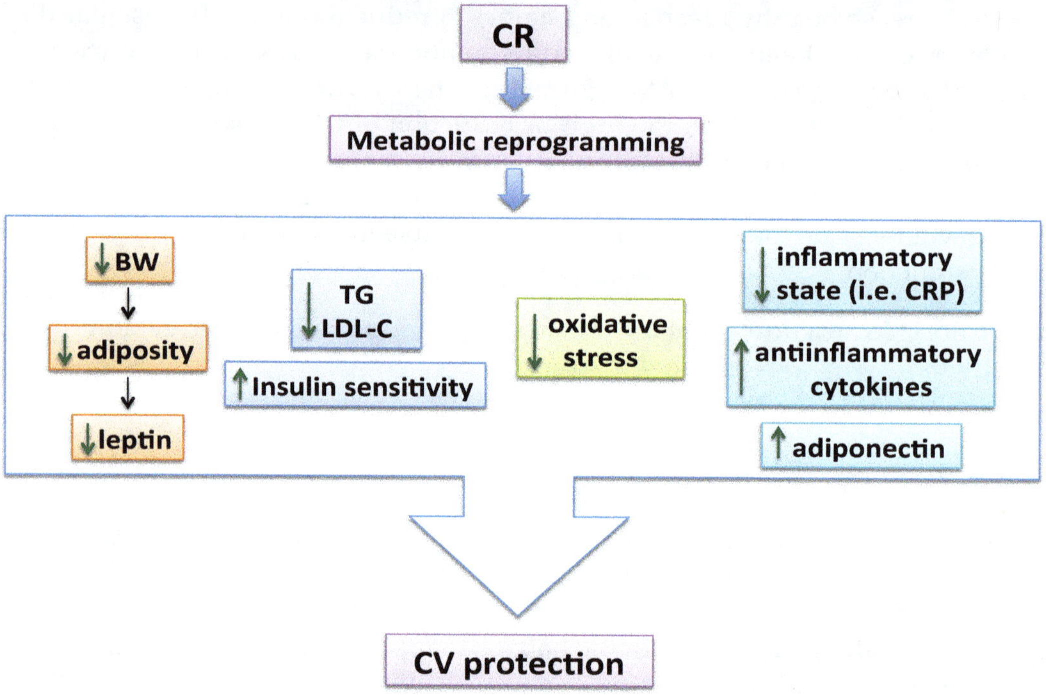

Figure 1. Main mechanisms by which CR exerts CV protection. Reducing the daily caloric intake induces a metabolic reprogramming in both healthy and obese individuals, subsequently leading to CV protection. This includes a reduction in BW and adiposity, thus lessening leptin levels. A decrease in TG and LDL-cholesterol levels together with less oxidative stress and inflammation and an increase in adiponectin levels are some of the main underlying mechanisms described (BW: body weight; CR: caloric restriction; CRP: high-sensitivity C-reactive protein; CV: cardiovascular; LDL-C: low-density lipoprotein -cholesterol; TG: triglycerides).

Interestingly, benefits of CR are not only observed in obese subjects. Long-term (3–15 years) CR in non-obese humans has a profound beneficial impact on CV risk factors, such as serum total cholesterol, LDL-cholesterol, high-density lipoprotein (HDL)-cholesterol, TG, and BP [20]. A decrease in the inflammatory state is reflected by the extremely low levels of high-sensitivity C-reactive protein (CRP) detected in these subjects [20]. Since CV risk factors increase with age, CR reveals as a promising strategy to prevent the development of CVD in both obese and non-obese individuals. However, it has to be noted that long-term interventions might not be equivalent to short-term interventions in the context of obesity and/or metabolic dysfunction, which may include increased resilience and/or improvements in indices of disease risk but are not associated with delayed aging (Figure 1).

3. CR Protocols Differ in Their Starting Point, Severity, Duration and Number of Phases

To assess and compare the effectiveness of CR protocols on CVD several aspects, such as CR severity, its duration, starting point and number of phases, need to be taken into account (Figure 2). A comparison of several approaches is shown in Table 1.

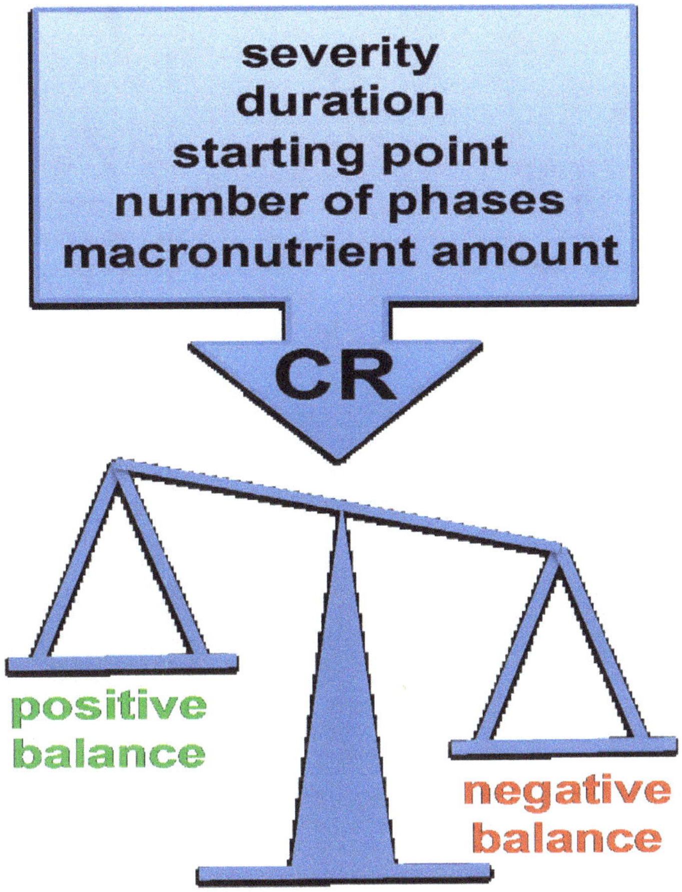

Figure 2. Critical aspects in a CR to achieve the desired effects. Although effects exerted by CR have been widely studied, there is no agreement in how a CR must be in order to prevent CV events. Numerous studies suggest that its severity, duration, starting point, number of phases and composition (*i.e.*, macronutrient amount) are important aspects to take into account. Modifying all these characteristics in different ways can exert a positive or a negative balance, thus affecting CV risk factors (CR: caloric restriction; CV: cardiovascular).

There is no agreement on how severe a CR must be in order to confer benefits in different organs and systems. In general, the *ad libitum* (AL) caloric intake is reduced around 20%–40% exerting positive effects without deleterious consequences [21]. However, numerous protocols include an alternate-day fasting, in which caloric intake reduction will be intermittent [22,23]. Most of the CR protocols reduce very intensively the energetic consumption for a long time. Some examples include a daily 30%–40% reduction for 12 months or longer [24,25]. Others use comparable approaches but only for four or five weeks, obtaining similar effects [26]. This suggests that a CR does not need to be prolonged for a long time to be effective, with the advantage that short-term CR is easier to include in clinical practice. In this context, a genomic analysis revealed that the results obtained after CR during four weeks were similar to those from longer CR (28 weeks). In this study, the short-term CR revealed the 70% of the effects observed under the long-term CR on liver gene expression with age [27]. However, other authors report different findings in other tissues, such as in white adipose tissue [28], probably due to variations in responding to fasting cycles. Overall, we feel that most of the studies do not reflect a realistic intervention since they include really severe protocols.

Table 1. Comparison of several caloric restriction (CR) protocols in rodents and humans.

Reference	Model	CR Protocol
Kondo *et al.*, 2009 [26]	C57/BL6 mice	35% CR for 4 weeks
Donato *et al.*, 2013 [29]	mice	10% CR (1 week) + 25% CR (1 week) + 40% CR throughout the life of the animal
Chen *et al.*, 2015 [30]	Wistar rats	20% CR or 40% CR for 12 weeks—only reduction of starch
Chou *et al.*, 2010 [31]	Wistar rats	40% CR for 2 weeks
Dolinsky *et al.*, 2010 [32]	Wistar and SHR rats	10% CR (2 weeks) + 40% CR (3 weeks)
Chandrasekar *et al.*, 2001 [33]	Fisher344 rats	40% CR for 10 months
Csiszar *et al.*, 2009 [34]	Fisher344 rats	40% CR (life-long; age-related studies)
Ahmet *et al.*, 2011 [24]	Fisher344 rats	40% CR for 22 months (age-related studies)
Zanetti *et al.*, 2010 [35]	Fisher344 rats	26% CR for 3 weeks (age-related studies)
Castello *et al.*, 2005 [36]	Sprague Dawley rats	40% CR for 4, 10 or 22 months (age-related studies)
Ozbek *et al.*, 2013 [37]	Sprague Dawley rats	40% CR for 3 months
Minamiyama *et al.*, 2007 [38]	type II diabetic rats (OLETF)	30% CR for 13 weeks
García-Prieto *et al.*, 2015 [39]	Zucker obese rats	20% CR for 2 weeks
Ketonen *et al.*, 2010 [40]	C57Bl/6J mice under HFD	30% CR for 50 days (with HFD)
Iacobellis *et al.*, 2008 [41]	patients	VLCD (900 kcal/day). Phase 1—complete meal replacement (12 weeks); phase 2—transition period including healthy foods and partial meal replacement (4–6 weeks); phase 3—long-term maintenance
Kitada *et al.*, 2013 [19]	overweight patients	25% CR for 7 weeks
Siklova-Vitkova *et al.*, 2012 [42]	obese patients	800 kcal/day (1 month) + weight stabilization period (low-calorie diet for 2 months + weight maintenance diet for 3 months)
Capel *et al*, 2009 [43]	obese patients	800 kcal/day (1 month) + weight stabilization period (low-calorie diet for 2 months + weight maintenance diet for 3–4 months)
Davì *et al.*, 2002 [9]	obese patients	1200 kcal/day for 12 weeks
Ziccardi *et al.*, 2002 [10]	obese patients	1300 kcal/day for 12 months
Raitakari *et al.*, 2004 [11]	obese patients	580 kcal/day for 6 weeks
Cooper *et al.*, 2012 [15]	obese patients	CR to produce a 8%–10% weight loss within 12 months with or without physical activity
Morel *et al.*, 2011 [44]	obese patients	600 kcal/day (1 month) + 1200 kcal/day (1 month)
Fontana *et al.*, 2007 [13]	overweight/obese patients	16% CR (3 months) + 20% CR (9 months)
Ho *et al.*, 2015 [18]	overweight/obese patients	CR to produce a 5%–7% weight loss within 12 months
Murakami *et al.*, 2007 [45]	overweight/obese patients	≈1200 kcal/day (women) or 1600 kcal/day (men) for 12 weeks with or without exercise program
Sasaki *et al.*, 2002 [8]	obese patients with hypertension	800 kcal/day for 2 weeks

AL: *ad libitum;* CR: caloric restriction; HFD: high-fat diet; SHR: spontaneously hypertensive rats; VLCD: very low-calorie diet.

Initially, it was thought that benefits appeared only after long periods of CR [46]. Nevertheless some of the beneficial effects promoted by CR, such as plasmatic glucose levels decrease, show up within the first week of the diet [47]. Important protection of endothelial function occurs in vascular aging models even under CR protocols for less than three weeks [35,48]. Other vascular aged-related complications, such as aortic stiffening and artery wall hypertrophy, need longer dietary treatments to be prevented [29].

Regarding the starting point of a CR, its effects on lifespan are higher if it is initiated at the weaning [49–51]. A study in 10-week-old spontaneously hypertensive rats (SHR), with a moderate hypertension, showed that a 10% CR for two weeks followed by a 40% CR for three additional weeks avoided the increase in BP levels [32]. However, starting the same protocol at older ages, when BP values were higher (>200 mmHg) could not reduce those values. This suggests that CR protocols might be more beneficial at early stages of vascular disease [32].

The different phases in which a CR can be subdivided play a substantial role in the achievements can be reached. In multiphase dietary interventions, the pattern of adipokine expression, secretion rate, and plasma levels is different with respect to the phase of the intervention, and to the cellular origin of the respective adipokine [42]. Adipocyte-derived adipokines (adiponectin, leptin, serum amyloid A, or haptoglobin) decrease (except for adiponectin), during the initial very low-calorie diet (VLCD), whereas they increase toward prediet levels during the weight stabilization phase. Similar results have been observed with low-calorie diets [52]. In contrast, expression and secretion rate of stromal-vascular fraction-derived adipokines (tumor necrosis factor α TNF-α, interleukins IL-6, IL-10, IL-8, monocyte chemoattractant protein-1, and plasminogen activator inhibitor-1, PAI-1) increased or remained unchanged during the initial VLCD but decreased during the weight stabilization phase [42]. During the various phases of a dietary weight loss program, adipose tissue macrophages and adipocytes show distinct patterns of gene regulation and association with insulin sensitivity, the regulation of gene expression being dependent on the severity and duration of CR [43].

In conclusion, the optimal CR protocol for each specific situation remains to be determined and standardization will be necessary to allow comparison of the beneficial effects of different dietary approaches on CVD.

4. Mechanisms by Which CR Exerts Vascular Protection in Metabolic Disorders

The improvement of vascular dysfunction associated with metabolic disorders might be due to changes in endothelial function, in the arterial wall structure, or in the paracrine effects of perivascular adipose tissue (PVAT).

4.1. Effects of CR on Endothelial Function

CR leads to an improvement of endothelial function in arteries from several models of aged [24,29,33,34,36,53] and obese rodents [38–40]. Underlying mechanisms include the increase of nitric oxide (NO) bioavailability [29,31,35,48] due to the enhancement of endothelial nitric oxide synthase (eNOS) expression and/or activity [29,37,54], together with the suppression of vascular oxidative stress associated to superoxide anion (O_2^-) production [29,31,34,38,40] and lipid peroxidation [38]. Vasoprotective effects of life-long CR both reduce the expression and activity of NADPH oxidase and O_2^- production, and enhance superoxide dismutase (SOD) activity [29].

Endothelial function improvement is also achieved by the reduction of inflammatory mediators, such as CRP, which is a moderately good predictor of acute vascular events related to obesity [55], IL-6 and TNF-α in mice [55], as well as decreases in nuclear factor NF-κB activity [33,34].

A key event associated with the improvement of endothelial function under CR is the activation of the AMPK-PI3K-Akt-eNOS signaling pathway. A dysregulation of this pathway in over-nutrition and obesity contributes to the development of endothelial dysfunction (for review, see [56]) in both diet-induced [57] and genetic models of obesity, such as Zucker *fa/fa* obese rats [58], Zucker diabetic fatty rats [59] or Otsuka Long Evans Tokushima Fatty rats [60]. CR triggers endothelial AMPK activation leading to (i) normalization of endothelial function and systolic BP reduction in Zucker obese rats [39]; (ii) an improvement of vascular compliance and BP reduction in hypertensive rats [32]; or (iii) revascularization in response to ischemia [26]. Moreover, activation of AMPK by CR reduces lipotoxicity associated with high-fat diets (HFD), insulin resistance, and obesity by decreasing the excessive exposure of the endothelium to free fatty-acids (FFAs) [61,62], thus exerting a protective effect on endothelial cells [61,62]. Obese patients subjected to CR that reported systolic BP reduction, as well as FFA and inflammatory marker level decrease, showed an increase of AMPK phosphorylation in peripheral blood mononuclear cells [19]. The fact that these changes are observed even with a moderate reduction in BW supports the predominant role of the negative energy balance to achieve CV benefits of CR.

Activation of the cellular sensing protein sirtuin-1 (SIRT1) is another mechanism proposed as key mediator of vascular benefits of CR [29,34]. Arterial aging is associated with changes in expression and/or activity of SIRT1 and mammalian target of rapamycin (mTOR), which are ameliorated by life-long CR. In the same line, serum obtained from CR patients activates SIRT1 in human cells *in vitro* [63]. There are, however, very few studies assessing the vascular role of SIRT1 activation by CR in obesity, and further research needs to be performed in this line.

4.2. Effects of CR on Arterial Wall Structure and Remodeling

Subclinical organ damage, such as vascular remodeling, precedes the occurrence of CV events in individuals with obesity and hypertension [64]. Life-long CR significantly reduces large elastic artery wall hypertrophy and prevents aortic stiffening in mice [29] due to a suppression of collagen production [29] and elastin fiber degradation [53]. Increases in elasticity after CR have also been described in arteries from young, but not from aged SHR [32]. This suggests that reversal of early changes in the arterial wall structure, at a time when vascular remodeling is emerging and still reversible, is essential for the prevention of vascular dysfunction.

Mechanisms underlying CR-induced changes in vascular remodeling have been mainly analyzed in models of aging. CR introduced early in life protects against aortic fibrosclerosis by decreasing oxidative damage and consequently reducing the levels of transforming growth factor beta-1 (TGFβ1). This change very likely occurs through a downregulation of the mitogen-activated protein kinases (MAPK), c-Jun N-terminal kinase (JNK) and activator protein-1 (AP-1) signaling pathways [36]. Whether the same mechanisms underlie the effects of CR on metabolic arterial wall remodeling remains to be further analyzed.

Both intervention and cross-sectional studies in humans demonstrate that short-term CR and reduced BW are associated with lower BP and carotid wall thickness [15,16,20,65]. A weight loss of around 8% results in a mean decrease of 0.07 mm in carotid artery diameter, whereas individuals who achieved at least a 5% weight loss showed a significant reduction in mean carotid intima:media thickness [15]. A meta-analysis of 43 studies on moderate weight loss (around 11%) due to CR, with or without exercise, demonstrates an improvement of some arterial compliance and stiffness parameters, such as cardio-ankle vascular and β-stiffness index, arterial compliance and distensibility, distal oscillatory compliance, proximal capacitive compliance, systemic arterial compliance or reflection time. However, other parameters, such as augmentation index, strain, augmentation pressure and pulse pressure were not significantly improved with weight loss [66]. All of these results demonstrate that an intensive dietary intervention at a time when vascular remodeling has only been initiated and is not irreversibly established might significantly reverse some of the key adverse vascular structural changes associated with excess weight in severely obese adults.

4.3. Effects of CR on PVAT Dysfunction in Obesity

Perivascular adipose tissue (PVAT) is the adipose tissue surrounding most blood vessels, except cerebral vessels. It might be white or brown adipose tissue and produces a number of vasoactive factors, adipokines and cytokines. A large body of evidence supports the paracrine influence of PVAT for the maintenance of vascular resistance under physiological and pathophysiological conditions [67]. PVAT releases a number of adipokines, inflammatory cytokines, and other vasoactive factors, which are variable in quantity and pattern depending on the PVAT amount [67]. In fact, obesity triggers an increase in PVAT throughout the vasculature [68,69], accompanied by an unbalance in favor of vasoconstrictor and pro-inflammatory substances, which leads to endothelial dysfunction and vascular damage [70–72]. Long-term HFD in mice leads to PVAT dysfunction, characterized by an increase in

NADPH oxidase activity and O_2^- release, as well as by a reduction in extracellular SOD expression, total SOD activity, eNOS levels, and NO availability [70]. Similarly, PVAT of New Zealand obese mice show increased O_2^- levels formation and decreased SOD expression, leading to an impaired hydrogen peroxide (H_2O_2) production, which contributes to vascular dysfunction reducing the anti-contractile effects of PVAT [73]. In Ossabaw obese swine H_2O_2-mediated vasodilatation was markedly attenuated by the presence of coronary PVAT [74]. Ma *et al.* [72] showed that PVAT induces endothelial dysfunction by dysregulation of the AMPK/mTOR pathway in the aorta of diet-induced obese rats, characterized by a downregulation of AMPK-eNOS pathway and a concurrent upregulation of mTOR. Moreover, obese periaortic PVAT high FFA levels could attenuate the anti-contractile properties of PVAT by a TNF-α-dependent [75].

An interesting issue, which deserves future investigation, is the impact of the diet composition on oxidative stress in PVAT. A fructose-rich diet, which decreases polyunsaturated FAs and increases saturated and monounsaturated FAs in PVAT impairs vascular function by a decrease in antioxidant enzymes and a reduction in glutathione content [76]. Altogether, these results indicate that obesity and the diet composition induce a switch in PVAT to a more pro-inflammatory, pro-oxidant and vasoconstrictor phenotype.

Since the beneficial or deleterious paracrine influence of PVAT is directly dependent on its amount [77,78], a key question is whether the proportion of adipose tissue loss induced by CR is uniform (overall adiposity) or predominant in specific adipose depots (*i.e.*, PVAT). Significant reduction in the thickness of epicardial fat (surrounding coronary arteries) has been described both in severely obese patients who underwent substantial weight loss after bariatric surgery [79], as well as after a short-term VLCD program [41]. Interestingly, the decrease of epicardial fat is substantially higher than changes in overall BW loss body mass index and waist circumference, and correlates with the improvement in both left ventricular mass and diastolic function. Interestingly, bariatric surgery also reverses the obesity-induced damage to PVAT anticontractile function by reducing adipocyte hypertrophy, PVAT inflammation and increasing both PVAT-derived NO and adiponectin availability [80]. We believe that these studies open a new approach for the management of vascular damage and CV risk associated with PVAT dysfunction in metabolic related disorders.

4.4. *Effects of CR on Vascular Actions of Leptin and Adiponectin*

Obesity is associated with hyperleptinemia and hypoadiponectinemia, both playing a key role in the pathogenesis of endothelial dysfunction [81]. Chronic hyperleptinemia has been linked to endothelial dysfunction and damage [82–84] stimulating the increase in NADPH oxidase activity and O_2^- production in the vascular wall, as well as promoting glutathione peroxidase activation to remove excessive H_2O_2 production. On the other hand, hypoadiponectinemia is closely associated with endothelial dysfunction in humans and adiponectin knock-out mice show a decrease in eNOS phosphorilation levels.

Different CR protocols in rats, markedly changes the adipokine production pattern leading to an increase in circulating levels of adiponectin, whereas leptin levels profoundly decrease in adipose tissue [85,86].

A role for adipokine levels in PVAT and their paracrine influence on the vascular wall might not be discarded. *Ob/ob* mice lacking leptin do not exhibit NO production in perivascular adipocytes. Interestingly, this is restored in PVAT after two-week subcutaneous leptin infusion, suggesting that NO release in PVAT seems to be mediated by leptin [87]. Hypoadiponectinemia in patients with T2D stimulates vascular NADPH oxidase expression, which is counterbalanced by upregulation of adiponectin expression in PVAT aimed at suppressing in a paracrine manner NADPH oxidase activity via a PI3K/Akt-mediated deactivation of Rac1 and the downregulation of $p22^{phox}$ gene expression [88]. These studies again stress the concept that PVAT-vessel interaction is a promising therapeutic target for the prevention of vascular complications of metabolic disorders. The effect of CR and dietary approaches on this interaction deserves future investigation.

5. Dietary Strategies Based on Macronutrients Modification

Not only the amount but also the quality of the nutrient intake contributes to benefits on vascular function [89–91]. However, any dietary change can be universally applied as positive at the CV level since their beneficial effects are different depending on the metabolic state of the individual. Although dietary interventions need to be personalized on the basis of patient requirements, some of the most widely approaches used in clinical practice regarding macronutrients content on the diet and its effects at vascular level are described in Sections 5.1 to 5.3 below.

5.1. Low-Carbohydrate Diets

In both overweight and obese patients, carbohydrate restricted diets are more effective than low-fat diets in terms of atherogenic dyslipemia and other metabolic syndrome characteristics such as inflammation, oxidative stress and CV risk markers (*i.e.*, apolipoproteins A-1 and B, LDL particle distribution, and FMD) [92–95]. Peripheral small artery vascular function is improved with low carbohydrate diets when there is a decrease in BW [96,97]. However, some authors report that the degree of weight loss in obese patients is not correlated to changes in BP, endothelial function and inflammatory markers [98]. Restricting dietary carbohydrate positively impacts lipid homeostasis and inflammatory markers (*i.e.*, TNF-α, IL-6, PAI-1) even when the saturated fat intake is higher due to the isocaloric replacement of carbohydrates [92–95]. Dysregulation of PAI-1 is involved in enhanced inflammation, vascular damage and subsequent thrombogenicity [99]. Thus, studies with different dietary interventions aim to establish PAI-1 as a possible therapeutic target for controlling CVD in obese patients [44,45]. Moreover, beneficial effects of carbohydrate restriction in combination with pharmacological treatments, *i.e.*, statins, have been described [98]. A decrease in approximately 400 kcal/day for six weeks (with carbohydrates representing the 11% of the daily intake) reduced CV risk markers such as serum TG, soluble E-selectin and intracellular adhesion molecule-1. Both systolic and diastolic BP decreased together with an increase in reactive hyperemia, indicating a better resistance vessel endothelial function, probably in a prostaglandins-mediated way and independent of NO increase [98,100].

However, there is no consensus regarding how much the carbohydrate amount of the diet must be reduced to be beneficial. A recent study comparing the effects of two low-carbohydrate diets for 12 weeks in rats (80% energy intake with 34% carbohydrate reduction *vs.* 60% energy intake with 68% carbohydrate reduction of the control diet) demonstrated that decreasing carbohydrate intake to a large extent even with a lower caloric intake has detrimental effects on lipid balance due to an increase in LDL and total cholesterol levels [30]. Indeed, dietary patterns characterized by a low amount of carbohydrate but reciprocally higher content in fat and protein are related to a poorer vascular reactivity in overweight and obese patients [97] and in patients with T2D and increased vascular risk [101]. This emphasizes the necessity of studying the impact of macronutrient composition and nature on CVD (Figure 3).

5.2. Higher Protein Content: Does It Make the Difference?

Diets low in carbohydrates have been proven to reduce BW in both overweight and obese patients [91,96,97,102] and to maintain weight when associated with a moderate increase in protein amount [103]. Low-fat/high-protein diets are more effective for long-term maintenance or further improvement of vascular function [104,105]. Thus, energy-restricted diets are generally compensated by protein content, usually with meal replacements [101,105]. Obese T2D subjects receiving either a meal replacement-based low-calorie diet (approximately 1000 kcal/day) or a low-fat, high-protein, reduced-carbohydrate diet (HP, intake decrease about 600 kcal/day) for eight weeks and either switching to or continuing with the HP diet for 44 additional weeks showed similar positive impacts on endothelial function and inflammatory markers [105]. Both diets reduced blood glucose, TG and LDL-cholesterol and improved endothelial function by lessening soluble E-selectin and increasing

FMD. However, only the HP diet decreased CRP and IL-6 levels, markers of inflammation related to vascular homeostasis. Controlled trials in which obese patients were assigned to two periods of a four-week hypocaloric diet (either high in proteins or a conventional one, 1200 kcal/day) [106] showed similar results in some metabolic risk markers after both diets. Interestingly, diets high in protein were associated with improvement in some cardiometabolic risk factors such as PAI-1, vascular endothelial growth factor, fasting plasma glucose and CRP despite the fact of its higher fat content. However, only the conventional hypocaloric diet decreased systolic BP, highlighting the importance of every macronutrient maintaining vascular homeostasis in obese patients [106]. Since high CRP precedes atheromatic events [107], lessening its levels could pave the way to better prevent CV disease. Some clinical trials (*i.e.*, the OmniHeart study) support the idea that a partial replacement of carbohydrates with either protein or monounsaturated fat has additional beneficial effects on the basis of a healthy diet at a vascular level independent of BW loss in both non-obese and obese patients with prehypertension or stage 1 hypertension [108]. Without reducing caloric intake (2100 kcal/day), these patients further reduced systolic and diastolic BP and decreased estimated risk of suffering coronary heart disease with both diets rich in protein or rich in unsaturated fat [108].

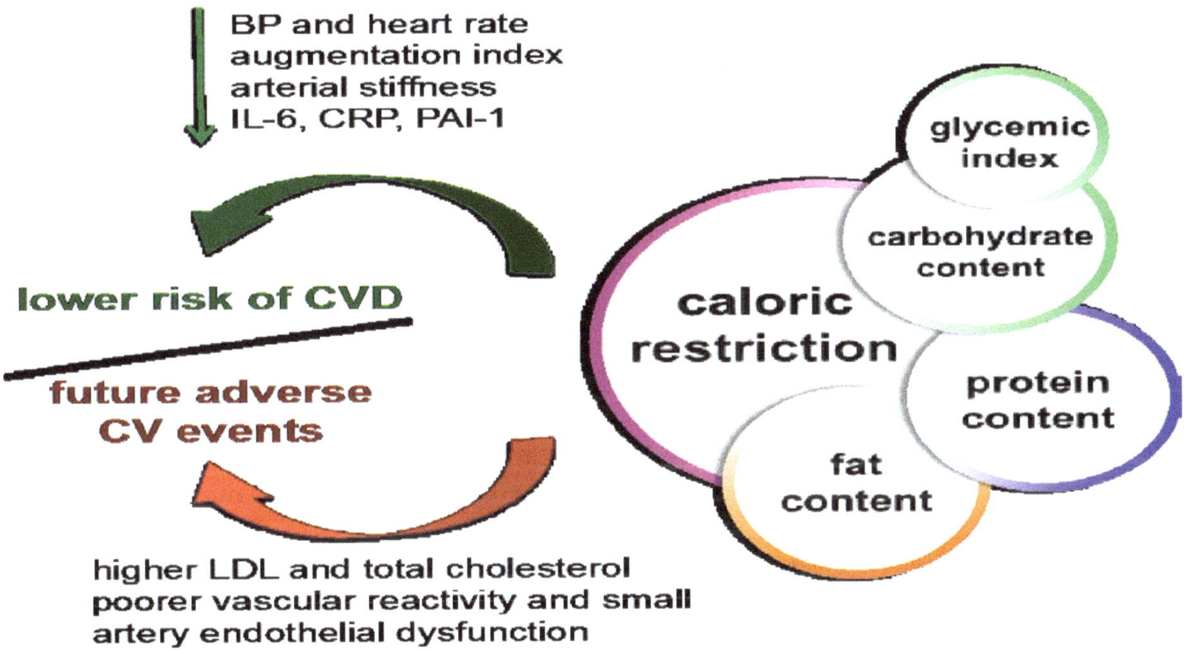

Figure 3. CV outcome of CR depends on macronutrient composition of the diet. Both the amount and the quality of each macronutrient of the diet are important in order to achieve positive effects at CV level. A proper balance in macronutrient amount is key to avoid future adverse CV events (BP: blood pressure; CR: caloric restriction; CRP: high-sensitivity C-reactive protein; CV: cardiovascular; CVD: cardiovascular disease; IL-6: interleukin 6; LDL: low-density lipoprotein; PAI-1: plasminogen activator inhibitor-1).

Besides the positive effects that a protein supplementation can exert, replacing carbohydrates with higher amounts of protein and fat lead to a low small artery reactive hyperaemia index, a marker of small artery endothelial function [101], which correlates with endothelial dysfunction [109], thus predicting future adverse CV events [110]. Hence, balancing the amount of each macronutrient of the diet might be of importance for achieving positive effects at the CV level (Figure 3).

5.3. Diet Glycemic Index Variation

Both the carbohydrate and fat content of a diet influences the occurrence of diabetes and CVD [102,111]. Although diets restricting carbohydrate consumption are a well-known strategy for weight loss with the subsequent improvement of metabolic-related complications in overweight and obese patients [102], recent studies show that following these diets for a long time does not always protect from CVD [101,112,113]. In this context, changing carbohydrate quality rather than quantity has emerged as a better approach to dealing with CV risk factors. Glycemic index (GI) is the quantification of the blood glucose response to a carbohydrate compared to a carbohydrate reference [114]. That is, foods with similar carbohydrate content can behave differently in terms of raising blood glucose. Thus, varying GI might be useful in the management of these diseases (Figure 3). The effects on metabolism exerted by different GI diets are diverse [89,91,115]. Control trials in which obese patients at increased CV risk were subjected to hypocaloric diets with different GI for three months showed a decrease in BW, plasma glucose, total cholesterol, LDL-cholesterol, TG, systolic BP and heart rate independent of the GI of the diet [91]. Interestingly, FMD was influenced, being higher after following the low GI diet [91], a fact observed in studies assessing the acute effects of different GI diets [89]. In this context, the EVIDENT study (2010, Spain) aims to establish an association between GI and vascular homeostasis by assessing arterial stiffness (via pulse wave velocity measurement) and augmentation index (vascular aging related to endothelial dysfunction) [116]. Their latest results show that an increase in GI correlates with an enhancement of augmentation index, thus increasing the risk of suffering a CVD [116]. Low GI diets can reduce oxidative stress [117] and inflammation [90], factors widely associated with endothelial dysfunction. In this context, low GI hypocaloric diets have been shown to decrease CRP blood levels in overweight patients [90]. However, some clinical trials claim that GI is not related to an improvement in CV risk factors on the basis of a healthy diet [118]. In this controlled feeding study, the effects of four different interventions on carbohydrate content from a healthy diet without losing weight were analyzed. No differences were observed between high and low GI diets regarding insulin sensitivity, lipid homeostasis and systolic BP [118]. All of these diverse results between studies may be due to changes in content of total carbohydrates and fibers, no concomitant weight loss and duration of the dietary treatment, although long-term studies with BW decrease conclude in a similar way [90,119].

6. Conclusions

All the described dietary modifications are effective by mitigating CV risk factors in obesity. However, despite all the efforts made to establish CR or a balanced diet as the main strategies to either prevent or treat CV complications related to metabolic disorders, there is no fully effective formula, and factors such as severity, duration, starting point, number of phases and composition need to be taken into account. It is important to note that an intensive dietary intervention at a time when vascular dysfunction has only been initiated and is not irreversibly established might significantly reverse some of the key adverse vascular changes associated with obesity.

On the other hand, many mechanisms underlying CR-induced changes in vascular dysfunction have been mainly analyzed in models of aging (*i.e.*, vascular remodeling). Whether the same mechanisms underlie the effects of CR on obesity related vascular dysfunction remains to be further analyzed. In addition, most of these regimens have the ability to attenuate some, but not all, of the components involved in this complicated multifactorial condition. Therefore, further research is needed to understand in depth the mechanisms involved in the positive effects of CR and macronutrient intake modification on vascular dysfunction associated with being overweight and obese.

Moreover, we need to define specific biomarkers to (i) assess and/or predict the effect CR on CV risk and (ii) design an optimal and more personalized dietary regime, taking into account individual differences in age, metabolic function and CV risk factors.

Acknowledgments: This work was supported by SAF2011-25303, GR921641-Santander, Fundación Mutua Madrileña and Fundación Eugenio Rodríguez Pascual.

Author Contributions: Both authors generated the concept of the review, and wrote and approved the text.

Abbreviations

The following abbreviations are used in this manuscript:

Akt	protein kinase B
AL	*ad libitum*
AMPK	adenosine monophosphate-activated protein kinase
AP-1	activator protein-1
BP	blood pressure
BW	body weight
CR	caloric restriction
CRP	high-sensitivity C-reactive protein
CV	cardiovascular
CVD	cardiovascular disease
eNOS	endothelial nitric oxide synthase
FA	fatty acid
FFAs	free fatty-acids
FMD	flow-mediated dilation
GI	glycemic index
H_2O_2	hydrogen peroxide
HDL	high-density lipoprotein
HFD	high-fat diet
HP	low-fat, high-protein, reduced-carbohydrate
IL	interleukin
JNK	c-Jun N-terminal kinase
LDL	low-density lipoprotein
MAPK	mitogen-activated protein kinases
MCP-1	monocyte chemoattractant protein-1
mTOR	mammalian target of rapamycin
NF-κB	nuclear factor κB
NO	nitric oxide
O_2^-	superoxide anion
PAI-1	plasminogen activator inhibitor-1
PI3K	phosphoinositide 3-kinase
PVAT	perivascular adipose tissue
SHR	spontaneously hypertensive rats
SIRT1	sirtuin-1
SOD	superoxide dismutase
T2D	type 2 diabetes
TG	triglycerides
TGFβ1	transforming growth factor beta-1
TNF-α	tumor necrosis factor α
VLCD	very low-calorie diet

References

1. Galassi, A.; Reynolds, K.; He, J. Metabolic syndrome and risk of cardiovascular disease: A meta-analysis. *Am. J. Med.* **2006**, *119*, 812–819. [CrossRef] [PubMed]
2. DeMarco, V.G.; Aroor, A.R.; Sowers, J.R. The pathophysiology of hypertension in patients with obesity. *Nat. Rev. Endocrinol.* **2014**, *10*, 364–376. [CrossRef] [PubMed]
3. Wing, R.R.; Lang, W.; Wadden, T.A.; Safford, M.; Knowler, W.C.; Bertoni, A.G.; Hill, J.O.; Brancati, F.L.; Peters, A.; Wagenknecht, L.; *et al.* Benefits of modest weight loss in improving cardiovascular risk factors in overweight and obese individuals with type 2 diabetes. *Diabetes Care* **2011**, *34*, 1481–1486. [CrossRef] [PubMed]

4. Sjöström, L.; Lindroos, A.K.; Peltonen, M.; Torgerson, J.; Bouchard, C.; Carlsson, B.; Dahlgren, S.; Larsson, B.; Narbro, K.; Sjöström, C.D.; *et al.* Lifestyle, diabetes, and cardiovascular risk factors 10 years after bariatric surgery. *N. Engl. J. Med.* **2004**, *351*, 2683–2693. [CrossRef] [PubMed]
5. Klein, S.; Fontana, L.; Young, V.L.; Coggan, A.R.; Kilo, C.; Patterson, B.W.; Mohammed, B.S. Absence of an effect of liposuction on insulin action and risk factors for coronary heart disease. *N. Engl. J. Med.* **2004**, *350*, 2549–2557. [CrossRef] [PubMed]
6. Fabbrini, E.; Tamboli, R.A.; Magkos, F.; Marks-Shulman, P.A.; Eckhauser, A.W.; Richards, W.O.; Klein, S.; Abumrad, N.N. Surgical removal of omental fat does not improve insulin sensitivity and cardiovascular risk factors in obese adults. *Gastroenterology* **2010**, *139*, 448–455. [CrossRef] [PubMed]
7. Stevens, V.J.; Obarzanek, E.; Cook, N.R.; Lee, I.M.; Appel, L.J.; Smith West, D.; Milas, N.C.; Mattfeldt-Beman, M.; Belden, L.; Bragg, C.; *et al.* Long-term weight loss and changes in blood pressure: Results of the trials of hypertension prevention, phase II. *Ann. Intern. Med.* **2001**, *134*, 1–11. [CrossRef] [PubMed]
8. Sasaki, S.; Higashi, Y.; Nakagawa, K.; Kimura, M.; Noma, K.; Hara, K.; Matsuura, H.; Goto, C.; Oshima, T.; Chayama, K. A low-calorie diet improves endothelium-dependent vasodilation in obese patients with essential hypertension. *Am. J. Hypertens.* **2002**, *15*, 302–309. [CrossRef]
9. Davì, G.; Guagnano, M.T.; Ciabattoni, G.; Basili, S.; Falco, A.; Marinopiccoli, M.; Nutini, M.; Sensi, S.; Patrono, C. Platelet activation in obese women: Role of inflammation and oxidant stress. *JAMA* **2002**, *288*, 2008–2014. [CrossRef] [PubMed]
10. Ziccardi, P.; Nappo, F.; Giugliano, G.; Esposito, K.; Marfella, R.; Cioffi, M.; D'Andrea, F.; Molinari, A.M.; Giugliano, D. Reduction of inflammatory cytokine concentrations and improvement of endothelial functions in obese women after weight loss over one year. *Circulation* **2002**, *105*, 804–809. [CrossRef] [PubMed]
11. Raitakari, M.; Ilvonen, T.; Ahotupa, M.; Lehtimäki, T.; Harmoinen, A.; Suominen, P.; Elo, J.; Hartiala, J.; Raitakari, O.T. Weight reduction with very-low-caloric diet and endothelial function in overweight adults: Role of plasma glucose. *Arterioscler. Thromb. Vasc. Biol.* **2004**, *24*, 124–128. [CrossRef] [PubMed]
12. Pereira, M.A.; Swain, J.; Goldfine, A.B.; Rifai, N.; Ludwig, D.S. Effects of a low-glycemic load diet on resting energy expenditure and heart disease risk factors during weight loss. *JAMA* **2004**, *292*, 2482–2490. [CrossRef] [PubMed]
13. Fontana, L.; Villareal, D.T.; Weiss, E.P.; Racette, S.B.; Steger-May, K.; Klein, S.; Holloszy, J.O.; Washington University School of Medicine CALERIE Group. Calorie restriction or exercise: Effects on coronary heart disease risk factors. A randomized, controlled trial. *Am. J. Physiol. Endocrinol. Metab.* **2007**, *293*, E197–E202. [CrossRef] [PubMed]
14. Jung, S.H.; Park, H.S.; Kim, K.S.; Choi, W.H.; Ahn, C.W.; Kim, B.T.; Kim, S.M.; Lee, S.Y.; Ahn, S.M.; Kim, Y.K.; *et al.* Effect of weight loss on some serum cytokines in human obesity: Increase in IL-10 after weight loss. *J. Nutr. Biochem.* **2008**, *19*, 371–375. [CrossRef] [PubMed]
15. Cooper, J.N.; Columbus, M.L.; Shields, K.J.; Asubonteng, J.; Meyer, M.L.; Sutton-Tyrrell, K.; Goodpaster, B.H.; DeLany, J.P.; Jakicic, J.M.; Barinas-Mitchell, E. Effects of an intensive behavioral weight loss intervention consisting of caloric restriction with or without physical activity on common carotid artery remodeling in severely obese adults. *Metabolism* **2012**, *61*, 1589–1597. [CrossRef] [PubMed]
16. Samaras, K.; Viardot, A.; Lee, P.N.; Jenkins, A.; Botelho, N.K.; Bakopanos, A.; Lord, R.V.; Hayward, C.S. Reduced arterial stiffness after weight loss in obese type 2 diabetes and impaired glucose tolerance: The role of immune cell activation and insulin resistance. *Diabetes Vasc. Dis. Res.* **2013**, *10*, 40–48. [CrossRef] [PubMed]
17. Soare, A.; Weiss, E.P.; Pozzilli, P. Benefits of caloric restriction for cardiometabolic health, including type 2 diabetes mellitus risk. *Diabetes Metab. Res. Rev.* **2014**, *30*, 41–47. [CrossRef] [PubMed]
18. Ho, T.P.; Zhao, X.; Courville, A.B.; Linderman, J.D.; Smith, S.; Sebring, N.; Della Valle, D.M.; Fitzpatrick, B.; Simchowitz, L.; Celi, F.S. Effects of a 12-month moderate weight loss intervention on insulin sensitivity and inflammation status in nondiabetic overweight and obese subjects. *Horm. Metab. Res.* **2015**, *47*, 289–296. [CrossRef] [PubMed]
19. Kitada, M.; Kume, S.; Takeda-Watanabe, A.; Tsuda, S.; Kanasaki, K.; Koya, D. Calorie restriction in overweight males ameliorates obesity-related metabolic alterations and cellular adaptations through anti-aging effects, possibly including AMPK and SIRT1 activation. *Biochim. Biophys. Acta* **2013**, *1830*, 4820–4827. [CrossRef] [PubMed]

20. Fontana, L.; Meyer, T.E.; Klein, S.; Holloszy, J.O. Long-term calorie restriction is highly effective in reducing the risk for atherosclerosis in humans. *Proc. Natl. Acad. Sci. USA* **2004**, *101*, 6659–6663. [CrossRef] [PubMed]
21. Piper, M.D.; Bartke, A. Diet and aging. *Cell Metab.* **2008**, *8*, 99–104. [CrossRef] [PubMed]
22. Varady, K.A.; Hellerstein, M.K. Alternate-day fasting and chronic disease prevention: A review of human and animal trials. *Am. J. Clin. Nutr.* **2007**, *86*, 7–13. [PubMed]
23. Heilbronn, L.K.; Smith, S.R.; Martin, C.K.; Anton, S.D.; Ravussin, E. Alternate-day fasting in nonobese subjects: Effects on body weight, body composition, and energy metabolism. *Am. J. Clin. Nutr.* **2005**, *81*, 69–73. [PubMed]
24. Ahmet, I.; Tae, H.J.; de Cabo, R.; Lakatta, E.G.; Talan, M.I. Effects of calorie restriction on cardioprotection and cardiovascular health. *J. Mol. Cell. Cardiol.* **2011**, *51*, 263–271. [CrossRef] [PubMed]
25. Colman, R.J.; Anderson, R.M.; Johnson, S.C.; Kastman, E.K.; Kosmatka, K.J.; Beasley, T.M.; Allison, D.B.; Cruzen, C.; Simmons, H.A.; Kemnitz, J.W.; *et al.* Caloric restriction delays disease onset and mortality in rhesus monkeys. *Science* **2009**, *325*, 201–204. [CrossRef] [PubMed]
26. Kondo, M.; Shibata, R.; Miura, R.; Shimano, M.; Kondo, K.; Li, P.; Ohashi, T.; Kihara, S.; Maeda, N.; Walsh, K.; *et al.* Caloric restriction stimulates revascularization in response to ischemia via adiponectin-mediated activation of endothelial nitric-oxide synthase. *J. Biol. Chem.* **2009**, *284*, 1718–1724. [CrossRef] [PubMed]
27. Cao, S.X.; Dhahbi, J.M.; Mote, P.L.; Spindler, S.R. Genomic profiling of short- and long-term caloric restriction effects in the liver of aging mice. *Proc. Natl. Acad. Sci. USA* **2001**, *98*, 10630–10635. [CrossRef] [PubMed]
28. Higami, Y.; Barger, J.L.; Page, G.P.; Allison, D.B.; Smith, S.R.; Prolla, T.A.; Weindruch, R. Energy restriction lowers the expression of genes linked to inflammation, the cytoskeleton, the extracellular matrix, and angiogenesis in mouse adipose tissue. *J. Nutr.* **2006**, *136*, 343–352. [PubMed]
29. Donato, A.J.; Walker, A.E.; Magerko, K.A.; Bramwell, R.C.; Black, A.D.; Henson, G.D.; Lawson, B.R.; Lesniewski, L.A.; Seals, D.R. Life-long caloric restriction reduces oxidative stress and preserves nitric oxide bioavailability and function in arteries of old mice. *Aging Cell* **2013**, *12*, 772–783. [CrossRef] [PubMed]
30. Chen, J.H.; Ouyang, C.; Ding, Q.; Song, J.; Cao, W.; Mao, L. A moderate low-carbohydrate low-calorie diet improves lipid profile, insulin sensitivity and adiponectin expression in rats. *Nutrients* **2015**, *7*, 4724–4738. [CrossRef] [PubMed]
31. Chou, S.H.; Lee, Y.C.; Huang, C.F.; Wang, Y.R.; Yu, H.P.; Lau, Y.T. Gender-specific effects of caloric restriction on the balance of vascular nitric oxide and superoxide radical. *Cardiovasc. Res.* **2010**, *87*, 751–759. [CrossRef] [PubMed]
32. Dolinsky, V.W.; Morton, J.S.; Oka, T.; Robillard-Frayne, I.; Bagdan, M.; Lopaschuk, G.D.; Des Rosiers, C.; Walsh, K.; Davidge, S.T.; Dyck, J.R. Calorie restriction prevents hypertension and cardiac hypertrophy in the spontaneously hypertensive rat. *Hypertension* **2010**, *56*, 412–421. [CrossRef] [PubMed]
33. Chandrasekar, B.; Nelson, J.F.; Colston, J.T.; Freeman, G.L. Calorie restriction attenuates inflammatory responses to myocardial ischemia-reperfusion injury. *Am. J. Physiol. Heart Circ. Physiol.* **2001**, *280*, H2094–H2102. [PubMed]
34. Csiszar, A.; Labinskyy, N.; Jimenez, R.; Pinto, J.T.; Ballabh, P.; Losonczy, G.; Pearson, K.J.; de Cabo, R.; Ungvari, Z. Anti-oxidative and anti-inflammatory vasoprotective effects of caloric restriction in aging: Role of circulating factors and SIRT1. *Mech. Ageing Dev.* **2009**, *130*, 518–527. [CrossRef] [PubMed]
35. Zanetti, M.; Gortan Cappellari, G.; Burekovic, I.; Barazzoni, R.; Stebel, M.; Guarnieri, G. Caloric restriction improves endothelial dysfunction during vascular aging: Effects on nitric oxide synthase isoforms and oxidative stress in rat aorta. *Exp. Gerontol.* **2010**, *45*, 848–855. [CrossRef] [PubMed]
36. Castello, L.; Froio, T.; Cavallini, G.; Biasi, F.; Sapino, A.; Leonarduzzi, G.; Bergamini, E.; Poli, G.; Chiarpotto, E. Calorie restriction protects against age-related rat aorta sclerosis. *FASEB J.* **2005**, *19*, 1863–1865. [CrossRef] [PubMed]
37. Ozbek, E.; Simsek, A.; Ozbek, M.; Somay, A. Caloric restriction increases internal iliac artery and penil nitric oxide synthase expression in rat: Comparison of aged and adult rats. *Arch. Ital. Urol. Androl.* **2013**, *85*, 113–117. [CrossRef] [PubMed]
38. Minamiyama, Y.; Bito, Y.; Takemura, S.; Takahashi, Y.; Kodai, S.; Mizuguchi, S.; Nishikawa, Y.; Suehiro, S.; Okada, S. Calorie restriction improves cardiovascular risk factors via reduction of mitochondrial reactive oxygen species in type II diabetic rats. *J. Pharmacol. Exp. Ther.* **2007**, *320*, 535–543. [CrossRef] [PubMed]

39. Garcia-Prieto, C.F.; Pulido-Olmo, H.; Ruiz-Hurtado, G.; Gil-Ortega, M.; Aranguez, I.; Rubio, M.A.; Ruiz-Gayo, M.; Somoza, B.; Fernandez-Alfonso, M.S. Mild caloric restriction reduces blood pressure and activates endothelial AMPK-PI3K-Akt-eNOS pathway in obese Zucker rats. *Vascul. Pharmacol.* **2015**, *65–66*, 3–12. [CrossRef] [PubMed]
40. Ketonen, J.; Pilvi, T.; Mervaala, E. Caloric restriction reverses high-fat diet-induced endothelial dysfunction and vascular superoxide production in C57Bl/6 mice. *Heart Vessel.* **2010**, *25*, 254–262. [CrossRef] [PubMed]
41. Iacobellis, G.; Singh, N.; Wharton, S.; Sharma, A.M. Substantial changes in epicardial fat thickness after weight loss in severely obese subjects. *Obesity (Silver Spring)* **2008**, *16*, 1693–1697. [CrossRef] [PubMed]
42. Siklova-Vitkova, M.; Klimcakova, E.; Polak, J.; Kovacova, Z.; Tencerova, M.; Rossmeislova, L.; Bajzova, M.; Langin, D.; Stich, V. Adipose tissue secretion and expression of adipocyte-produced and stromavascular fraction-produced adipokines vary during multiple phases of weight-reducing dietary intervention in obese women. *J. Clin. Endocrinol. Metab.* **2012**, *97*, E1176–E1181. [CrossRef] [PubMed]
43. Capel, F.; Klimcakova, E.; Viguerie, N.; Roussel, B.; Vitkova, M.; Kovacikova, M.; Polak, J.; Kovacova, Z.; Galitzky, J.; Maoret, J.J.; *et al.* Macrophages and adipocytes in human obesity: Adipose tissue gene expression and insulin sensitivity during calorie restriction and weight stabilization. *Diabetes* **2009**, *58*, 1558–1567. [CrossRef] [PubMed]
44. Morel, O.; Luca, F.; Grunebaum, L.; Jesel, L.; Meyer, N.; Desprez, D.; Robert, S.; Dignat-George, F.; Toti, F.; Simon, C.; *et al.* Short-term very low-calorie diet in obese females improves the haemostatic balance through the reduction of leptin levels, PAI-1 concentrations and a diminished release of platelet and leukocyte-derived microparticles. *Int. J. Obes.* **2011**, *35*, 1479–1486. [CrossRef] [PubMed]
45. Murakami, T.; Horigome, H.; Tanaka, K.; Nakata, Y.; Ohkawara, K.; Katayama, Y.; Matsui, A. Impact of weight reduction on production of platelet-derived microparticles and fibrinolytic parameters in obesity. *Thromb. Res.* **2007**, *119*, 45–53. [CrossRef] [PubMed]
46. Robertson, L.T.; Mitchell, J.R. Benefits of short-term dietary restriction in mammals. *Exp. Gerontol.* **2013**, *48*, 1043–1048. [CrossRef] [PubMed]
47. Cartee, G.D.; Dean, D.J. Glucose transport with brief dietary restriction: Heterogenous responses in muscles. *Am. J. Physiol.* **1994**, *266*, E946–E952. [PubMed]
48. Mattagajasingh, I.; Kim, C.S.; Naqvi, A.; Yamamori, T.; Hoffman, T.A.; Jung, S.B.; DeRicco, J.; Kasuno, K.; Irani, K. SIRT1 promotes endothelium-dependent vascular relaxation by activating endothelial nitric oxide synthase. *Proc. Natl. Acad. Sci. USA* **2007**, *104*, 14855–14860. [CrossRef] [PubMed]
49. Weindruch, R.; Walford, R.L. Dietary restriction in mice beginning at 1 year of age: Effect on life-span and spontaneous cancer incidence. *Science* **1982**, *215*, 1415–1418. [CrossRef] [PubMed]
50. Weindruch, R.; Gottesman, S.R.; Walford, R.L. Modification of age-related immune decline in mice dietarily restricted from or after midadulthood. *Proc. Natl. Acad. Sci. USA* **1982**, *79*, 898–902. [CrossRef] [PubMed]
51. Forster, M.J.; Morris, P.; Sohal, R.S. Genotype and age influence the effect of caloric intake on mortality in mice. *FASEB J.* **2003**, *17*, 690–692. [CrossRef] [PubMed]
52. Arvidsson, E.; Viguerie, N.; Andersson, I.; Verdich, C.; Langin, D.; Arner, P. Effects of different hypocaloric diets on protein secretion from adipose tissue of obese women. *Diabetes* **2004**, *53*, 1966–1971. [CrossRef] [PubMed]
53. Fornieri, C.; Taparelli, F.; Quaglino, D.; Contri, M.B.; Davidson, J.M.; Algeri, S.; Ronchetti, I.P. The effect of caloric restriction on the aortic tissue of aging rats. *Connect. Tissue Res.* **1999**, *40*, 131–143. [CrossRef] [PubMed]
54. Zanetti, M.; Barazzoni, R.; Vadori, M.; Stebel, M.; Biolo, G.; Guarnieri, G. Lack of direct effect of moderate hyperleptinemia to improve endothelial function in lean rat aorta: Role of calorie restriction. *Atherosclerosis* **2004**, *175*, 253–259. [CrossRef] [PubMed]
55. Heilbronn, L.K.; Clifton, P.M. C-reactive protein and coronary artery disease: Influence of obesity, caloric restriction and weight loss. *J. Nutr. Biochem.* **2002**, *13*, 316–321. [CrossRef]
56. Garcia-Prieto, C.F.; Gil-Ortega, M.; Aranguez, I.; Ortiz-Besoain, M.; Somoza, B.; Fernandez-Alfonso, M.S. Vascular ampk as an attractive target in the treatment of vascular complications of obesity. *Vascul. Pharmacol.* **2015**, *67–69*, 10–20. [CrossRef] [PubMed]

57. García-Prieto, C.F.; Hernández-Nuño, F.; Rio, D.D.; Ruiz-Hurtado, G.; Aránguez, I.; Ruiz-Gayo, M.; Somoza, B.; Fernández-Alfonso, M.S. High-fat diet induces endothelial dysfunction through a down-regulation of the endothelial AMPK-PI3K-Akt-eNOS pathway. *Mol. Nutr. Food Res.* **2015**, *59*, 520–532. [CrossRef] [PubMed]
58. Lobato, N.S.; Filgueira, F.P.; Prakash, R.; Giachini, F.R.; Ergul, A.; Carvalho, M.H.; Webb, R.C.; Tostes, R.C.; Fortes, Z.B. Reduced endothelium-dependent relaxation to anandamide in mesenteric arteries from young obese Zucker rats. *PLoS ONE* **2013**, *8*, e63449. [CrossRef] [PubMed]
59. Blume, C.; Benz, P.M.; Walter, U.; Ha, J.; Kemp, B.E.; Renné, T. Amp-activated protein kinase impairs endothelial actin cytoskeleton assembly by phosphorylating vasodilator-stimulated phosphoprotein. *J. Biol. Chem.* **2007**, *282*, 4601–4612. [CrossRef] [PubMed]
60. Lee, W.J.; Lee, I.K.; Kim, H.S.; Kim, Y.M.; Koh, E.H.; Won, J.C.; Han, S.M.; Kim, M.S.; Jo, I.; Oh, G.T.; *et al.* Alpha-lipoic acid prevents endothelial dysfunction in obese rats via activation of AMP-activated protein kinase. *Arterioscler. Thromb. Vasc. Biol.* **2005**, *25*, 2488–2494. [CrossRef] [PubMed]
61. Dagher, Z.; Ruderman, N.; Tornheim, K.; Ido, Y. Acute regulation of fatty acid oxidation and amp-activated protein kinase in human umbilical vein endothelial cells. *Circ. Res.* **2001**, *88*, 1276–1282. [CrossRef]
62. McCarty, M.F. Ampk activation as a strategy for reversing the endothelial lipotoxicity underlying the increased vascular risk associated with insulin resistance syndrome. *Med. Hypotheses* **2005**, *64*, 1211–1215. [CrossRef] [PubMed]
63. Allard, J.S.; Heilbronn, L.K.; Smith, C.; Hunt, N.D.; Ingram, D.K.; Ravussin, E.; de Cabo, R.; Team, P.C. *In vitro* cellular adaptations of indicators of longevity in response to treatment with serum collected from humans on calorie restricted diets. *PLoS ONE* **2008**, *3*, e3211. [CrossRef] [PubMed]
64. Briones, A.M.; Aras-Lopez, R.; Alonso, M.J.; Salaices, M. Small artery remodeling in obesity and insulin resistance. *Curr. Vasc. Pharmacol.* **2014**, *12*, 427–437. [CrossRef] [PubMed]
65. Walford, R.L.; Harris, S.B.; Gunion, M.W. The calorically restricted low-fat nutrient-dense diet in biosphere 2 significantly lowers blood glucose, total leukocyte count, cholesterol, and blood pressure in humans. *Proc. Natl. Acad. Sci. USA* **1992**, *89*, 11533–11537. [CrossRef] [PubMed]
66. Petersen, K.S.; Clifton, P.M.; Lister, N.; Keogh, J.B. Effect of weight loss induced by energy restriction on measures of arterial compliance: A systematic review and meta-analysis. *Atherosclerosis* **2016**, *247*, 7–20. [CrossRef] [PubMed]
67. Fernandez-Alfonso, M.S.; Gil-Ortega, M.; Garcia-Prieto, C.F.; Aranguez, I.; Ruiz-Gayo, M.; Somoza, B. Mechanisms of perivascular adipose tissue dysfunction in obesity. *Int. J. Endocrinol.* **2013**, *2013*, 402053. [CrossRef] [PubMed]
68. Iacobellis, G.; Ribaudo, M.C.; Assael, F.; Vecci, E.; Tiberti, C.; Zappaterreno, A.; di Mario, U.; Leonetti, F. Echocardiographic epicardial adipose tissue is related to anthropometric and clinical parameters of metabolic syndrome: A new indicator of cardiovascular risk. *J. Clin. Endocrinol. Metab.* **2003**, *88*, 5163–5168. [CrossRef] [PubMed]
69. Somoza, B.; Guzman, R.; Cano, V.; Merino, B.; Ramos, P.; Diez-Fernandez, C.; Fernandez-Alfonso, M.S.; Ruiz-Gayo, M. Induction of cardiac uncoupling protein-2 expression and adenosine 5′-monophosphate-activated protein kinase phosphorylation during early states of diet-induced obesity in mice. *Endocrinology* **2007**, *148*, 924–931. [CrossRef] [PubMed]
70. Gil-Ortega, M.; Condezo-Hoyos, L.; García-Prieto, C.F.; Arribas, S.M.; González, M.C.; Aranguez, I.; Ruiz-Gayo, M.; Somoza, B.; Fernández-Alfonso, M.S. Imbalance between pro and anti-oxidant mechanisms in perivascular adipose tissue aggravates long-term high-fat diet-derived endothelial dysfunction. *PLoS ONE* **2014**, *9*, e95312.
71. Greenstein, A.S.; Khavandi, K.; Withers, S.B.; Sonoyama, K.; Clancy, O.; Jeziorska, M.; Laing, I.; Yates, A.P.; Pemberton, P.W.; Malik, R.A.; *et al.* Local inflammation and hypoxia abolish the protective anticontractile properties of perivascular fat in obese patients. *Circulation* **2009**, *119*, 1661–1670. [CrossRef] [PubMed]
72. Ma, L.; Ma, S.; He, H.; Yang, D.; Chen, X.; Luo, Z.; Liu, D.; Zhu, Z. Perivascular fat-mediated vascular dysfunction and remodeling through the AMPK/mTOR pathway in high-fat diet-induced obese rats. *Hypertens Res.* **2010**, *33*, 446–453. [CrossRef] [PubMed]
73. Fésüs, G.; Dubrovska, G.; Gorzelniak, K.; Kluge, R.; Huang, Y.; Luft, F.C.; Gollasch, M. Adiponectin is a novel humoral vasodilator. *Cardiovasc. Res.* **2007**, *75*, 719–727. [CrossRef] [PubMed]

74. Owen, M.K.; Witzmann, F.A.; McKenney, M.L.; Lai, X.; Berwick, Z.C.; Moberly, S.P.; Alloosh, M.; Sturek, M.; Tune, J.D. Perivascular adipose tissue potentiates contraction of coronary vascular smooth muscle: Influence of obesity. *Circulation* **2013**, *128*, 9–18. [CrossRef] [PubMed]
75. Sun, X.; Hou, N.; Han, F.; Guo, Y.; Hui, Z.; Du, G.; Zhang, Y. Effect of high free fatty acids on the anti-contractile response of perivascular adipose tissue in rat aorta. *J. Mol. Cell. Cardiol.* **2013**, *63*, 169–174. [CrossRef] [PubMed]
76. Rebolledo, A.; Rebolledo, O.R.; Marra, C.A.; Garcia, M.E.; Roldan Palomo, A.R.; Rimorini, L.; Gagliardino, J.J. Early alterations in vascular contractility associated to changes in fatty acid composition and oxidative stress markers in perivascular adipose tissue. *Cardiovasc. Diabetol.* **2010**, *9*, 65. [CrossRef] [PubMed]
77. Verlohren, S.; Dubrovska, G.; Tsang, S.Y.; Essin, K.; Luft, F.C.; Huang, Y.; Gollasch, M. Visceral periadventitial adipose tissue regulates arterial tone of mesenteric arteries. *Hypertension* **2004**, *44*, 271–276. [CrossRef] [PubMed]
78. Gálvez, B.; de Castro, J.; Herold, D.; Dubrovska, G.; Arribas, S.; González, M.C.; Aranguez, I.; Luft, F.C.; Ramos, M.P.; Gollasch, M.; *et al.* Perivascular adipose tissue and mesenteric vascular function in spontaneously hypertensive rats. *Arterioscler. Thromb. Vasc. Biol.* **2006**, *26*, 1297–1302. [CrossRef] [PubMed]
79. Willens, H.J.; Byers, P.; Chirinos, J.A.; Labrador, E.; Hare, J.M.; de Marchena, E. Effects of weight loss after bariatric surgery on epicardial fat measured using echocardiography. *Am. J. Cardiol.* **2007**, *99*, 1242–1245. [CrossRef] [PubMed]
80. Aghamohammadzadeh, R.; Greenstein, A.S.; Yadav, R.; Jeziorska, M.; Hama, S.; Soltani, F.; Pemberton, P.W.; Ammori, B.; Malik, R.A.; Soran, H.; *et al.* Effects of bariatric surgery on human small artery function: Evidence for reduction in perivascular adipocyte inflammation, and the restoration of normal anticontractile activity despite persistent obesity. *J. Am. Coll. Cardiol.* **2013**, *62*, 128–135. [CrossRef] [PubMed]
81. Rahmouni, K.; Correia, M.L.; Haynes, W.G.; Mark, A.L. Obesity-associated hypertension: New insights into mechanisms. *Hypertension* **2005**, *45*, 9–14. [CrossRef] [PubMed]
82. Blanquicett, C.; Graves, A.; Kleinhenz, D.J.; Hart, C.M. Attenuation of signaling and nitric oxide production following prolonged leptin exposure in human aortic endothelial cells. *J. Investig. Med.* **2007**, *55*, 368–377. [CrossRef] [PubMed]
83. Knudson, J.D.; Dincer, U.D.; Zhang, C.; Swafford, A.N., Jr.; Koshida, R.; Picchi, A.; Focardi, M.; Dick, G.M.; Tune, J.D. Leptin receptors are expressed in coronary arteries, and hyperleptinemia causes significant coronary endothelial dysfunction. *Am. J. Physiol. Heart Circ. Physiol.* **2005**, *289*, H48–H56. [CrossRef] [PubMed]
84. Bouloumie, A.; Marumo, T.; Lafontan, M.; Busse, R. Leptin induces oxidative stress in human endothelial cells. *FASEB J.* **1999**, *13*, 1231–1238. [PubMed]
85. Shinmura, K.; Tamaki, K.; Bolli, R. Short-term caloric restriction improves ischemic tolerance independent of opening of ATP-sensitive K^+ channels in both young and aged hearts. *J. Mol. Cell. Cardiol.* **2005**, *39*, 285–296. [CrossRef] [PubMed]
86. Zhu, M.; Miura, J.; Lu, L.X.; Bernier, M.; DeCabo, R.; Lane, M.A.; Roth, G.S.; Ingram, D.K. Circulating adiponectin levels increase in rats on caloric restriction: The potential for insulin sensitization. *Exp. Gerontol.* **2004**, *39*, 1049–1059. [CrossRef] [PubMed]
87. Gil-Ortega, M.; Stucchi, P.; Guzmán-Ruiz, R.; Cano, V.; Arribas, S.; González, M.C.; Ruiz-Gayo, M.; Fernández-Alfonso, M.S.; Somoza, B. Adaptative nitric oxide overproduction in perivascular adipose tissue during early diet-induced obesity. *Endocrinology* **2010**, *151*, 3299–3306. [CrossRef] [PubMed]
88. Antonopoulos, A.S.; Margaritis, M.; Coutinho, P.; Shirodaria, C.; Psarros, C.; Herdman, L.; Sanna, F.; De Silva, R.; Petrou, M.; Sayeed, R.; *et al.* Adiponectin as a link between type 2 diabetes and vascular NADPH oxidase activity in the human arterial wall: The regulatory role of perivascular adipose tissue. *Diabetes* **2015**, *64*, 2207–2219. [CrossRef] [PubMed]
89. Lavi, T.; Karasik, A.; Koren-Morag, N.; Kanety, H.; Feinberg, M.S.; Shechter, M. The acute effect of various glycemic index dietary carbohydrates on endothelial function in nondiabetic overweight and obese subjects. *J. Am. Coll. Cardiol.* **2009**, *53*, 2283–2287. [CrossRef] [PubMed]
90. Gögebakan, O.; Kohl, A.; Osterhoff, M.A.; van Baak, M.A.; Jebb, S.A.; Papadaki, A.; Martinez, J.A.; Handjieva-Darlenska, T.; Hlavaty, P.; Weickert, M.O.; *et al.* Effects of weight loss and long-term weight maintenance with diets varying in protein and glycemic index on cardiovascular risk factors: The diet, obesity, and genes (diogenes) study: A randomized, controlled trial. *Circulation* **2011**, *124*, 2829–2838. [CrossRef] [PubMed]

91. Buscemi, S.; Cosentino, L.; Rosafio, G.; Morgana, M.; Mattina, A.; Sprini, D.; Verga, S.; Rini, G.B. Effects of hypocaloric diets with different glycemic indexes on endothelial function and glycemic variability in overweight and in obese adult patients at increased cardiovascular risk. *Clin. Nutr.* **2013**, *32*, 346–352. [CrossRef] [PubMed]
92. Volek, J.S.; Fernandez, M.L.; Feinman, R.D.; Phinney, S.D. Dietary carbohydrate restriction induces a unique metabolic state positively affecting atherogenic dyslipidemia, fatty acid partitioning, and metabolic syndrome. *Prog. Lipid Res.* **2008**, *47*, 307–318. [CrossRef] [PubMed]
93. Volek, J.S.; Phinney, S.D.; Forsythe, C.E.; Quann, E.E.; Wood, R.J.; Puglisi, M.J.; Kraemer, W.J.; Bibus, D.M.; Fernandez, M.L.; Feinman, R.D. Carbohydrate restriction has a more favorable impact on the metabolic syndrome than a low fat diet. *Lipids* **2009**, *44*, 297–309. [CrossRef] [PubMed]
94. Volek, J.S.; Ballard, K.D.; Silvestre, R.; Judelson, D.A.; Quann, E.E.; Forsythe, C.E.; Fernandez, M.L.; Kraemer, W.J. Effects of dietary carbohydrate restriction *versus* low-fat diet on flow-mediated dilation. *Metabolism* **2009**, *58*, 1769–1777. [CrossRef] [PubMed]
95. Forsythe, C.E.; Phinney, S.D.; Fernandez, M.L.; Quann, E.E.; Wood, R.J.; Bibus, D.M.; Kraemer, W.J.; Feinman, R.D.; Volek, J.S. Comparison of low fat and low carbohydrate diets on circulating fatty acid composition and markers of inflammation. *Lipids* **2008**, *43*, 65–77. [CrossRef] [PubMed]
96. Clifton, P.M.; Keogh, J.B.; Foster, P.R.; Noakes, M. Effect of weight loss on inflammatory and endothelial markers and fmd using two low-fat diets. *Int. J. Obes.* **2005**, *29*, 1445–1451. [CrossRef] [PubMed]
97. Wycherley, T.P.; Brinkworth, G.D.; Keogh, J.B.; Noakes, M.; Buckley, J.D.; Clifton, P.M. Long-term effects of weight loss with a very low carbohydrate and low fat diet on vascular function in overweight and obese patients. *J. Intern. Med.* **2010**, *267*, 452–461. [CrossRef] [PubMed]
98. Ballard, K.D.; Quann, E.E.; Kupchak, B.R.; Volk, B.M.; Kawiecki, D.M.; Fernandez, M.L.; Seip, R.L.; Maresh, C.M.; Kraemer, W.J.; Volek, J.S. Dietary carbohydrate restriction improves insulin sensitivity, blood pressure, microvascular function, and cellular adhesion markers in individuals taking statins. *Nutr. Res.* **2013**, *33*, 905–912. [CrossRef] [PubMed]
99. Alessi, M.C.; Juhan-Vague, I. PAI-1 and the metabolic syndrome: Links, causes, and consequences. *Arterioscler. Thromb. Vasc. Biol.* **2006**, *26*, 2200–2207. [CrossRef] [PubMed]
100. Tagawa, T.; Imaizumi, T.; Endo, T.; Shiramoto, M.; Harasawa, Y.; Takeshita, A. Role of nitric oxide in reactive hyperemia in human forearm vessels. *Circulation* **1994**, *90*, 2285–2290. [CrossRef] [PubMed]
101. Merino, J.; Kones, R.; Ferré, R.; Plana, N.; Girona, J.; Aragonés, G.; Ibarretxe, D.; Heras, M.; Masana, L. Negative effect of a low-carbohydrate, high-protein, high-fat diet on small peripheral artery reactivity in patients with increased cardiovascular risk. *Br. J. Nutr.* **2013**, *109*, 1241–1247. [CrossRef] [PubMed]
102. Hite, A.H.; Berkowitz, V.G.; Berkowitz, K. Low-carbohydrate diet review: Shifting the paradigm. *Nutr. Clin. Pract.* **2011**, *26*, 300–308. [CrossRef] [PubMed]
103. Larsen, T.M.; Dalskov, S.M.; van Baak, M.; Jebb, S.A.; Papadaki, A.; Pfeiffer, A.F.; Martinez, J.A.; Handjieva-Darlenska, T.; Kunešová, M.; Pihlsgård, M.; *et al.* Diets with high or low protein content and glycemic index for weight-loss maintenance. *N. Engl. J. Med.* **2010**, *363*, 2102–2113. [CrossRef] [PubMed]
104. Brinkworth, G.D.; Noakes, M.; Parker, B.; Foster, P.; Clifton, P.M. Long-term effects of advice to consume a high-protein, low-fat diet, rather than a conventional weight-loss diet, in obese adults with type 2 diabetes: One-year follow-up of a randomised trial. *Diabetologia* **2004**, *47*, 1677–1686. [CrossRef] [PubMed]
105. Khoo, J.; Ling, P.S.; Tan, J.; Teo, A.; Ng, H.L.; Chen, R.Y.; Tay, T.L.; Tan, E.; Cheong, M. Comparing the effects of meal replacements with reduced-fat diet on weight, sexual and endothelial function, testosterone and quality of life in obese asian men. *Int. J. Impot. Res.* **2014**, *26*, 61–66. [CrossRef] [PubMed]
106. Rizkalla, S.W.; Prifti, E.; Cotillard, A.; Pelloux, V.; Rouault, C.; Allouche, R.; Laromiguière, M.; Kong, L.; Darakhshan, F.; Massiera, F.; *et al.* Differential effects of macronutrient content in 2 energy-restricted diets on cardiovascular risk factors and adipose tissue cell size in moderately obese individuals: A randomized controlled trial. *Am. J. Clin. Nutr.* **2012**, *95*, 49–63. [CrossRef] [PubMed]
107. Ridker, P.M. High-sensitivity C-reactive protein: Potential adjunct for global risk assessment in the primary prevention of cardiovascular disease. *Circulation* **2001**, *103*, 1813–1818. [CrossRef] [PubMed]
108. Appel, L.J.; Sacks, F.M.; Carey, V.J.; Obarzanek, E.; Swain, J.F.; Miller, E.R.; Conlin, P.R.; Erlinger, T.P.; Rosner, B.A.; Laranjo, N.M.; *et al.* Effects of protein, monounsaturated fat, and carbohydrate intake on blood pressure and serum lipids: Results of the omniheart randomized trial. *JAMA* **2005**, *294*, 2455–2464. [CrossRef] [PubMed]

109. Bonetti, P.O.; Pumper, G.M.; Higano, S.T.; Holmes, D.R.; Kuvin, J.T.; Lerman, A. Noninvasive identification of patients with early coronary atherosclerosis by assessment of digital reactive hyperemia. *J. Am. Coll. Cardiol.* **2004**, *44*, 2137–2141. [CrossRef] [PubMed]
110. Rubinshtein, R.; Kuvin, J.T.; Soffler, M.; Lennon, R.J.; Lavi, S.; Nelson, R.E.; Pumper, G.M.; Lerman, L.O.; Lerman, A. Assessment of endothelial function by non-invasive peripheral arterial tonometry predicts late cardiovascular adverse events. *Eur. Heart J.* **2010**, *31*, 1142–1148. [CrossRef] [PubMed]
111. Siri-Tarino, P.W.; Sun, Q.; Hu, F.B.; Krauss, R.M. Saturated fat, carbohydrate, and cardiovascular disease. *Am. J. Clin. Nutr.* **2010**, *91*, 502–509. [CrossRef] [PubMed]
112. Lagiou, P.; Sandin, S.; Lof, M.; Trichopoulos, D.; Adami, H.O.; Weiderpass, E. Low carbohydrate-high protein diet and incidence of cardiovascular diseases in swedish women: Prospective cohort study. *BMJ* **2012**, *344*, e4026. [CrossRef] [PubMed]
113. Noto, H.; Goto, A.; Tsujimoto, T.; Noda, M. Low-carbohydrate diets and all-cause mortality: A systematic review and meta-analysis of observational studies. *PLoS ONE* **2013**, *8*, e55030. [CrossRef] [PubMed]
114. Jenkins, D.J.; Wolever, T.M.; Taylor, R.H.; Barker, H.; Fielden, H.; Baldwin, J.M.; Bowling, A.C.; Newman, H.C.; Jenkins, A.L.; Goff, D.V. Glycemic index of foods: A physiological basis for carbohydrate exchange. *Am. J. Clin. Nutr.* **1981**, *34*, 362–366. [PubMed]
115. McMillan-Price, J.; Petocz, P.; Atkinson, F.; O'neill, K.; Samman, S.; Steinbeck, K.; Caterson, I.; Brand-Miller, J. Comparison of 4 diets of varying glycemic load on weight loss and cardiovascular risk reduction in overweight and obese young adults: A randomized controlled trial. *Arch. Intern. Med.* **2006**, *166*, 1466–1475. [CrossRef] [PubMed]
116. Recio-Rodriguez, J.I.; Gomez-Marcos, M.A.; Patino-Alonso, M.C.; Rodrigo-De Pablo, E.; Cabrejas-Sánchez, A.; Arietaleanizbeaskoa, M.S.; Repiso-Gento, I.; Gonzalez-Viejo, N.; Maderuelo-Fernandez, J.A.; Agudo-Conde, C.; *et al.* Glycemic index, glycemic load, and pulse wave reflection in adults. *Nutr. Metab. Cardiovasc. Dis.* **2015**, *25*, 68–74. [CrossRef] [PubMed]
117. Hu, Y.; Block, G.; Norkus, E.P.; Morrow, J.D.; Dietrich, M.; Hudes, M. Relations of glycemic index and glycemic load with plasma oxidative stress markers. *Am. J. Clin. Nutr.* **2006**, *84*, 70–76, quiz 266–267. [PubMed]
118. Sacks, F.M.; Carey, V.J.; Anderson, C.A.; Miller, E.R.; Copeland, T.; Charleston, J.; Harshfield, B.J.; Laranjo, N.; McCarron, P.; Swain, J.; *et al.* Effects of high vs low glycemic index of dietary carbohydrate on cardiovascular disease risk factors and insulin sensitivity: The omnicarb randomized clinical trial. *JAMA* **2014**, *312*, 2531–2541. [CrossRef] [PubMed]
119. Schwingshackl, L.; Hoffmann, G. Long-term effects of low glycemic index/load *vs.* High glycemic index/load diets on parameters of obesity and obesity-associated risks: A systematic review and meta-analysis. *Nutr. Metab. Cardiovasc. Dis.* **2013**, *23*, 699–706. [CrossRef]

5

Relationships of Dietary Histidine and Obesity in Northern Chinese Adults, an Internet-Based Cross-Sectional Study

Yan-Chuan Li [1,†], Chun-Long Li [2,†], Jia-Yue Qi [1], Li-Na Huang [3], Dan Shi [1], Shan-Shan Du [1], Li-Yan Liu [1], Ren-Nan Feng [1,*] and Chang-Hao Sun [1,*]

1 Department of Nutrition and Food Hygiene, School of Public Health, Harbin Medical University, No. 157 Baojian Road, Nangang District, Harbin 150086, China; liyanchuan2013@foxmail.com (Y.-C.L.); qijiayue678@163.com (J.-Y.Q.); shidanhmu@foxmail.com (D.S.); dushanshan1007@163.com (S.-S.D.); yanziliu2100@163.com (L.-Y.L.)

2 Department of General Surgery, The Second Affiliated Hospital of Harbin Medical University, Harbin 150086, China; chunlong81@163.com

3 Liaoning Institute for Food Control, Shenyang 110015, China; lnspjcy@163.com

* Correspondence: fengrennan@163.com (R.-N.F.); changhao2002sun@gmail.com (C.-H.S.)

† These authors contributed equally to this work.

Abstract: Our previous studies have demonstrated that histidine supplementation significantly ameliorates inflammation and oxidative stress in obese women and high-fat diet-induced obese rats. However, the effects of dietary histidine on general population are not known. The objective of this Internet-based cross-sectional study was to evaluate the associations between dietary histidine and prevalence of overweight/obesity and abdominal obesity in northern Chinese population. A total of 2376 participants were randomly recruited and asked to finish our Internet-based dietary questionnaire for the Chinese (IDQC). Afterwards, 88 overweight/obese participants were randomly selected to explore the possible mechanism. Compared with healthy controls, dietary histidine was significantly lower in overweight ($p < 0.05$) and obese ($p < 0.01$) participants of both sexes. Dietary histidine was inversely associated with body mass index (BMI), waist circumference (WC) and blood pressure in overall population and stronger associations were observed in women and overweight/obese participants. Higher dietary histidine was associated with lower prevalence of overweight/obesity and abdominal obesity, especially in women. Further studies indicated that higher dietary histidine was associated with lower fasting blood glucose (FBG), homeostasis model assessment of insulin resistance (HOMA-IR), 2-h postprandial glucose (2 h-PG), tumor necrosis factor-α (TNF-α), interleukin-1β (IL-1β), interleukin-6 (IL-6), C-reactive protein (CRP), malonaldehyde (MDA) and vaspin and higher glutathione peroxidase (GSH-Px), superoxide dismutase (SOD) and adiponectin of overweight/obese individuals of both sexes. In conclusion, higher dietary histidine is inversely associated with energy intake, status of insulin resistance, inflammation and oxidative stress in overweight/obese participants and lower prevalence of overweight/obesity in northern Chinese adults.

Keywords: dietary histidine; overweight/obesity; insulin resistance; inflammation; oxidative stress

1. Introduction

The rising prevalence of overweight and obesity has become a major global health challenge [1]. Obesity is a major risk factor for a series of metabolic disorders and chronic diseases, including insulin resistance, metabolic syndrome, type 2 diabetes, hypertension, cardiovascular diseases and certain cancer [2–5]. Accumulating evidence has proved that nutritional factors are strongly associated with the development, treatment and prevention of chronic diseases, such as obesity, hyperlipidemia, diabetes mellitus and cardiovascular diseases [6–9]. Therefore, it is urgent to improve etiologic research on diet by investigating nutrient and food intakes and reasonable dietary guidelines should be proposed by the government.

Histidine, a precursor for the synthesis of histamine, is abundant in red meat and fish and is an important amino acid for humans. It has been reported that lower plasma concentration of histidine is associated with protein-energy wasting, inflammation and oxidative stress in chronic kidney disease patients [10]. Previous animal studies confirmed that histidine supplementation could reduce body weight and ameliorates inflammation and oxidative stress of adipose tissue in a high-fat diet induced female obese rat model [11]. Moreover, dietary histidine also suppresses food intake and fat accumulation in rats [12]. In our previous study, we had found that serum histidine concentrations in obese women were significantly lower than those in non-obese women and had negative relationships with inflammation and oxidative stress [13]. The recovery of serum histidine concentrations through histidine supplementation could improve insulin resistance, reduce body mass index (BMI) and fat mass, and suppress inflammation and oxidative stress in obese women [14]. Only one cross-sectional study in Japanese adolescents showed a significantly negative correlation between energy intake and ratio of histidine to protein intake [15].

Although the central roles of dietary histidine for regulation of energy intake have already been established in animal and in vitro studies, to our knowledge, no study has analyzed the associations between dietary histidine and prevalence of obesity in general population. Moreover, whether chronic intake of dietary histidine is associated with insulin resistance, inflammation and oxidative stress in overweight/obese individuals is still unclear. The contribution of dietary histidine is not yet fully confirmed. Therefore, we assessed dietary histidine intakes of 2376 participants and examined relationships between dietary histidine and obesity in this population in this study. Furthermore, a subgroup study of 88 overweight/obese subjects (44 men and 44 women) was performed to explore the possible mechanism of the anti-obesity effect of histidine.

2. Materials and Methods

2.1. *Development and Validation of the IDQC*

To investigate dietary habits accurately, many methods for dietary assessment have been used by researchers. The food frequency questionnaire (FFQ) provides us a convenient and economic method to assess the general dietary intakes in a large population [16]. However, traditional face-to-face FFQs are impossible to conduct in a large population during a short period as the face-to-face FFQs always consume much time [17]. Previously, a convenient tool named Internet-based dietary questionnaire for the Chinese (IDQC) has been designed and validated at Harbin Medical University previously by experts of nutrition, epidemiology and bio-statistics [18].

Commonly eaten foods were divided into 16 categories (i.e., grains, potatoes, legumes, vegetables, fungus, fruits, seeds and nuts, livestock, poultry, dairy, eggs, fish, snacks, sugar, condiments, and beverages). Reference images of each food item's weight/volume were created as references to assist the participants in making accurate estimation of food portions. Each participant had to choose the frequency and amount of each subtype of food groups. Finally, the questionnaire was uploaded to a secure website, which is free of access [19].

The IDQC has been validated as a convenient dietary assessment tool in our previous study [18]. Briefly, 644 recruited participants had completed the IDQC, the intakes of the food groups and nutrients in the IDQC were validated against those in the 3-day dietary records. The IDQC has been confirmed as an accurate tool for dietary assessment, because it has good consistency to results of 3-day dietary records. Therefore, the IDQC can be used for dietary assessment in large population.

2.2. Participants, Exclusive Criteria, Power Calculation and Study Design

We randomly invited 3626 participants from the Health Examination Center of the Second Affiliated Hospital of Harbin Medical University. Of the 3626 invited participants, 2995 agreed to participate in our study, register an account and finish the IDQC. Firstly, online demographic questionnaires were completed by all participants; the details of which were provided in our previous published manuscript [20]. The exclusive criteria were as follows: (1) incomplete information on the IDQC; (2) extreme daily energy intake (<800 kcal (3349 kJ) or >5000 kcal (20,934 kJ) for males; <600 kcal (2512 kJ) or >4000 kcal (16,747 kJ) for females); (3) low BMI (BMI < 18.5); and (4) diabetes diagnosis or being on a diet in the past 6 months. In total, 619 were excluded for the above reasons (Figure 1).

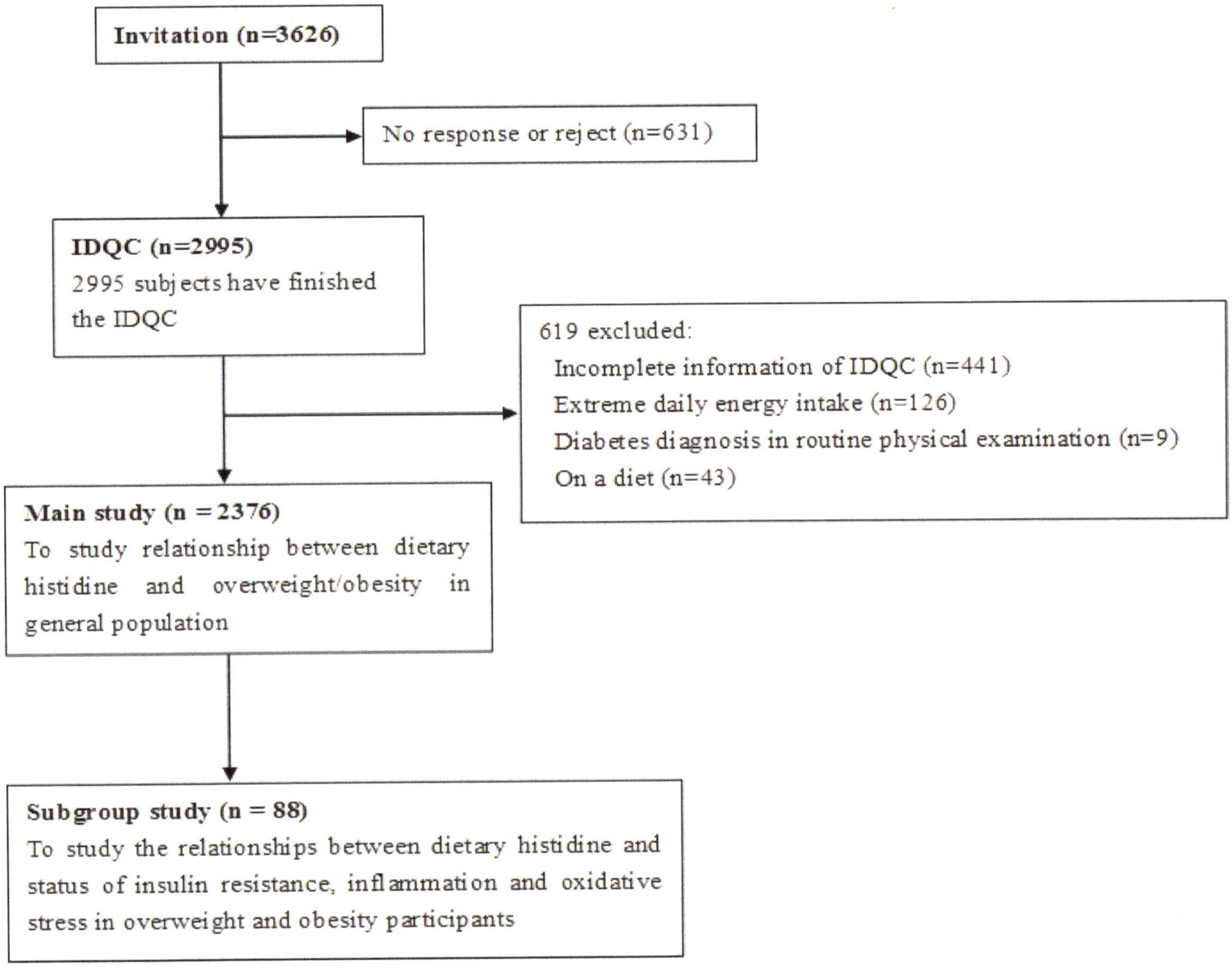

Figure 1. Flow of the study population.

For power calculation, considering the 9.9 cm standard deviation of waist circumference (WC) in the overall population, a sample size of 594 in each quartile will be sufficient to detect a difference of 2.4 cm between quartiles. Moreover, this sample size is also sufficient to detect a difference of 1.0 kg/m^2 in BMI, at 99% power and 5% level of significance.

To explore possible mechanisms of the anti-obesity effect of histidine, 88 overweight/obese subjects were randomly selected by stratified sampling for subgroup study. Except for dietary histidine (% protein), body weight, BMI, WC, and drinking and smoking habits, there is no difference between included participants and excluded participants. Characteristics are presented in Table S1. An oral glucose tolerance test (OGTT) was performed and metabolic profile, status of inflammation and oxidative stress were also examined. A flow chart of the study population is shown in Figure 1. This study was conducted according to the guidelines of the Declaration of Helsinki and all procedures involving humans were approved by the Human Research Ethics Committee of the Harbin Medical University (approval code [2015]006). Online informed consent was obtained from all participants.

2.3. Estimation of Dietary Nutrients Intake

After the online demographic questionnaire, all participants were asked to complete the IDQC for the past 4 months, and details of the IDQC are provided in our previous published manuscript [20]. The intake detail (frequency and amount) of each kind of food was obtained and average daily intakes of all nutrients were then calculated according to the China Food Composition Tables [21]. China Food Composition Tables is an important reference book for researchers of nutrition and public health of China. In this book, commonly eaten Chinese foods are evaluated and average nutrient contents (including energy, macro nutrients, trace elements, amino acids, and fatty acids) of these foods are measured by researchers and provided in the book. In our study, the histidine amount is total dietary source histidine (including protein, peptide and free form of histidine).

2.4. Anthropometric Measurements

All participants were asked to stand on an anthropometer without heavy clothing and shoes. Body weight and height were measured to the nearest 0.1 kg and 0.1 cm. For WC measurement, the same standard was applied for each individual. WC was measured using a flexible anthropometric tape on the horizontal plane between the lowest rib and the iliac crest, to the nearest 0.1 cm. Blood pressure was measured using a standard mercury sphygmomanometer. Each participant was seated comfortably for 10 min in a quiet room. Korotkoff sounds I and V were criteria for systolic blood pressure (SBP) and diastolic blood pressure (DBP), respectively. SBP and DBP were measured twice and the mean values were calculated. All anthropometric measurements were performed by standardized and trained personnel and have good reproducibility.

2.5. Definition of Overweight/Obesity and Abdominal Obesity

BMI was defined as weight in kilograms divided by the square of height in meters (kg/m^2). As this study was performed in Chinese population, the BMI cut-off points of Chinese subjects (overweight: 24.0–27.9; obesity $\geqslant$ 28.0) were used [22]. Abdominal obesity was defined as WC $\geqslant$ 85 cm in men and WC $\geqslant$ 80 cm in women, according to the 2006 Guidelines on Preservation and Control Overweight and Obesity in Chinese Adults classification [23].

2.6. Collection and Laboratory Analysis of Serum

Eighty-eight participants were instructed to fast overnight (more than 12 h) and fasting blood samples were collected in the morning. After fasting blood samples were obtained, each participant was asked to take 75 g glucose (dissolved in 200 mL of warm water), and after 2 h, postprandial blood samples were obtained. Blood samples were centrifuged at 3000 rpm for 15 min to obtain serum and serum were stored at -80 °C immediately. Fasting and 2 h-postprandial blood glucose levels were measured with a hand-held glucose monitoring system (One-Touch Ultra 2; Life Scan, Milpitas, CA, USA). Serum insulin concentration was measured by ROCHE Elecsys 2010 Chemiluminescence Immune Analyzer (Roche Diagnostics, Mannheim, Germany). Fasting and 2 h-postprandial serum triglyceride (TG,) total cholesterol (TC), high destiny lipoprotein (HDL) and low destiny protein (LDL) were determined using a ROCHE Modular P800 Automatic Biochemical Analyzer (Roche Diagnostics, Mannheim, Germany). Homeostasis model assessment of insulin resistance (HOMA-IR) index was calculated as previously described [24]. Serum tumor necrosis factor-α (TNF-α), interleukin-1β (IL-1β), interleukin-6 (IL-6), C-reactive protein (CRP), adiponectin and vaspin concentrations were assayed using ELISA with commercial kits (TNF-α, IL-1β, IL-6, and vaspin, catalog number CSB-E04740h, CSB-E08053h, CSB-E04638h, CSB-E09771h, Cusabio, China; CRP, catalog number BC-1119, Biocheck, USA; adiponectin, catalog number ab99968, Abcam, UK). Serum superoxide dismutase (SOD), glutathione peroxidase (GSH-Px), malonaldehyde (MDA) were measured with enzymatic methods using commercial kits (Jiancheng Technology, Nanjing, China). Coefficients of variations (CVs) of lab measurements are presented in Supplementary Materials.

2.7. Statistical Analysis

For descriptive statistics, means and SDs (or frequencies and percentages) were calculated across BMI categories (normal weight: BMI < 24.0; overweight: 24.0–27.9; obese: ⩾28.0) and compared using one-way analysis of variance (one-way ANOVA) or chi-square test, as appropriate. Dietary histidine of different BMI categories was further analyzed by means of analysis of covariance (ANCOVA).

Considering the high correlation between histidine and total protein intake ($r = 0.925$), and that nutrient densities can be used to reduce the likelihood of multicollinearity [25], we used histidine (percent total protein intake) in our study. Bivariate correlation analysis (without variants adjusted) and partial correlation analysis was performed to assess the association of branched-chain amino acid (BCAA) and BMI, WC, SBP and DBP (adjusting for age, dietary carbohydrate, fat, protein, cholesterol and fiber intake), fasting blood glucose (FBG), insulin, HOMA-IR, TC, TG, HDL, LDL, 2-h postprandial glucose (2 h-PG), 2 h-insulin, 2 h-TC, 2 h-TG, 2 h-HDL, 2 h-LDL, GSH-Px, SOD, MDA, TNF-α, IL-1β, IL-6, CRP, adiponectin and vaspin (adjusting for age, BMI, dietary carbohydrate, fat, protein, cholesterol and fiber intake).

To estimate the Odds ratio (OR) and 95% confidence interval (CI) of overweight/obesity and abdominal obesity between quartiles of dietary histidine, logistic regression model was used. Age, education, income, labor, exercise status, dietary carbohydrate, fat, protein, cholesterol, fiber intake and smoking habits in three models. The statistical analyses were carried out using SAS software (version 9.1; SAS Institute, Cary, NC, USA). By statistician and $p < 0.05$ was considered statistically significant.

3. Results

3.1. Descriptive Statistics

The characteristics of participants by dietary histidine quartiles are summarized in Table 1. Compared with those in the first quartile of dietary histidine, participants of the 4th quartile were more likely to be youthful and had lower body weight, BMI, WC, and higher percentage of women. The highest prevalence of current smoking was observed in the 2nd quartile of dietary histidine. Income, education, labor and physical exercise status were also different between histidine quartiles (all $p < 0.05$). SBP and DBP of the 4th quartile were also significantly lower than those in the 1st quartile of dietary histidine. The prevalence of overweight/obesity was 37.4% and the prevalence of abdominal obesity was 28.5% among our participants.

For dietary intake, total protein, total amino acids, total fat, cholesterol and fiber of the 3rd and 4th quartiles were significantly higher than the 1st quartile. Dietary carbohydrates of the 1st quartile was significantly higher than the 3rd and 4th quartiles. Total energy intake was also different between histidine quartiles ($p = 0.048$).

Table 1. Characteristics and dietary intake of participants by quartile of histidine intake.

	Quartiles of Histidine (% Total Protein Intake)				*p*
	1	**2**	**3**	**4**	
Histidine, % total protein intake	<1.38	1.38–1.59	1.59–1.77	>1.77	
Participants, *n*	594	594	594	594	
BMI categories					<0.001
<24.0, *n* (%)	327 (55.1)	352 (59.3)	384 (64.6)	424 (71.4)	
24.0–28.0, *n* (%)	191 (32.2)	182 (30.6)	165 (27.8)	141 (23.7)	
⩾28.0, *n* (%)	76 (12.8)	60 (10.1)	45 (7.6)	29 (4.9)	
Abdominal obesity					0.020
Yes, *n* (%)	191 (32.1)	174 (29.3)	168 (28.3)	143 (24.1)	
No, *n* (%)	403 (67.9)	420 (70.7)	426 (71.7)	451 (75.9)	
Age, year	34.7 ± 14.9	34.6 ± 16.3	33.3 ± 15.5	29.9 ± 14.5	<0.001
Gender					0.018
Men, *n* (%)	319 (53.7)	296 (49.8)	266 (44.8)	283 (47.6)	
Women, *n* (%)	275 (46.3)	298 (50.2)	328 (55.2)	311 (52.4)	
Body weight, kg	67.6 ± 12.5	66.1 ± 11.6	65.4 ± 11.3	64.2 ± 11.4	<0.001
BMI, kg/m^2	23.8 ± 3.7	23.3 ± 3.3	23.2 ± 3.3	22.8 ± 3.1	<0.001
WC, cm	80.6 ± 10.3	79.2 ± 9.7	79.0 ± 9.5	78.2 ± 9.8	<0.001
Income per month					<0.001
<2000 yuan, *n* (%)	355 (59.8)	366 (61.6)	374 (63.0)	442 (74.4)	
2000–5000 yuan, *n* (%)	223 (37.5)	207 (34.8)	203 (34.2)	123 (20.7)	
⩾5000 yuan, *n* (%)	16 (2.7)	21 (3.5)	17 (2.9)	29 (4.9)	
Education					0.021
Under college, *n* (%)	175 (29.5)	145 (24.4)	132 (22.2)	122 (20.5)	
Bachelor, *n* (%)	398 (67.0)	424 (71.4)	437 (73.6)	449 (75.6)	
Master or doctor, *n* (%)	21 (3.5)	25 (4.2)	25 (4.2)	23 (3.9)	
Labor					<0.001
Light, *n* (%)	164 (27.6)	179 (30.1)	149 (25.1)	135 (22.7)	
Medium, *n* (%)	391 (65.8)	397 (66.8)	430 (72.4)	453 (76.3)	
Heavy, *n* (%)	39 (6.6)	18 (3.0)	15 (2.5)	6 (1.0)	
Exercise					<0.001
<10 h/week, *n* (%)	281 (47.3)	223 (3.8)	182 (30.6)	137 (23.1)	
10–20 h/week, *n* (%)	300 (50.5)	315 (53.0)	317 (53.4)	334 (56.2)	
⩾20 h/week, *n* (%)	13 (2.2)	56 (9.4)	95 (16.0)	123 (20.7)	
Smoking					0.046
Non-smoker, *n* (%)	493 (83.0)	494 (83.2)	530 (89.2)	507 (85.4)	
Current smoker, *n* (%)	73 (12.3)	75 (12.6)	49 (8.2)	61 (10.3)	
Quit smoking, *n* (%)	28 (4.7)	25 (4.2)	15 (2.5)	26 (4.4)	
Drinking					0.44
Non-drinker, *n* (%)	475 (80.0)	489 (82.3)	495 (83.7)	480 (80.8)	
Current drinker, *n* (%)	119 (20.0)	105 (17.7)	99 (16.7)	114 (19.2)	
SBP (mmHg)	119.1 ± 12.9	119.0 ± 14.1	117.7 ± 12.4	115.1 ± 11.4	<0.001
DBP (mmHg)	78.9 ± 8.7	78.7 ± 9.1	77.9 ± 8.9	76.2 ± 8.4	<0.001
Dietary intakes					
Energy, kcal/day	2448.4 ± 824.5	2534.2 ± 867.6	2430.5 ± 865.5	2399.9 ± 896.0	0.048
Total protein, g/day	79.7 ± 30.5	92.7 ± 35.2	93.8 ± 37.9	95.0 ± 41.7	<0.001
Total amino acids, g/day	36.9 ± 16.8	54.2 ± 20.7	61.3 ± 24.7	69.8 ± 30.5	<0.001
Histidine, g/day	0.9 ± 0.4	1.4 ± 0.5	1.6 ± 0.6	1.8 ± 0.8	<0.001
Total fat, g/day	60.8 ± 28.2	78.5 ± 35.3	83.4 ± 37.6	81.2 ± 43.0	<0.001
Total carbohydrate, g/day	406.9 ± 146.3	382.5 ± 137.9	345.2 ± 133.4	341.9 ± 141.9	<0.001
Cholesterol, mg/day	405.7 ± 309.9	495.8 ± 338.9	489.6 ± 309.6	435.8 ± 349.0	<0.001
Fiber, g/day	15.7 ± 7.6	20.9 ± 10.6	21.7 ± 11.1	22.6 ± 13.0	<0.001

Abbreviations: BMI, body mass index; WC, waist circumference; SBP, systolic blood pressure; DBP, diastolic blood pressure; *p* are for differences across quartiles of histidine intake. Data are expressed as mean ± SD or frequencies and percentages, as appropriate.

3.2. *Dietary Histidine of Overweight and Obesity Participants Was Lower than Healthy Controls*

We firstly performed this comparison to find the differences in dietary histidine among three BMI categories (normal weight < 24.0, overweight 24.0–28.0, and obesity ⩾ 28.0). In the overall male and female populations, dietary histidine of overweight and obese groups were all significantly lower than normal group ($p < 0.05$ between normal and overweight group, $p < 0.01$ between normal and obese group). Moreover, dietary histidine of obese group was significantly lower than overweight group ($p < 0.05$). Confounding factors such as age, education, income, labor, exercise status, dietary carbohydrate, fat, protein, fiber and cholesterol intake and smoking habits were controlled in this study (Figure 2).

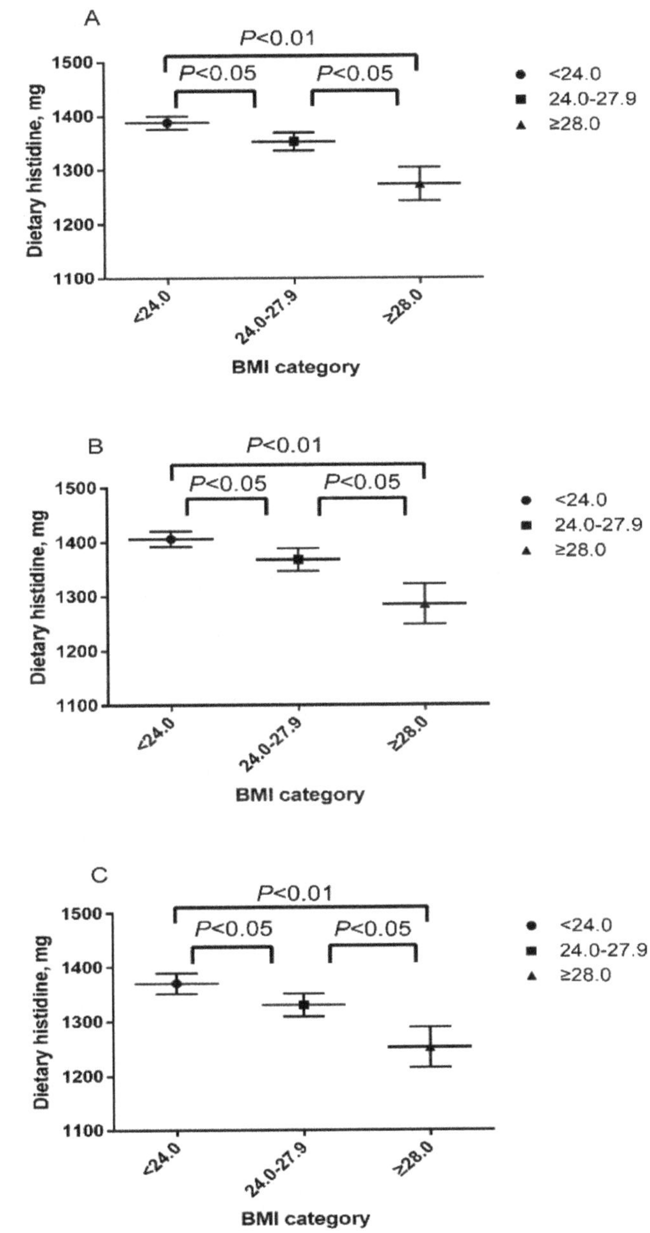

Figure 2. Dietary histidine of different body mass index (BMI) categories: (**A**) the overall population; (**B**) male participants; and (**C**) female participants. Confounding factors such as age, labor, exercise status, dietary carbohydrate, fat, protein, fiber and cholesterol intake and smoking habits were controlled.

3.3. *Correlations between Dietary Histidine and Body Weight, BMI, WC, SBP and DBP*

Bivariate correlation analysis and partial correlation analysis was used to examine these associations of dietary histidine with body weight, BMI, WC, SBP and DBP. Potential covariates (age, dietary carbohydrate, fat, protein, fiber and cholesterol intake) were adjusted in the partial correlation analysis. As shown in Table 2, we found negative correlations between dietary histidine and body weight, BMI, WC, SBP and DBP ($r = -0.076, -0.129, -0.132, -0.106$ and -0.092, respectively, all $p < 0.01$). Because of higher histidine intake in males (male: 1.6 ± 0.8 g vs. female: 1.3 ± 0.6 g, $p < 0.01$), we examined these associations in both gender, the significance was stronger in women. Furthermore, considering the higher histidine intake in normal BMI participants (Figure 2), we examined these associations in different BMI categories. We found negative correlations between dietary histidine and BMI, WC, SBP and DBP in overweight and obese participants, but no significant correlation of dietary histidine and BMI, WC, and DBP were observed in normal BMI participants.

Table 2. Correlations between dietary histidine and energy intake, body weight, BMI, WC and blood pressure.

	Unadjusted		Adjusted *			Unadjusted		Adjusted *	
	r	*p*	*r*	*p*		*r*	*p*	*r*	*p*
Overall					Normal BMI				
Energy intake	−0.031	NS	−0.053	<0.05	Energy intake	−0.032	NS	−0.027	NS
Body weight	−0.093	<0.001	−0.076	<0.01	Body weight	−0.042	NS	−0.029	NS
BMI	−0.126	<0.001	−0.129	<0.001	BMI	−0.046	NS	−0.037	NS
WC	−0.127	<0.001	−0.132	<0.001	WC	−0.061	NS	−0.071	NS
SBP	−0.119	<0.001	−0.106	<0.001	SBP	−0.109	<0.001	−0.056	<0.05
DBP	−0.104	<0.001	−0.092	<0.001	DBP	−0.079	<0.01	−0.052	NS
Men					Overweight				
Energy intake	−0.022	NS	−0.034	NS	Energy intake	−0.055	NS	−0.058	NS
Body weight	−0.061	<0.05	−0.064	<0.05	Body weight	−0.094	NS	−0.042	NS
BMI	−0.102	<0.01	−0.095	<0.05	BMI	−0.137	<0.001	−0.133	<0.001
WC	−0.096	<0.05	−0.093	<0.05	WC	−0.114	<0.05	−0.125	<0.05
SBP	−0.143	<0.001	−0.076	<0.05	SBP	−0.104	<0.01	−0.097	<0.05
DBP	−0.112	<0.001	−0.086	<0.01	DBP	−0.112	<0.01	−0.092	<0.05
Women					Obesity				
Energy intake	−0.065	<0.05	−0.056	<0.05	Energy intake	−0.068	<0.05	−0.073	<0.05
Body weight	−0.096	<0.05	−0.088	<0.01	Body weight	−0.119	<0.05	−0.104	<0.05
BMI	−0.136	<0.001	−0.147	<0.001	BMI	−0.131	<0.01	−0.147	<0.001
WC	−0.138	<0.01	−0.153	<0.001	WC	−0.143	<0.01	−0.142	<0.01
SBP	−0.066	<0.05	0.113	<0.01	SBP	−0.117	<0.01	−0.113	<0.05
DBP	−0.065	<0.05	−0.109	<0.01	DBP	−0.143	<0.05	−0.131	<0.05

Abbreviations: BMI, body mass index; WC, waist circumference; SBP, systolic blood pressure; DBP, diastolic blood pressure; NS, no significance. * Adjusting for dietary carbohydrate, fat, protein, fiber and cholesterol intake.

3.4. *Higher Dietary Histidine Intake Is Associated with Lower Prevalence of Overweight/Obesity and Abdominal Obesity in Northern Chinese*

With adjustment for potential dietary and non-dietary cofounders (age, gender; income; education; labor; physical exercise; dietary carbohydrate, fat, protein, fiber and cholesterol intake; and smoking status), higher dietary histidine was inversely associated with prevalence of overweight/obesity and Abdominal obesity. As shown in Tables 3 and 4, compared with the 1st quartile, the multivariable-adjusted ORs of overweight/obesity for the 3rd and 4th quartile were 0.745 (0.572, 0.969) and 0.650 (0.482, 0.876), respectively (all $p < 0.05$). After being stratified by gender, the significance still exists in the 4th quartile of men and the 2nd, 3rd and 4th quartile of women (all $p < 0.05$). For abdominal obesity, the multivariable-adjusted ORs for the 2nd, 3rd and 4th quartile were 0.716 (0.539, 0.952), 0.809 (0.597, 0.995) and 0.754 (0.545, 0.943), respectively (all $p < 0.05$). After being stratified by gender, the significance is stronger in women (all $p < 0.01$) but no significant correlation was observed in men.

Table 3. Multivariable-adjusted Odds ratio (OR) and 95% confidence interval (CI) of overweight/obesity by quartile of dietary histidine.

All				
Histidine Quartiles	**Quartile 1**	**Quartile 2**	**Quartile 3**	**Quartile 4**
Dietary histidine (% protein)	<1.38	1.38–1.59	1.59–1.77	>1.77
Participants, *n*	594	594	594	594
Overweight/obesity, *n* (%)	267 (44.9)	242 (40.7)	210 (35.4)	170 (28.6)
Crude	1	0.768 (0.610, 0.968) *	0.736 (0.584, 0.928) *	0.537 (0.423, 0.681) **
Model 1	1	0.772 (0.602, 0.990) *	0.752 (0.586, 0.966) *	0.646 (0.500, 0.834) **
Model 2	1	0.777 (0.587, 1.029)	0.744 (0.572, 0.968) *	0.649 (0.481, 0.875) **
Model 3	1	0.772 (0.583, 1.023)	0.745 (0.572, 0.969) *	0.650 (0.482, 0.876) **
Men				
Histidine Quartiles	**Quartile 1**	**Quartile 2**	**Quartile 3**	**Quartile 4**
Dietary histidine (% protein)	<1.35	1.35–1.57	1.57–1.76	>1.76
Participants, *n*	291	291	291	291
Overweight/obesity, *n* (%)	132 (45.4)	117 (40.2)	98 (33.7)	85 (29.2)
Crude	1	0.926 (0.671, 1.278)	0.826 (0.592, 1.154)	0.608 (0.434, 0.853) **
Model 1	1	0.919 (0.655, 1.289)	0.843 (0.594, 1.197)	0.599 (0.490, 0.998) *
Model 2	1	0.973 (0.676, 1.388)	0.828 (0.561, 1.288)	0.578 (0.468, 0.991) *
Model 3	1	0.969 (0.672, 1.396)	0.838 (0.577, 1.302)	0.575 (0.456, 0.988) *
Women				
Histidine Quartiles	**Quartile 1**	**Quartile 2**	**Quartile 3**	**Quartile 4**
Dietary histidine (% protein)	<1.40	1.40–1.61	1.61–1.77	>1.77
Participants, *n*	303	303	303	303
Overweight/obesity, *n* (%)	135 (44.6)	125 (41.3)	112 (37.0)	85 (28.1)
Crude	1	0.639 (0.461, 0.884) **	0.624 (0.448, 0.871) **	0.463 (0.330, 0.649) **
Model 1	1	0.642 (0.445, 0.925) *	0.574 (0.393, 0.837) **	0.549 (0.376, 0.803) **
Model 2	1	0.607 (0.403, 0.915) *	0.557 (0.375, 0.827) **	0.515 (0.333, 0.796) **
Model 3	1	0.612 (0.406, 0.923) *	0.556 (0.374, 0.826) **	0.518 (0.335, 0.801) **

Model 1: adjusting for age, education, income, labor and exercise status. Model 2: Model 1 + dietary carbohydrate, fat, protein, fiber and cholesterol intake were adjusted. Model 3: Model 2 + smoking habits were adjusted. * $p < 0.05$; ** $p < 0.01$ compared with the 1st quartile.

3.5. Correlations between Dietary Histidine and Status of Insulin Resistance, Inflammation and Oxidative Stress in Overweight/Obese Participants

Considering the stronger correlations between dietary histidine and BMI and WC in overweight/obese participants, 88 overweight/obese individuals were selected for subgroup study to explore the possible mechanism. Characteristics of subgroup study population are provided in Table S1. Overweight and obesity are always accompanied by abnormal postprandial metabolism, chronic low-grade inflammation and oxidative stress [20]. Therefore, serum biochemistry indexes and biomarkers of inflammation and oxidative stress were measured. Partial correlation analysis was used to examine these associations of dietary histidine with status of insulin resistance, inflammation and oxidative stress, independent of total energy intake. Potential covariates (age, BMI, dietary carbohydrate, fat, protein, fiber and cholesterol intake) were adjusted in the model. As shown in Table 5, higher dietary histidine is associated with lower FBG, HOMA-IR, 2 h-PG, MDA, TNF-α, IL-1β, IL-6, CRP, MDA and vaspin and higher GSH-Px, SOD and adiponectin of overweight/obese individuals of both sexes (all $p < 0.05$).

Table 4. Multivariable-adjusted Odds ratio (OR) and 95% confidence interval (CI) of abdominal obesity by quartile of dietary histidine.

All				
Histidine Quartiles	**Quartile 1**	**Quartile 2**	**Quartile 3**	**Quartile 4**
Dietary histidine (% protein)	<1.38	1.38–1.59	1.59–1.77	>1.77
Participants, *n*	594	594	594	594
Abdominal obesity, *n* (%)	191 (32.1)	174 (29.3)	168 (28.3)	143 (24.1)
Crude	1	0.771 (0.603, 0.987) *	0.752 (0.587, 0.963) *	0.614 (0.477, 0.792) **
Model 1	1	0.733 (0.563, 0.956) *	0.774 (0.594, 0.996) *	0.742 (0.565, 0.974) *
Model 2	1	0.723 (0.545, 0.059) *	0.782 (0.579, 0.998) *	0.761 (0.552, 0.985) *
Model 3	1	0.716 (0.539, 0.952) *	0.809 (0.597, 0.995) *	0.754 (0.545, 0.943) *
Men				
Histidine Quartiles	**Quartile 1**	**Quartile 2**	**Quartile 3**	**Quartile 4**
Dietary histidine (% protein)	<1.35	1.35–1.57	1.57–1.76	>1.76
Participants, *n*	291	291	291	291
Abdominal obesity, *n* (%)	120 (41.2)	118 (40.5)	114 (39.2)	102 (35.1)
Crude	1	0.972 (0.698, 1.353)	0.918 (0.659, 1.279)	0.769 (0.550, 1.075)
Model 1	1	0.943 (0.663, 1.341)	0.923 (0.648, 1.315)	0.908 (0.634, 1.301)
Model 2	1	0.948 (0.650, 1.383)	0.940 (0.627, 1.410)	0.928 (0.600, 1.435)
Model 3	1	0.929 (0.636, 1.357)	0.959 (0.639, 1.441)	0.916 (0.592, 1.419)
Women				
Histidine Quartiles	**Quartile 1**	**Quartile 2**	**Quartile 3**	**Quartile 4**
Dietary histidine (% protein)	<1.40	1.40–1.61	1.61–1.77	>1.77
Participants, *n*	303	303	303	303
Abdominal obesity, *n* (%)	71 (23.4)	56 (18.5)	54 (17.8)	41 (13.5)
Crude	1	0.639 (0.461, 0.884) **	0.624 (0.448, 0.871) **	0.463 (0.330, 0.649) **
Model 1	1	0.499 (0.313, 0.794) **	0.539 (0.280, 0.938) *	0.507 (0.314, 0.816) **
Model 2	1	0.477 (0.293, 0.777) **	0.476 (0.278, 0.802) **	0.472 (0.272, 0.821) **
Model 3	1	0.478 (0.294, 0.778) **	0.501 (0.320, 0.840) **	0.473 (0.272, 0.822) **

Model 1: adjusting for age, education, income, labor and exercise status. Model 2: Model 1 + dietary carbohydrate, fat, protein, fiber and cholesterol intake were adjusted. Model 3: Model 2 + smoking habits were adjusted. *: $p < 0.05$; **: $p < 0.01$ compared with the 1st quartile.

Table 5. Associations between dietary histidine and metabolic profile, inflammation and oxidative stress in overweight/obese participants.

	Overall		Men		Women	
Parameters	r *	p	r *	p	r *	p
FBG	−0.179	<0.05	−0.171	<0.05	−0.214	<0.05
Insulin	−0.122	NS	−0.111	NS	−0.098	NS
HOMA-IR	−0.233	<0.05	−0.221	<0.05	−0.237	<0.05
TC	−0.103	NS	−0.089	NS	−0.109	NS
TG	−0.122	NS	−0.106	NS	−0.127	NS
HDL	0.074	NS	0.033	NS	0.098	NS
LDL	0.081	NS	0.089	NS	0.076	NS
2 h-PG	−0.171	<0.05	−0.167	NS	−0.189	<0.05
2 h-Insulin	−0.112	NS	−0.078	NS	−0.131	NS
2 h-TC	−0.081	NS	−0.065	NS	−0.057	NS
2 h-TG	−0.056	NS	−0.034	NS	−0.078	NS
2 h-HDL	0.098	NS	0.035	NS	0.101	NS
2 h-LDL	0.035	NS	0.008	NS	0.041	NS
GSH-Px	0.265	<0.05	0.231	<0.05	0.283	<0.05
SOD	0.167	<0.05	0.149	NS	0.198	<0.05
MDA	−0.202	<0.05	−0.187	<0.05	−0.231	<0.05
TNF-α	−0.271	<0.05	−0.265	<0.05	−0.273	<0.05

Table 5. *Cont.*

	Overall		Men		Women	
Parameters	r *	p	r *	p	r *	p
IL-1β	−0.178	<0.05	−0.172	<0.05	−0.189	<0.05
IL-6	−0.182	<0.05	−0.166	<0.05	−0.198	<0.05
CRP	−0.242	<0.05	−0.178	<0.05	−0.267	<0.05
Adiponectin	0.188	<0.05	0.176	<0.05	0.195	<0.05
Vaspin	−0.217	<0.05	−0.231	<0.05	−0.203	<0.05

Abbreviations: FBG, fasting blood glucose; HOMA-IR, homeostasis model assessment of insulin resistance; TC, total cholesterol; TG, triglyceride; HDL, high destiny lipoprotein; LDL, low destiny lipoprotein; 2 h-PG, 2 h-postprandial glucose; GSH-Px, glutathione peroxidase; SOD, superoxide dismutase; MDA, malonaldehyde; TNF-α, tumor necrosis factor-α; IL-1β, interleukin-1β; IL-6, interleukin-6; CRP, C-reactive protein; NS, no significance. * Adjusting for dietary carbohydrate, fat, protein, fiber and cholesterol intake.

4. Discussion

This is the first Internet-based cross-sectional study to investigate associations between dietary histidine and prevalence of overweight/obesity and abdominal obesity in northern Chinese adults. We firstly reported that higher dietary histidine intake was associated with lower prevalence of overweight/obesity and abdominal obesity and lower BMI, waist circumference and blood pressure in northern Chinese population, which was firstly found using an Internet-based FFQ study. Moreover, we firstly reported that in overweight/obese individuals, higher dietary histidine is associated with lower FBG, HOMA-IR, 2 h-PG, MDA, TNF-α, IL-1β, IL-6, CRP, MDA and vaspin and higher GSH-Px, SOD and adiponectin.

In this study, we firstly found that dietary histidine is inversely associated with SBP and DBP in northern Chinese population, but no direct evidence was found to support our finding. Only one cross-sectional study reported a positive association between histidine and blood pressure in adolescents [25]. However, the relationship between obesity and hypertension is well established and the mechanisms through which obesity directly causes hypertension are still an area that requires more research [26]. The negative association between dietary histidine and blood pressure can be explained by anti-obesity effect of histidine.

Insulin resistance is the central feature of the metabolic syndrome and is considered as a critical link between obesity and many chronic diseases [27]. To effectively control these chronic diseases, the positive prevention of insulin resistance in obese individuals is extremely important. It has been reported that histidine supplementation could improve insulin resistance in obese women [14]. In the present study, we firstly found that dietary histidine is inversely associated with FBG, HOMA-IR and 2 h-PG in obese individuals, but no significant correlation between dietary histidine and fasting/postprandial insulin was found. These results indicated that dietary histidine also might improve insulin resistance in overweight and obese individuals. However, limited sample size may influence this effect and further studies are needed to confirm this association in normal weight individuals.

It has been confirmed that concentrations of pro-inflammatory cytokines such as TNF-α, IL-6 and CRP are elevated in obese subjects [28] and elevated TNF-α, IL-6 are associated with obesity related insulin resistance [29]. CRP is the most important inflammation biomarker in humans; it is elevated in status of systemic inflammation and is also related to insulin resistance and metabolic syndrome [30]. Therefore, the suppression of pro-inflammation cytokines is considered as an effective strategy for reducing the risk of obesity-related diseases. In animal models of diabetes, histidine supplementation could reduce the levels of IL-6, TNF-α and CRP [31]. Our previous studies in a high-fat diet induced female obese rat model also confirmed that histidine supplementation could ameliorate inflammation and oxidative stress of adipose tissue [11]. In an in vitro study, Son et al. [32] reported that histidine inhibited the hydrogen peroxide- (H_2O_2-) and TNF-α-induced IL-8 secretion at the transcriptional level in intestinal epithelial cells. In a previous study, we had found lower serum histidine concentrations in obese women than non-obese women. In obese women, serum histidine was negatively associated with inflammation and oxidative stress [13]. Histidine supplementation could improve IR, reduce BMI, fat mass and suppress inflammation and oxidative stress in obese women [14]. In the present study, we firstly found that dietary histidine was inversely associated with TNF-α, IL-1β, IL-6 and CRP, which indicated that dietary histidine also might improve inflammation in overweight and obese individuals. However, this correlation in normal weight individuals is unclear.

Adiponectin is a novel adipocytokine that has been suggested to play a role in the development of insulin resistance and atherosclerosis [33]. Circulating adiponectin levels were decreased in parallel with the development of insulin resistance in rhesus monkeys [34], which indicates that reduced plasma adiponectin levels might play a role in the progress of insulin resistance. In the present study, we also found positive correlation between dietary histidine and serum adiponectin in overweight/obese induviduals. Dietary histidine may increase secretion of adiponectin by suppressing inflammation and oxidative stress in white adipose tissue. Further studies are needed to verify this correlation in normal weight individuals.

Vaspin (visceral adipose tissue-derived serpin) was firstly found in an abdominal obesity with T2DM animal model and was shown as a new adipocytokine to influence insulin sensitivity of white adipose tissues in obese rats. Interestingly, the serum level of vaspin shows increasing trend in prediabetic stage, but decreased with the development of diabetes along with a sharp body weight loss [35]. Circulating vaspin is strongly associated with BMI and insulin sensitivity [36]. A meta-analysis also reporting vaspin levels in subjects with obesity and type 2 diabetes mellitus was higher than healthy controls [37]. In the present study, we firstly found that dietary histidine was inversely associated with serum vaspin in overweight/obese participants. However, the mechanism is unknown.

Oxidative stress is considered as one main cause of insulin resistance and many chronic diseases are characterized by excessive oxidative stress [38]. Therefore, the suppression of oxidative stress is an effective strategy for reducing the risk of obesity-related diseases. Previous study found that the concentrations of SOD in the serum and the mRNA expression of copper zinc superoxide dismutase (CuZnSOD) in the white adipose tissue were increased and the concentrations of MDA in the serum were decreased by histidine supplementation in high-fat diet-induced female obese rat model [11]. In the present study, we quantified three oxidative biomarkers, GSH-Px, SOD and MDA, and the results revealed that the concentrations of GSH-Px and SOD in the serum was positively associated with dietary histidine and the concentrations MDA in the serum was inversely associated with dietary histidine, which provides more evidence that histidine is a potential antioxidant in obese individuals.

For the gender and BMI difference of histidine in our study, we found that negative correlations between dietary histidine and BMI and WC were stronger in overweight and obese participants. Moreover, the association between dietary histidine and overweight/obesity and abdominal obesity is much stronger in women. Several potential mechanisms might account for this finding. In this study, lower histidine intake was observed in female participants and overweight/obese individuals, which may lead to lower serum histidine and stronger response to dietary histidine. Moreover, previous studies found that women were more sensitive to dietary histidine and energy intake than men [15,39], but the mechanisms are still unclear and further studies are needed.

The primary limitation of this study is the cross-sectional and retrospective design. We must acknowledge that reverse causality may be exists as cross-sectional studies were insufficient to confirm the causal relationship between dietary factors and occurrence of disease [17]. Long term cohort studies for this issue are needed to verify the casual relationship; Secondly, current study was only performed in a northern Chinese population. Consider of the large population and vast territory of China, we must be rigorous when extrapolating this result to the general population. Moreover, beneficial effects of dietary histidine such as lower fasting blood glucose, insulin resistance, inflammation and oxidative stress may be associated with histidine peptides (carnosine, anserine and balenine), which has been shown in recent studies of carnosine supplementation in animals [40] and more recently in humans [41]. However, in our study, data of dietary histidine peptides were lacking. In spite of these limitations, this study provides a lot of practical significance, especially in nutritional counseling. As nutrition is important for prevention of obesity and reduction of excess body weight, reasonable dietary intervention should be useful for the prevention of overweight/obesity. For overweight/obese clients, advice of consuming more histidine-rich foods may be useful for weight control.

5. Conclusions

In summary, our study adds evidence supporting the inverse associations between dietary histidine and obesity, possibly through reduction of energy intake and improvements of insulin resistance, inflammation and oxidative stress. To confirm the casual associations, long-term cohort studies of this issue are needed.

Acknowledgments: The study was supported by the National Natural Science Fund of China (No. 81202184, 81573133), Natural Science Fund of Heilongjiang Province (No. JJ2016ZR1154, No. H2016018) and Financial Grant from China Postdoctoral Science Foundation (2013M531076).

Author Contributions: R.-N.F. and C.-H.S. were responsible for the study concept and design; Y.-C.L., J.-Y.Q., and D.S. performed the experiment and collected the data; Y.-C.L. carried out the analysis and interpretation of data; Y.-C.L. and C.-L.L. wrote the paper; L.-N.H., S.-S.D., L.-Y.L. and C.-L.L. contributed to the critical revision of the manuscript; R.-N.L. and C.-H.S. were responsible for obtaining funds and supervision.

References

1. Ng, M.; Fleming, T.; Robinson, M.; Thomson, B.; Graetz, N.; Margono, C.; Mullany, E.C.; Biryukov, S.; Abbafati, C.; Abera, S.F.; et al. Global, regional, and national prevalence of overweight and obesity in children and adults during 1980–2013: A systematic analysis for the global burden of disease study 2013. *Lancet* **2014**, *384*, 766–781. [CrossRef]
2. Kim, S.K.; Kim, H.J.; Hur, K.Y.; Choi, S.H.; Ahn, C.W.; Lim, S.K.; Kim, K.R.; Lee, H.C.; Huh, K.B.; Cha, B.S. Visceral fat thickness measured by ultrasonography can estimate not only visceral obesity but also risks of cardiovascular and metabolic diseases. *Am. J. Clin. Nutr.* **2004**, *79*, 593–599. [PubMed]
3. Wolongevicz, D.M.; Zhu, L.; Pencina, M.J.; Kimokoti, R.W.; Newby, P.K.; D'Agostino, R.B.; Millen, B.E. Diet quality and obesity in women: The framingham nutrition studies. *Br. J. Nutr.* **2010**, *103*, 1223–1229. [CrossRef] [PubMed]
4. De Simone, G.; Devereux, R.B.; Chinali, M.; Roman, M.J.; Best, L.G.; Welty, T.K.; Lee, E.T.; Howard, B.V. Strong Heart Study Investigators. Risk factors for arterial hypertension in adults with initial optimal blood pressure: The strong heart study. *Hypertension* **2006**, *47*, 162–167. [CrossRef] [PubMed]
5. De Pergola, G.; Silvestris, F. Obesity as a major risk factor for cancer. *J. Obes.* **2013**, *2013*, 291546. [CrossRef] [PubMed]
6. Hu, F.B.; Liu, Y.; Willett, W.C. Preventing chronic diseases by promoting healthy diet and lifestyle: Public policy implications for China. *Obes. Rev.* **2011**, *12*, 552–559. [CrossRef] [PubMed]
7. Estruch, R.; Ros, E.; Martinez-Gonzalez, M.A. Mediterranean diet for primary prevention of cardiovascular disease. *N. Engl. J. Med.* **2013**, *369*, 676–677. [CrossRef] [PubMed]
8. Choi, J.H.; Woo, H.D.; Lee, J.H.; Kim, J. Dietary patterns and risk for metabolic syndrome in Korean women: A cross-sectional study. *Medicine (Baltimore)* **2015**, *94*, e1424. [CrossRef] [PubMed]
9. Gardner, C.D.; Kiazand, A.; Alhassan, S.; Kim, S.; Stafford, R.S.; Balise, R.R.; Kraemer, H.C.; King, A.C. Comparison of the atkins, zone, ornish, and learn diets for change in weight and related risk factors among overweight premenopausal women: The a to z weight loss study: A randomized trial. *JAMA* **2007**, *297*, 969–977. [CrossRef] [PubMed]
10. Watanabe, M.; Suliman, M.E.; Qureshi, A.R.; Garcia-Lopez, E.; Barany, P.; Heimburger, O.; Stenvinkel, P.; Lindholm, B. Consequences of low plasma histidine in chronic kidney disease patients: Associations with inflammation, oxidative stress, and mortality. *Am. J. Clin. Nutr.* **2008**, *87*, 1860–1866. [PubMed]
11. Sun, X.; Feng, R.; Li, Y.; Lin, S.; Zhang, W.; Li, Y.; Sun, C.; Li, S. Histidine supplementation alleviates inflammation in the adipose tissue of high-fat diet-induced obese rats via the nf-kappab- and ppargamma-involved pathways. *Br. J. Nutr.* **2014**, *112*, 477–485. [CrossRef] [PubMed]

12. Kasaoka, S.; Tsuboyama-Kasaoka, N.; Kawahara, Y.; Inoue, S.; Tsuji, M.; Ezaki, O.; Kato, H.; Tsuchiya, T.; Okuda, H.; Nakajima, S. Histidine supplementation suppresses food intake and fat accumulation in rats. *Nutrition* **2004**, *20*, 991–996. [CrossRef] [PubMed]
13. Niu, Y.C.; Feng, R.N.; Hou, Y.; Li, K.; Kang, Z.; Wang, J.; Sun, C.H.; Li, Y. Histidine and arginine are associated with inflammation and oxidative stress in obese women. *Br. J. Nutr.* **2012**, *108*, 57–61. [CrossRef] [PubMed]
14. Feng, R.N.; Niu, Y.C.; Sun, X.W.; Li, Q.; Zhao, C.; Wang, C.; Guo, F.C.; Sun, C.H.; Li, Y. Histidine supplementation improves insulin resistance through suppressed inflammation in obese women with the metabolic syndrome: A randomised controlled trial. *Diabetologia* **2013**, *56*, 985–994. [CrossRef] [PubMed]
15. Okubo, H.; Sasaki, S. Histidine intake may negatively correlate with energy intake in human: A cross-sectional study in Japanese female students aged 18 years. *J. Nutr. Sci. Vitaminol. (Tokyo)* **2005**, *51*, 329–334. [CrossRef] [PubMed]
16. Sublette, M.E.; Segal-Isaacson, C.J.; Cooper, T.B.; Fekri, S.; Vanegas, N.; Galfalvy, H.C.; Oquendo, M.A.; Mann, J.J. Validation of a food frequency questionnaire to assess intake of n-3 polyunsaturated fatty acids in subjects with and without major depressive disorder. *J. Am. Diet. Assoc.* **2011**, *111*, 117–123.e1-2. [CrossRef] [PubMed]
17. Haftenberger, M.; Heuer, T.; Heidemann, C.; Kube, F.; Krems, C.; Mensink, G.B. Relative validation of a food frequency questionnaire for national health and nutrition monitoring. *Nutr. J.* **2010**, *9*, 36. [CrossRef] [PubMed]
18. Du, S.S.; Jiang, Y.S.; Chen, Y.; Li, Z.; Zhang, Y.F.; Sun, C.H.; Feng, R.N. Development and applicability of an internet-based diet and lifestyle questionnaire for college students in china: A cross-sectional study. *Medicine (Baltimore)* **2015**, *94*, e2130. [CrossRef] [PubMed]
19. Yingyangjiayuan. Available online: http://www.yyjy365.org/diet (accessed on 23 March 2012).
20. Li, Y.C.; Li, Y.; Liu, L.Y.; Chen, Y.; Zi, T.Q.; Du, S.S.; Jiang, Y.S.; Feng, R.N.; Sun, C.H. The ratio of dietary branched-chain amino acids is associated with a lower prevalence of obesity in young northern Chinese adults: An internet-based cross-sectional study. *Nutrients* **2015**, *7*, 9573–9589. [CrossRef] [PubMed]
21. Yang, Y.; Wang, G.; Guo, X. *China Food Composition Tables*; Peking University Medical Press: Beijing, China, 2009.
22. Zhou, B.F. Effect of body mass index on all-cause mortality and incidence of cardiovascular diseases—Report for meta-analysis of prospective studies open optimal cut-off points of body mass index in Chinese adults. *Biomed. Environ. Sci.* **2002**, *15*, 245–252. [PubMed]
23. Hu, J.; Wallace, D.C.; Jones, E.; Liu, H. Cardiometabolic health of Chinese older adults with diabetes living in Beijing, China. *Public Health Nurs.* **2009**, *26*, 500–511. [CrossRef] [PubMed]
24. Matthews, D.R.; Hosker, J.P.; Rudenski, A.S.; Naylor, B.A.; Treacher, D.F.; Turner, R.C. Homeostasis model assessment: Insulin resistance and beta-cell function from fasting plasma glucose and insulin concentrations in man. *Diabetologia* **1985**, *28*, 412–419. [CrossRef] [PubMed]
25. De Moraes, A.C.; Bel-Serrat, S.; Manios, Y.; Molnar, D.; Kafatos, A.; Cuenca-Garcia, M.; Huybrechts, I.; Sette, S.; Widhalm, K.; Stehle, P.; et al. Dietary protein and amino acids intake and its relationship with blood pressure in adolescents: The Helena study. *Eur. J. Public Health* **2015**, *25*, 450–456. [CrossRef] [PubMed]
26. Kotsis, V.; Stabouli, S.; Papakatsika, S.; Rizos, Z.; Parati, G. Mechanisms of obesity-induced hypertension. *Hypertens. Res.* **2010**, *33*, 386–393. [CrossRef] [PubMed]
27. Kahn, S.E.; Hull, R.L.; Utzschneider, K.M. Mechanisms linking obesity to insulin resistance and type 2 diabetes. *Nature* **2006**, *444*, 840–846. [CrossRef] [PubMed]
28. Greenberg, A.S.; Obin, M.S. Obesity and the role of adipose tissue in inflammation and metabolism. *Am. J. Clin. Nutr.* **2006**, *83*, 461S–465S. [PubMed]
29. Kern, P.A.; Ranganathan, S.; Li, C.; Wood, L.; Ranganathan, G. Adipose tissue tumor necrosis factor and interleukin-6 expression in human obesity and insulin resistance. *Am. J. Physiol. Endocrinol. Metab.* **2001**, *280*, E745–E751. [PubMed]
30. Gonzalez, A.S.; Guerrero, D.B.; Soto, M.B.; Diaz, S.P.; Martinez-Olmos, M.; Vidal, O. Metabolic syndrome, insulin resistance and the inflammation markers c-reactive protein and ferritin. *Eur. J. Clin. Nutr.* **2006**, *60*, 802–809. [CrossRef] [PubMed]

31. Lee, Y.T.; Hsu, C.C.; Lin, M.H.; Liu, K.S.; Yin, M.C. Histidine and carnosine delay diabetic deterioration in mice and protect human low density lipoprotein against oxidation and glycation. *Eur. J. Pharmacol.* **2005**, *513*, 145–150. [CrossRef] [PubMed]
32. Son, D.O.; Satsu, H.; Shimizu, M. Histidine inhibits oxidative stress- and tnf-alpha-induced interleukin-8 secretion in intestinal epithelial cells. *FEBS Lett.* **2005**, *579*, 4671–4677. [CrossRef] [PubMed]
33. Lihn, A.S.; Pedersen, S.B.; Richelsen, B. Adiponectin: Action, regulation and association to insulin sensitivity. *Obes. Rev.* **2005**, *6*, 13–21. [CrossRef] [PubMed]
34. Hotta, K.; Funahashi, T.; Bodkin, N.L.; Ortmeyer, H.K.; Arita, Y.; Hansen, B.C.; Matsuzawa, Y. Circulating concentrations of the adipocyte protein adiponectin are decreased in parallel with reduced insulin sensitivity during the progression to type 2 diabetes in rhesus monkeys. *Diabetes* **2001**, *50*, 1126–1133. [CrossRef] [PubMed]
35. Hida, K.; Wada, J.; Eguchi, J.; Zhang, H.; Baba, M.; Seida, A.; Hashimoto, I.; Okada, T.; Yasuhara, A.; Nakatsuka, A.; et al. Visceral adipose tissue-derived serine protease inhibitor: A unique insulin-sensitizing adipocytokine in obesity. *Proc. Natl. Acad. Sci. USA* **2005**, *102*, 10610–10615. [CrossRef] [PubMed]
36. Youn, B.S.; Kloting, N.; Kratzsch, J.; Lee, N.; Park, J.W.; Song, E.S.; Ruschke, K.; Oberbach, A.; Fasshauer, M.; Stumvoll, M.; et al. Serum vaspin concentrations in human obesity and type 2 diabetes. *Diabetes* **2008**, *57*, 372–377. [CrossRef] [PubMed]
37. Feng, R.; Li, Y.; Wang, C.; Luo, C.; Liu, L.; Chuo, F.; Li, Q.; Sun, C. Higher vaspin levels in subjects with obesity and type 2 diabetes mellitus: A meta-analysis. *Diabetes Res. Clin. Pract.* **2014**, *106*, 88–94. [CrossRef] [PubMed]
38. Ndisang, J.F.; Vannacci, A.; Rastogi, S. Oxidative stress and inflammation in obesity, diabetes, hypertension, and related cardiometabolic complications. *Oxid. Med. Cell. Longev.* **2014**, *2014*. [CrossRef] [PubMed]
39. Kasaoka, S.; Kawahara, Y.; Inoue, S.; Tsuji, M.; Kato, H.; Tsuchiya, T.; Okuda, H.; Nakajima, S. Gender effects in dietary histidine-induced anorexia. *Nutrition* **2005**, *21*, 855–858. [CrossRef] [PubMed]
40. Nagai, K.; Tanida, M.; Niijima, A.; Tsuruoka, N.; Kiso, Y.; Horii, Y.; Shen, J.; Okumura, N. Role of L-carnosine in the control of blood glucose, blood pressure, thermogenesis, and lipolysis by autonomic nerves in rats: Involvement of the circadian clock and histamine. *Amino Acids* **2012**, *43*, 97–109. [CrossRef] [PubMed]
41. Courten, B.; Jakubova, M.; de Courten, M.P.; Kukurova, I.J.; Vallova, S.; Krumpolec, P.; Valkovic, L.; Kurdiova, T.; Garzon, D.; Barbaresi, S.; et al. Effects of carnosine supplementation on glucose metabolism: Pilot clinical trial. *Obesity (Silver Spring)* **2016**, *24*, 1027–1034. [CrossRef] [PubMed]

6

Postprandial Effect of a High-Fat Meal on Endotoxemia in Arab Women with and without Insulin-Resistance-Related Diseases

Dara A. Al-Disi [1,2], Nasser M. Al-Daghri [3,4,†,*], Nasiruddin Khan [3,4], Assim A. Alfadda [5,6], Reem M. Sallam [5,6,7], Mohammed Alsaif [2], Shaun Sabico [1,3,4], Gyanendra Tripathi [1] and Philip G. McTernan [1,†,*]

1 Division of Biomedical Sciences, Warwick Medical School, University of Warwick, Coventry CV2 2DX, UK; dara.aldesi@warwick.ac.uk (D.A.A.-D.); s.l.sabico@warwick.ac.uk (S.S.); g.tripathi@warwick.ac.uk (G.T.)

2 Department of Community Health Sciences, College of Applied Medical Sciences, King Saud University, Riyadh 11451, Saudi Arabia; malsaif@ksu.edu.sa

3 Biomarkers Research Program, Riyadh Biochemistry Department, College of Science, King Saud University, Riyadh 11451, Saudi Arabia; nasiruddin2006@gmail.com

4 Prince Mutaib Chair for Biomarkers of Osteoporosis, Biochemistry Department, College of Science, King Saud University, Riyadh 11451, Saudi Arabia

5 Obesity Research Center, College of Medicine, King Saud University, Riyadh 11461, Saudi Arabia; dralfadda@hotmail.com (A.A.A.); sallam_reem@yahoo.com (R.M.S.)

6 Department of Medicine, College of Medicine, King Saud University, Riyadh 11461, Saudi Arabia

7 Clinical Chemistry Unit, Department of Pathology, College of Medicine, King Saud University, Riyadh 11461, Saudi Arabia

* Correspondence: aldaghri2011@gmail.com (N.M.A.-D.); p.g.mcternan@warwick.ac.uk (P.G.M.)

† These authors contributed equally to this work.

Abstract: This study determined the effects of a high-fat meal on circulating endotoxin and cardiometabolic indices in adult Arab women. The cohort consisted of 92 consenting Saudi women (18 non-diabetic (ND)) control subjects; Age 24.4 ± 7.9 year; body mass index (BMI) 22.2 ± 2.2 Kg/m^2), 24 overweight/obese (referred to as overweight-plus (overweight$^+$)) subjects (Age 32.0 ± 7.8 year; BMI 28.5 ± 1.5 Kg/m^2) and 50 type 2 diabetes mellitus (T2DM) patients (Age 41.5 ± 6.2 year; BMI 35.2 ± 7.7 Kg/m^2). All were given a high-fat meal (standardized meal: 75 g fat, 5 g carbohydrate, 6 g protein) after an overnight fast of 12–14 h. Anthropometrics were obtained and fasting blood glucose, lipids, and endotoxin were serially measured for four consecutive postprandial hours. Endotoxin levels were significantly elevated prior to a high-fat meal in the overweight$^+$ and T2DM than the controls ($p < 0.05$). Furthermore, the postprandial cardiometabolic changes led to a more detrimental risk profile in T2DM subjects than other groups, with serial changes most notable in glucose, triglycerides, high density lipoprotein-cholesterol (HDL-cholesterol), and insulin levels (p-values < 0.05). The same single meal given to subjects with different metabolic states had varying impacts on cardiometabolic health. Endotoxemia is exacerbated by a high-fat meal in Arab subjects with T2DM, accompanied by a parallel increase in cardiometabolic risk profile, suggesting disparity in disease pathogenesis of those with or without T2DM through the altered cardiometabolic risk profile rather than variance in metabolic endotoxinaemia with a high-fat meal.

Keywords: endotoxin; type 2 diabetes mellitus; Arab women; high fat meal

---

1. Introduction

The nutritional transition and the rapid urbanization in the Middle East has introduced energy-dense refined carbohydrates and increased saturated fat intake [1]. This transition has paralleled the increase in lifestyle-related chronic diseases such as obesity and type 2 diabetes mellitus (T2DM) [2,3].

Whilst obesity represents the single most influential risk factor for T2DM, weight gain itself is a result of a complex interaction between genetic, epigenetic, and environmental factors. Amongst the latter, a carbohydrate-rich high-fat diet can quickly drive the increased obesity mediated T2DM [4]. The major metabolic consequence of a high-fat diet is the negative effect on insulin action, where the regulatory mechanisms of body weight become impaired through lipotoxic effects as well as the increased low grade chronic systemic inflammatory response [5,6].

Previous models of diet-induced and genetic obesity has shown that adipose tissue presents an important source of pro-inflammatory adipocytokines, such as tumor necrosis factor α (TNF-α), interleukin-1 (IL-1), and interleukin-6 (IL-6) during weight gain [7,8]. These adipocytokines can have a simultaneous dual impact leading to insulin resistance through activation of the pro-inflammatory mechanisms as well as a direct impact on insulin signaling capacity [9]. As such, the development of the insulin resistance through a sustained energy dense diet promotes hyperinsulinaemic conditions, coupled with increased adipose tissue and ectopic fat accumulation [10].

The impact of a high-fat diet at the molecular level remains to be fully understood. However, postprandial lipidaemia has emerged as a potential candidate to promote an inflammatory response. Studies have shown that the ingestion of a single high-fat meal can mediate systemic increases of a wide range of inflammatory factors with noted activation of nuclear factor-κB (NF-κB) in leukocytes [11–14], a key transcription factor in the inflammatory cascade that regulates the transcription of numerous pro-inflammatory cytokines and adipocytokines [15,16]. To date, the cause of these postprandial inflammatory events remains poorly understood. One potential candidate factor is bacterial endotoxin (lipopolysaccharide (LPS)), a potent inflammatory bacterial antigen that is present in large quantities in the human gut [17]. Endotoxin circulates in the blood of healthy human subjects at low concentrations (between 1 and 200 pg/mL) [18]. However, clinical studies have implicated gut-derived endotoxin as a "primary insult" that activates the inflammatory state, contributing to metabolic disease, with cross sectional data showing elevated systemic endotoxin levels in obesity, T2DM, coronary artery disease and fatty liver disease with the ability to be influenced by changes in diet [19–23].

The aim of this study was therefore to determine the influence of a high-fat meal on changes in circulating endotoxin and whether this is altered in different metabolic disease states amongst Arab adult women.

2. Experimental Section

The study comprised of three groups of subjects: non-T2DM, lean subjects (control; Body Mass Index (BMI) 22.2 $\pm$ 2.2 Kg/m^2; n = 18), overweight/obese (referred to as overweight-plus (overweight$^+$)) subjects (overweight$^+$ 28.5 $\pm$ 1.5 Kg/m^2) subjects (n = 24), and patients with early onset of T2DM (BMI: 35.2 $\pm$ 7.7 Kg/m^2; n = 50). All subjects were Saudi pre-menopausal women, randomly selected from different primary care centers (PCCs) of Riyadh, Saudi Arabia, nonsmokers, with a normal resting electrocardiogram (ECG) and blood pressure, and with no history of vascular disease. In addition, subjects with known long-standing diabetes and/or receiving anti-diabetic medication, those with fasting glucose levels > 11 mmol/L, or with fasting triglycerides levels > 4 mmol/L were excluded from the study. Ethical approval was granted by the Ethics Committee of King Saud University (No. 10-173), Riyadh, Kingdom of Saudi Arabia, prior to the commencement of the research and all patients gave written consent.

Screening fasting blood tests at baseline were performed to qualify subjects for the study and to assess glucose control as well as lipid profiles. In addition, all subjects had their weight, height, waist and hip circumferences measured. Weight (in kilograms) was measured in light clothing to the nearest 0.1 kg. Height was measured using a digital stadiometer to the nearest centimeter. Waist circumference was measured at the level of the iliac crest at the end of normal respiration, and hip was measured at the widest circumference around the buttocks using measuring tape. BMI, as well as waist-to-hip ratios (WHR), were calculated. Blood samples were taken from the right or left antecubital vein in the sitting position. Blood pressure was checked with a blood pressure monitor on the left arm using a standard protocol. All subjects ($n = 92$) with and without T2DM were given a high-fat meal (standardized meal: 75 g fat, 5 g carbohydrate, 6 g protein per m^2 body surface area corresponding to 700 Kcal/m^2 [24]) after an overnight fast of 12–14 h.

2.1. *In Vivo* Assessment of the Biochemical Profile

Blood samples were drawn via cannula at baseline (0 h) and postprandially (1, 2, 3, and 4 h), and endotoxin and lipid levels were measured. Serum glucose and lipid profile were measured routinely using a glucose oxidase method in an autoanalyzer (Konelab, Espoo, Finland). Serum-free insulin concentrations were determined by electro-chemiluminescence method (COBAS-E-411; Roche Diagnostics, Mannheim, Germany). Homeostasis model assessment for insulin resistance (HOMA-IR) was then calculated for all patients using the HOMA formula:

$$\text{HOMA-IR} = \text{fasting insulin (mU/L)} \times \text{fasting plasma glucose (mmol/L)}/22.5 \text{ [25].} \quad (1)$$

2.2. *Analysis of Circulating Endotoxin*

Serum endotoxin was analyzed using a commercially available QCL-1000 LAL End Point Assay (Lonza, Allendale, NJ, USA). The assay, and the values given by the manufacturer for intra-assay coefficient of variation (CV) (3.9% ± 0.46%) and inter-assay CV (9.6% ± 0.75%), have been validated as detailed previously by this research group [16].

2.3. *Statistical Analysis*

Data were analyzed using SPSS version 16.5 (SPSS, Chicago, IL, USA). All continuous variables were presented as mean ± standard deviation and were normalized prior to parametric analyses. For comparison between groups, Analysis of Variance (ANOVA) with Tukey *post-hoc* analysis and Kruskal-Wallis (for triglycerides) were used. For comparison overtime, repeated measures ANOVA and Friedman's two-way analysis of variance (for triglycerides, insulin, HOMA-IR and endotoxin) were used. For associations between endotoxin and variables of interest postprandial, Spearman bivariate correlations were utilized. Significance was set at $p < 0.05$.

3. Results

The clinical and metabolic characteristics were determined (Table 1) according to groups. Subjects with T2DM had a mean duration of diabetes of 2.04 years. Furthermore, it noted that there were significant differences in age and BMI across the cohort (Table 1). As expected, the T2DM group also had the highest anthropometric indices (BMI, waist and hip circumferences as well as WHR) than the overweight$^+$ group and controls, with the overweight$^+$ group being significantly higher than the controls in all indices as well. As anticipated, subjects with T2DM had significantly higher serum glucose levels (7.9 ± 2.73 mmol/L) than the overweight$^+$ (4.7 ± 0.41 mmol/L, $p < 0.01$) and control subjects (4.81 ± 0.86 mmol/L, $p < 0.001$). The subjects with T2DM also had significantly higher serum triglycerides (1.9 ± 1.0 mmol/L), total cholesterol (5.4 ± 1.07 mmol/L) and low density lipoprotein-cholesterol (LDL-cholesterol) (3.66 ± 0.8 mmol/L), as well as the lowest in mean high density lipoprotein-cholesterol (HDL-cholesterol) (0.96 ± 0.21 mmol/L) (all $p < 0.001$). Serum glucose and lipid levels of the overweight+ and control groups were not significantly different from one another (Table 1).

Table 1. Clinical and metabolic characteristics of subjects according to group.

	Control	Overweight+	T2DM	*p*-Value
N	18	24	50	
Age (years)	24.4 ± 7.9	32.0 ± 7.8 *	41.5 ± 6.2 *!	<0.001
T2DM Duration (years)	–	–	2.04 (0–9)	
BMI (Kg/m^2)	22.2 ± 2.2	28.5 ± 1.5 *	35.2 ± 7.7 *!	<0.001
Waist (cm)	80.6 ± 7.2	95.8 ± 7.4 *	112.3 ± 13.4 *!	<0.001
Hip (cm)	98.7 ± 7.3	109.7 ± 5.0 *	117.1 ± 11.6 *!	<0.001
WHR	0.8 ± 0.05	0.9 ± 0.05 *	1.0 ± 0.07 *!	<0.001
Glucose (mmol/L)	4.8 ± 0.9	4.7 ± 0.4	7.9 ± 2.7 *!	<0.001
LDL-Cholesterol (mmol/L)	2.8 ± 0.6	2.8 ± 0.7	3.7 ± 0.8 *!	<0.001
Triglycerides (mmol/L) #	1.0 ± 0.4	1.3 ± 0.8	1.9 ± 1.0 *!	0.001
Total Cholesterol (mmol/L)	4.2 ± 0.7	4.5 ± 01.0	5.4 ± 1.1 *!	0.003
HDL-Cholesterol (mmol/L)	1.3 ± 0.2	1.1 ± 0.4	0.96 ± 0.2 *!	<0.001

Data presented as mean ± standard error; # denotes non-Gaussian distribution; *p*-values at extreme right denotes over-all significance according to group; "*" denotes significance as compared with control subjects; "!" denotes significance as compared with overweight+ group; "–" denotes absence of T2DM in subjects; *p*-value significant at < 0.05. Analysis of Variance (ANOVA) with Tukey *post-hoc* analysis and Kruskal-Wallis (for triglycerides) tests were used (T2DM: Type 2 diabetes Mellitus; BMI: Body mass index; WHR: Waist hip ratio; LDL: Low density lipoprotein; HDL: High density lipoprotein).

3.1. *Effects of High-Fat Meal in Different Groups*

Blood samples were taken over time following a high-fat meal to assess changes in metabolic indices and endotoxin changes in the three cohorts. In the T2DM group, mean glucose level was highest at 0 h and lowest after 4 h, which was significantly lower than other hours with a noted stepwise reduction over time (Table 2). In both the control and overweight+ groups, no significant changes in glucose were noted over time (Table 2). In contrast to glucose levels, the triglyceride levels for all groups followed an increasing trend over time. The triglyceride levels in the subjects with T2DM was highest postprandially between 3 and 4 h, and was significantly higher than hours 0–2 ($p < 0.01$). In the overweight+ group, triglyceride levels were highest at 3 h than 4 h, with a stepwise increase from baseline over time until 3 h. Comparing all groups, the subjects with T2DM had significantly higher mean triglyceride levels as compared with either the overweight+ or control groups ($p < 0.01$). No significant changes were noted with total cholesterol over time.

In the subjects with T2DM, HDL-cholesterol was lowest after 4 h and was significantly lower than hours 0–3 ($p < 0.01$) with, again, a stepwise reduction in HDL-cholesterol level (Table 2). Similarly, the HDL-cholesterol levels in the overweight+ group were lowest at hour 4 than the previous hours 0–2 ($p < 0.01$). In contrast, the HDL-cholesterol levels of the control group were significantly higher than both the T2DM and overweight+ groups ($p < 0.01$).

In the T2DM group, LDL-cholesterol levels at baseline were significantly higher than hours 1–4 ($p < 0.05$). In the overweight+ group, LDL-cholesterol levels at baseline were significantly higher than hours 2–4 ($p < 0.05$). In the control group, LDL-cholesterol levels at baseline was significantly lower than hours 1 and 2 ($p < 0.05$) returning to baseline levels after that. T2DM had significantly higher LDL-cholesterol levels than either the control or overweight+ group.

Table 2. Metabolic changes pre- and post-high-fat meal.

	0 h	1 h	2 h	3 h	4 h
GLUCOSE (mmol/L)					
T2DM (N = 50)	7.9 ± 2.7	7.8 ± 2.5	7.5 ± 2.5 *	7.29 ± 2.7 *!§	7.0 ± 2.8 *!§†
Overweight⁺ (N = 24)	4.7 ± 0.4	4.6 ± 0.4	4.6 ± 0.4	4.6 ± 0.39	4.63 ± 0.7
Control (N = 18)	4.8 ± 0.86	5.1 ± 2.3	5.02 ± 1.7	4.76 ± 1.51	4.79 ± 1.6
TRIGLYCERIDES (mmol/L) #					
T2DM (N = 50)	1.9 ± 1.0	1.8 ± 0.7	2.4 ± 0.9 *!	2.7 ± 1.1 *!§	2.7 ± 1.3 *!§
Overweight⁺ (N = 24)	1.3 ± 0.8	1.4 ± 0.8	1.7 ± 0.9 *!	2.0 ± 1.1 *!§	1.9 ± 1.3 *!§
Control (N = 18)	1.0 ± 0.4	1.2 ± 0.6	1.4 ± 0.9	1.44 ± 0.91	1.54 ± 1.0
TOTAL CHOLESTEROL (mmol/L)					
T2DM (N = 50)	5.4 ± 1.1	5.3 ± 1.0	5.4 ± 1.1	5.3 ± 1.1	5.4 ± 1.1
Overweight⁺ (N = 24)	4.5 ± 1.0	4.5 ± 0.9	4.4 ± 0.8	4.4 ± 0.8	4.4 ± 1.0
Control (N = 18)	4.2 ± 0.7	4.1 ± 0.7	4.1 ± 0.6	4.1 ± 0.6	4.2 ± 0.7
HDL-CHOLESTEROL (mmol/L)					
T2DM (N = 50)	1.0 ± 0.2	1.0 ± 0.2	0.9 ± 0.2	0.9 ± 0.2 *!	0.89 ± 0.2 *!§†
Overweight⁺ (N = 24)	1.2 ± 0.3	1.1 ± 0.3	1.1 ± 0.3	1.1 ± 0.4 *!	1.1 ± 0.4 *!§
Control (N = 18)	1.3 ± 0.2	1.2 ± 0.3	1.2 ± 0.3	1.2 ± 0.3	1.2 ± 0.3
LDL-CHOLESTEROL (mmol/L)					
T2DM (N = 50)	3.7 ± 0.8	3.6 ± 0.8	3.4 ± 0.9 *	3.2 ± 0.9 *	3.3 ± 0.9 *
Overweight⁺ (N = 24)	2.8 ± 0.7	2.7 ± 0.6	2.5 ± 0.6 *	2.4 ± 0.6 *	2.4 ± 0.6 *
Control (N = 18)	2.7 ± 0.6	2.6 ± 0.6*	2.6 ± 0.6 *	2.6 ± 0.6	2.7 ± 0.6
Endotoxin (EU/mL)					
T2DM (N = 50)	3.4 ± 0.8	3.0 ± 0.8	3.4 ± 0.9 !	3.5 ± 0.9 !	3.6 ± 0.9 !
Overweight⁺ (N = 24)	3.0 ± 0.5	2.9 ± 1.4	3.5 ± 0.9	3.8 ± 1.6	3.5 ± 1.9
Control (N = 18)	1.5 ± 0.1	1.8 ± 0.1 *	1.7 ± 0.8 *	1.9 ± 0.2 *	2.1 ± 0.2 *
Insulin (IU/mL) #					
T2DM (N = 50)	11.7 ± 5.5	21.9 ± 17.7 *	19.3 ± 12.6 *	16.2 ± 12.3 *	14.3 ± 8.2 *
Overweight⁺ (N = 24)	5.0 ± 3.4	15.6 ± 16.2 *	16.9 ± 16.0 *	13.1 ± 8.0 *	10.3 ± 5.3 *
Control (N = 18)	5.8 ± 0.64	10.3 ± 1.7	9.6 ± 3.4	8.2 ± 1.6	10.2 ± 2.6
HOMA-IR #					
T2DM (N = 50)	3.7 ± 2.0	8.7 ± 12.0 *‡	6.6 ± 6.0 *‡	5.6 ± 5.4 ‡	3.9 ± 2.4
Overweight⁺ (N = 24)	1.12 ± 0.7	3.5 ± 4.1 *	3.9 ± 4.1 *	2.8 ± 1.9 *	2.1 ± 1.2
Control (N = 18)	1.3 ± 0.2	1.9 ± 0.4	2.1 ± 0.7 *	1.9 ± 0.4	2.2 ± 0.6

# denotes Non-Gaussian distribution; * denotes significance compared with 0 hour; ! denotes significance compared with 1; § denotes significance compared with 2; † denotes significance compared with 3; ‡ denotes significance compared with 4; p significant at ≤ 0.05. Repeated measures ANOVA and Friedman's two-way analysis of variance (for triglycerides, insulin, HOMA-IR and endotoxin) were the tests used (T2DM: Type 2 diabetes Mellitus; Overweight⁺: overweight/obese subjects referred to as overweight-plus; LDL: Low density lipoprotein; HDL: High density lipoprotein; HOMA-IR: Homeostasis model assessment for insulin resistance; ANOVA: analysis of Variance).

The highest endotoxin levels were noted at hour 4 in all groups and was statistically significant compared with hour 1 in the T2DM group and baseline in the control group ($p < 0.01$). No significant changes were observed in the overweight⁺ group. Both the T2DM and overweight⁺ groups had significantly higher endotoxin levels than the control subjects. Insulin levels were also noted to change over time in the subjects with T2DM, with the highest peak insulin levels noted at hours 1–2, lowest at hours 3–4, and baseline fasted insulin levels being significantly lower as compared to insulin levels across time ($p < 0.01$). This similar pattern was observed in the overweight⁺ and control groups, with the baseline noting the lowest insulin levels over time. Between groups, the insulin level in the T2DM group was significantly higher than either the overweight⁺ or control group as expected ($p < 0.01$).

Lastly, in both the T2DM and overweight$^+$ groups, HOMA-IR was lowest at baseline at the fourth hour with the T2DM group showing the highest mean HOMA-IR post 1 h feed and the overweight$^+$ group at hour 2. No significant changes in HOMA-IR were observed in the control group over time. Between groups, the HOMA-IR in subjects with T2DM was significantly higher than those of the overweight$^+$ and control groups ($p < 0.01$).

3.2. Associations of Metabolic Parameters to Endotoxin after a High-Fat Meal

In all subjects, endotoxin was positively associated with LDL cholesterol ($R = 0.38$; $p < 0.05$) and this was observed 3 h after a high-fat meal. In the subjects with T2DM, endotoxin was significantly associated with triglycerides at 3 and 4 h postprandial (R values 0.52 and 0.50; $p < 0.05$, respectively). In the overweight$^+$ subjects, endotoxin was highly associated with triglycerides ($R = 0.63$; $p < 0.05$) and total cholesterol ($R = 0.71$; $p < 0.05$) at baseline. Whilst in the control subjects no associations were observed at baseline or over time (Table 3).

4. Discussion

The present results affirm and extend our knowledge on the impact of a high-fat meal in different metabolic states. Specifically, circulating endotoxin levels were significantly raised during a high-fat meal in overweight$^+$ and T2DM metabolic states, with the impact of cardiometabolic changes imposing a more detrimental risk profile in T2DM subjects than either the overweight$^+$ or the non-diabetic lean control subjects as assessed by glucose, triglycerides, insulin and HOMA-IR and lower HDL postprandially. The results also highlighted that the same single meal given to subjects in different metabolic states had a different impact on cardiometabolic health. As such, daily repetition of this type of meal could have a much more damaging effect in the subjects with T2DM, closely followed by the overweight$^+$ subjects; whilst lean and non-diabetic subjects appear to better handle the insult of a high-fat meal, metabolically.

Despite the impact of the meal it was also identified that prior to the high-fat meal, the presence of sub-chronic inflammation was already apparent, with circulating endotoxin being highest in subjects with T2DM, affirming prior studies that suggest that endotoxin levels are altered in the presence of insulin-resistant diseases [16,19–22,26]. Previous studies have also shown that a high-fat meal, regardless of the individual's metabolic status, can induce inflammatory changes [27,28]. In this study, circulating endotoxin, a potential mediator of a low grade chronic inflammatory response, was comparably raised in both the overweight$^+$ and T2DM states, unlike previous studies in South Asians [26], suggesting that Arabs in the overweight$^+$ state may at least be at even higher metabolic risk, which could help to explain the country's current higher metabolic disease per capita.

Elevated endotoxin levels amongst Middle-Eastern patients with T2DM are also consistent across ethnic groups, such as Africans [29], Chinese [30], Caucasians [16,31], and South Asians [22,23]. Whilst endotoxin is seen as an important mediator of sub-clinical inflammation, Piya and colleagues have suggested that, ultimately, the gut flora may act as an essential determinant of the sub-chronic inflammation induced by obesity and T2DM, and that endotoxin may act as a systemic insult that triggers the inflammatory cascade [32]. In Saudi women, a high-fat meal given to both overweight+ and T2DM groups increased endotoxin levels from a higher baseline in these groups without a clear difference between them, in contrast to previous studies in South Asians [26]. Animal studies have shown that continuous infusion of endotoxin increases gut permeability, as does high-fat dietary feeding, therefore, one possible explanation for the difference could be due to the dietary differences in fat consumption that the obese subjects eat in Saudi Arabia as compared in UK [33].

Table 3. Bivariate associations between lipids, glucose and endotoxin.

Glucose					Triglycerides					Total Cholesterol					HDL-Cholesterol					LDL-Cholesterol				
0	1	2	3	4	0	1	2	3	4	0	1	2	3	4	0	1	2	3	4	0	1	2	3	4
ALL SUBJECTS																								
−0.17	0.04	0.13	0.08	0.00	−0.13	0.10	0.14	0.22	0.20	0.16	−0.08	0.00	−0.07	−0.21	−0.16	0.15	−0.01	−0.08	−0.06	0.22	−0.06	0.05	0.38	−0.12
T2DM SUBJECTS (N = 50)																								
−0.20	0.23	0.29	0.23	0.08	−0.12	0.32	0.26	0.52	0.50	0.18	0.04	0.02	0.0	−0.08	−0.28	-0.15	−0.14	−0.30	−0.05	0.30	0.02	0.005	−0.06	−0.19
OVERWEIGHT⁺ SUBJECTS (N = 24)																								
0.23	0.14	0.08	0.0	−0.18	0.63	0.04	0.08	0.26	0.25	0.71	−0.08	0.10	−0.13	−0.33	−0.13	0.41	0.13	−0.07	−0.18	0.36	0.14	0.43	0.64	0.28
CONTROL SUBJECTS (N = 18)																								
−0.36	0.15	0.22	0.24	0.14	−0.20	0.16	0.30	−0.14	−0.17	–	0.01	0.14	−0.05	−0.26	−0.28	−0.20	−0.39	−0.16	−0.31	−0.02	0.08	0.24	0.07	−0.09

Data presented as coefficient (R); bold and red denotes significance at $p < 0.05$. Spearman correlation tests were used (T2DM: Type 2 diabetes Mellitus; Overweight^{+}: overweight/obese subjects referred to as overweight-plus; Control Subjects: Non-daibetic lean individiuals; LDL: Low density lipoprotein; HDL: High density lipoprotein). "–" denotes absence of T2DM in subjects.

Animal studies involving *ob/ob* and *db/db* mice have demonstrated a leaky gut which is considered to be related to the impact insulin resistance on gut endothelium [33]. As such, our overweight$^+$ and T2DM subjects may have a more frequent snack habit, which consequentially affects how they subsequently handled the high-fat meal, which could be different from the white Caucasians given such a diet. Furthermore, ethnicity may clearly impact on individual sub-clinical inflammatory risk. Previous studies have shown that endotoxin can be stratified by gender and ethnicity; therefore, these data could help explain why different ethnicities have a variable cardiometabolic risk due to post-feeding increases in endotoxin [21].

The current study also considered the impact of a high-fat meal on elevating glucose and cholesterol levels, both considered important in the development of coronary artery disease, coupled with obesity and T2DM. The changes observed postprandially in the lipid profile and insulin in this study, resulted in lipidaemia regardless of their metabolic status and this is consistent with previous studies [26,34–36]. Prior analysis of the effects of a high saturated fat meal in other studies indicates that lipidaemia can mediate deleterious changes at the proteome and genome levels producing a pro-coagulant state [37]. Furthermore, it appears from other studies that triglycerides show the most dynamic changes during the postprandial phase compared to other lipids, regardless of the individual's metabolic status, although it appears dependent on the type of fat diet used [38]. Clinically, this is relevant. As observed in the present and other studies, higher postprandial hypertriglyceridemia and hyperlipidemia are observed amongst subjects with T2DM than their healthier counterparts [39]. Therefore, dietary strategies defining the type of dietary fat for patients, to lower saturated fat content, appears important to lead to better management of the insulin response and increased fat oxidation, both important determinants of cardiometabolic risk in overweight and T2DM patients [40].

The different cardiometabolic risk factor changes in pre- and post-feeding showed that the T2DM group had significantly higher glucose, triglycerides, insulin, and HOMA-IR, as well as significantly lower HDL-cholesterol throughout the high-fat challenge as compared with overweight$^+$ and control subjects. Whilst these significant differences were expected, since the baseline levels of T2DM subjects were already higher than other groups, the persistence of dysmetabolism in the T2DM group suggests that already deranged baseline glycemic and lipid parameters could be exacerbated further following a fat intake [41,42]. The postprandial increments in glucose and lipids observed confirms previous studies with women and even adolescents with T2DM [43–45] and also reaffirms the requirement to effectively manage postprandial glucose and lipid response in T2DM subjects through diet intervention to lower cardiovascular disease risk [42,46,47].

The authors acknowledge the significant variation in the mean age of the groups and this may have limited the present findings, taking into account the evidence that postprandial lipemia may be associated with age [48]. Nevertheless, comparisons were done mostly within groups and not independent of one another whilst observing for postprandial similarities and differences in patterns according to groups. Furthermore, the small and unequal sample size per group may have affected the few significant associations elicited out of a hundred possible correlations conducted, suggesting that these associations need to be further validated using a larger cohort per group.

5. Conclusions

In conclusion, our findings highlight that subjects with increased adiposity and or T2DM are at increased cardiometabolic risk given a high-fat meal, but particularly so in the subjects with T2DM. Furthermore, irrespective of their diabetic status, endotoxin levels, postprandial, were higher than control subjects. As such, the findings suggest that the disparity in lipidaemia, as opposed to endotoxin, post-meal, may exacerbate the pathogenesis of cardiovascular disease in Arab women in the long-term on this type of diet. Therefore, dietary interventions that can reduce the glycaemic and lipidomic response, as well as improving the gut microbiota for better gut barrier function, appears important in Saudi patients who have increased weight gain or a T2DM status.

Acknowledgments: This study has been funded by the National Plan for Science and Technology (NPST) in Riyadh, Saudi Arabia, Grant No: 11-MED1907-02, as well as a PhD scholarship for Dara Al-Disi provided by the Ministry of Higher Education in King Saud University in conjunction with King Saud University.

Author Contributions: Dara A. Al-Disi, Nasser M. Al-Daghri and Philip G. McTernan conceived the study; Dara A. Al-Disi, Nasiruddin Khan recruited the subjects; Philip G. McTernan and Gyanendra Tripathi performed sample analysis; Shaun Sabico performed data analysis; Dara A. Al-Disi and Shaun Sabico drafted the manuscript; Assim A. Alfadda, Reem M. Sallam, Gyanendra Tripathi, Mohammed Alsaif and Philip G. McTernan provided intellectual input in the final outcome of the manuscript.

References

1. Musaiger, A.O.; Al-Hazzaa, H.M. Prevalence and risk factors associated with nutrition-related noncommunicable diseases in the Eastern Mediterranean region. *Int. J. Gen. Med.* **2012**, *5*, 199–217. [CrossRef] [PubMed]
2. Al-Shoshan, A.A. The affluent diet and its consequences: Saudi Arabia—A case in point. *World Rev. Nutr. Diet.* **1992**, *69*, 113–165. [PubMed]
3. Amuna, P.; Zotor, F.B. Epidemiological and nutrition transition in developing countries: Impact on human health and development. *Proc. Nutr. Soc.* **2008**, *67*, 82–90. [CrossRef] [PubMed]
4. Hu, F.B. Globalization of diabetes: The role of diet, lifestyle, and genes. *Diabetes Care* **2011**, *34*, 1249–1257. [CrossRef] [PubMed]
5. Magnan, C.; Collins, S.; Berthault, M.F.; Kassis, N.; Vincent, M.; Gilber, M.; Pénicaud, L.; Ktorza, A.; Assimacopoulos-Jeannet, F. Lipid infusion lowers sympathetic nervous activity and leads to increased β-cell responsiveness to glucose. *J. Clin. Investig.* **1999**, *103*, 413–419. [CrossRef] [PubMed]
6. Wellen, K.E.; Hotamisligil, G.S. Inflammation, stress, and diabetes. *J. Clin. Investig.* **2005**, *115*, 1111–1119. [CrossRef] [PubMed]
7. Hotamisligil, G.S.; Shargill, N.S.; Spiegelman, B.M. Adipose expression of tumor necrosis factor-alpha: Direct role in obesity-linked insulin resistance. *Science* **1993**, *259*, 87–91. [CrossRef] [PubMed]
8. Weisberg, S.P.; McCann, D.; Desai, M.; Rosenbaum, M.; Leibel, R.L.; Ferrante, A.W. Obesity is associated with macrophage accumulation in adipose tissue. *J. Clin. Investig.* **2003**, *112*, 1796–1808. [CrossRef] [PubMed]
9. Hotamisligil, G.S.; Peraldi, P.; Budavari, A.; Ellis, R.; White, M.F.; Spiegelman, B.M. IRS-1-mediated inhibition of insulin receptor tyrosine kinase activity in TNF-alpha- and obesity-induced insulin resistance. *Science* **1996**, *271*, 665–668. [CrossRef] [PubMed]
10. Jung, U.J.; Choi, M.S. Obesity and its metabolic complications: The role of adipokines and the relationship between obesity, inflammation, insulin resistance, dyslipidemia and nonalcoholic fatty liver disease. *Int. J. Mol. Sci.* **2014**, *15*, 6184–6223. [CrossRef] [PubMed]
11. Aljada, A.; Mohanty, P.; Ghanim, H.; Abdo, T.; Tripathy, D.; Chaudhuri, A.; Dandona, P. Increase in intranuclear nuclear factor κB and decrease in inhibitor κB in mononuclear cells after a mixed meal: Evidence for a proinflammatory effect. *Am. J. Clin. Nutr.* **2004**, *79*, 682–690. [PubMed]
12. Blanco-Colio, L.M.; Valderrama, M.; Alvarez-Sala, L.A.; Bustos, C.; Ortego, M.; Hernández-Presa, M.A.; Cancelas, P.; Gómez-Gerique, J.; Millán, J.; Egido, J. Red Wine Intake Prevents Nuclear Factor-κB Activation in Peripheral Blood Mononuclear Cells of Healthy Volunteers During Postprandial Lipemia. *Circulation* **2000**, *102*, 1020–1026. [CrossRef] [PubMed]
13. Van Oostrom, A.J.; Rabelink, T.J.; Verseyden, C.; Sijmonsma, T.P.; Plokker, H.W.; De Jaegere, P.P.; Cabezas, M.C. Activation of leukocytes by postprandial lipemia in healthy volunteers. *Atherosclerosis* **2004**, *177*, 175–182. [CrossRef] [PubMed]
14. Van Oostrom, A.J.; Sijmonsma, T.P.; Verseyden, C.; Jansen, E.H.; de Koning, E.J.; Rabelink, T.J.; Castro-Cabezas, M. Postprandial recruitment of neutrophils may contribute to endothelial dysfunction. *J. Lipid Res.* **2003**, *44*, 576–583. [CrossRef] [PubMed]
15. Youssef-Elabd, E.M.; McGee, K.C.; Tripathi, G.; Aldaghri, N.; Abdalla, M.S.; Sharada, H.M.; Ashour, E.; Amin, A.I.; Ceriello, A.; O'Hare, J.P. Acute and chronic saturated fatty acid treatment as a key instigator of the TLR-mediated inflammatory response in human adipose tissue, *in vitro*. *J. Nutr. Biochem.* **2012**, *23*, 39–50. [CrossRef] [PubMed]

16. Creely, S.J.; McTernan, P.G.; Kusminski, C.M.; Da Silva, N.; Khanolkar, M.; Evans, M.; Harte, A.; Kumar, S. Lipopolysaccharide activates an innate immune system response in human adipose tissue in obesity and type 2 diabetes. *Am. J. Physiol. Endocrinol. Metab.* **2007**, *292*, E740–E747. [CrossRef] [PubMed]
17. Berg, R.D. The indigenous gastrointestinal microflora. *Trends Microbiol.* **1996**, *4*, 430–435. [CrossRef]
18. Wiedermann, C.J.; Kiechl, S.; Dunzendorfer, S.; Schratzberger, P.; Egger, G.; Oberhollenzer, F.; Willeit, J. Association of endotoxemia with carotid atherosclerosis and cardiovascular disease: Prospective results from the Bruneck study. *J. Am. Coll. Cardiol.* **1999**, *34*, 1975–1981. [CrossRef]
19. Baker, A.R.; Harte, A.L.; Howell, N.; Pritlove, D.C.; Ranasinghe, A.M.; da Silva, N.F.; Youssef, E.M.; Khunti, K.; Davies, M.J.; Bonser, R.S.; *et al.* Epicardial Adipose Tissue as a Source of Nuclear Factor-κB and c-Jun *N*-Terminal Kinase Mediated Inflammation in Patients with Coronary Artery Disease. *J. Clin. Endocrinol. Metab.* **2009**, *94*, 261–267. [CrossRef] [PubMed]
20. Al-Attas, O.S.; Al-Daghri, N.M.; Al-Rubeaan, K.; da Silva, N.F.; Sabico, S.L.; Kumar, S.; McTernan, P.G.; Harte, A.L. Changes in endotoxin levels in T2DM subjects on anti-diabetic therapies. *Cardiovasc. Diabetol.* **2009**, *8*, 20. [CrossRef] [PubMed]
21. Miller, M.A.; McTernan, P.G.; Harte, A.L.; da Silva, N.F.; Strazzullo, P.; Alberti, K.; Kumar, S.; Cappuccio, F.P. Ethnic and sex differences in circulating endotoxin levels: A novel marker of atherosclerotic and cardiovascular risk in a British multi-ethnic population. *Atherosclerosis* **2009**, *203*, 494–502. [CrossRef] [PubMed]
22. Harte, A.L.; da Silva, N.F.; Creely, S.J.; McGee, K.C.; Billyard, T.; Youssef-Elabd, E.M.; Tripathi, G.; Ashour, E.; Abdalla, M.S.; Sharada, H.M.; *et al.* Elevated endotoxin levels in non-alcoholic fatty liver disease. *J. Inflamm. (Lond.)* **2010**, *7*. [CrossRef] [PubMed]
23. Dixon, A.N.; Valsamakis, G.; Hanif, M.W.; Field, A.; Boutsiadis, A.; Harte, A.; McTernan, P.G.; Barnett, A.H.; Kumar, S. Effect of the orlistat on serum endotoxin lipopolysaccharide and adipocytokines in South Asian individuals with impaired glucose tolerance. *Int. J. Clin. Pract.* **2008**, *62*, 1124–1129. [CrossRef] [PubMed]
24. Ceriello, A.; Taboga, C.; Tonutti, L.; Quagliaro, L.; Piconi, L.; Bais, B.; Da Ros, R.; Motz, E. Evidence for an independent and cumulative effect of postprandial hypertriglyceridemia and hyperglycemia on endothelial dysfunction and oxidative stress generation: Effects of short- and long-term simvastatin treatment. *Circulation* **2002**, *106*, 1211–1218. [CrossRef] [PubMed]
25. Bonora, E.; Formentini, G.; Calcaterra, F.; Lombardi, S.; Marini, F.; Zenari, L.; Saggiani, F.; Poli, M.; Perbellini, S.; Raffaelli, A. HOMA-estimated insulin resistance is an independent predictor of cardiovascular disease in type 2 diabetic subjects prospective data from the Verona Diabetes Complications Study. *Diabetes Care* **2002**, *25*, 1135–1141. [CrossRef] [PubMed]
26. Shen, J.; Obin, M.S.; Zhao, L. The gut microbiota, obesity and insulin resistance. *Mol. Aspects. Med.* **2013**, *34*, 39–58. [CrossRef] [PubMed]
27. Harte, A.L.; Varma, M.C.; Tripathi, G.; McGee, K.C.; Al-Daghri, N.M.; Al-Attas, O.S.; Sabico, S.; O'Hare, J.P.; Ceriello, A.; Saravanan, P.; *et al.* High fat intake leads to acute postprandial exposure to circulating endotoxin in type 2 diabetic subjects. *Diabetes Care* **2012**, *5*, 375–382. [CrossRef] [PubMed]
28. Herieka, M.; Erridge, C. High-fat meal induced postprandial inflammation. *Mol. Nutr. Food Res.* **2014**, *58*, 136–146. [CrossRef] [PubMed]
29. Hawkesworth, S.; Moore, S.; Fulford, A.; Barclay, G.; Darboe, A.; Mark, H.; Nyan, O.; Prentice, A. Evidence for metabolic endotoxemia in obese and diabetic Gambian women. *Nutr. Diabetes* **2013**, *3*, e83. [CrossRef] [PubMed]
30. Liu, Y.; Zhao, T.; Hou, L. Change and correlated factors of fasting level of the plasma endotoxin in subjects with different glucose tolerances and body mass indices. *Sichuan Da Xue Xue Bao Yi Xue Ban* **2013**, *44*, 769–773, 778. [PubMed]
31. Monte, S.V.; Caruana, J.A.; Ghanim, H.; Sia, C.L.; Korzeniewski, K.; Schentag, J.J.; Dandona, P. Reduction in endotoxemia, oxidative and inflammatory stress, and insulin resistance after Roux-en-Y gastric bypass surgery in patients with morbid obesity and type 2 diabetes mellitus. *Surgery* **2012**, *151*, 587–593. [CrossRef] [PubMed]
32. Piya, M.K.; Harte, A.L.; McTernan, P.G. Metabolic endotoxaemia: Is it more than just a gut feeling? *Curr. Opin. Lipidol.* **2013**, *24*, 78–85. [CrossRef] [PubMed]

33. Brun, P.; Castagliuolo, I.; Di Leo, V.; Buda, A.; Pinzani, M.; Palù, G.; Martines, D. Increased intestinal permeability in obese mice: New evidence in the pathogenesis of nonalcoholic steatohepatitis. *Am. J. Physiol. Gastrointest. Liver Physiol.* **2007**, *292*, G518–G525. [CrossRef] [PubMed]
34. Wojczynski, M.K.; Glasser, S.P.; Oberman, A.; Kabagambe, E.K.; Hopkins, P.N.; Tsai, M.Y.; Straka, R.J.; Ordovas, J.M.; Arnett, D.K. High-fat meal effect on LDL, HDL, and VLDL particle size and number in the Genetics of Lipid-Lowering drugs and diet network (GOLDN): An interventional study. *Lipids Health Dis.* **2011**, *10*, 181. [CrossRef] [PubMed]
35. Camargo, A.; Meneses, M.E.; Pérez-Martínez, P.; Delgado-Lista, J.; Rangel-Zúñiga, O.A.; Marín, C.; Almadén, Y.; Yubero-Serrano, E.M.; González-Guardia, L.; Fuentes, F. Dietary fat modifies lipid metabolism in the adipose tissue of metabolic syndrome patients. *Genes Nutr.* **2014**, *9*, 1–9. [CrossRef] [PubMed]
36. Meher, D.; Dutta, D.; Ghosh, S.; Mukhopadhyay, P.; Chowdhury, S.; Mukhopadhyay, S. Effect of a mixed meal on plasma lipids, insulin resistance and systemic inflammation in non-obese Indian adults with normal glucose tolerance and treatment naïve type-2 diabetes. *Diabetes Res. Clin. Pract.* **2014**, *104*, 97–102. [CrossRef] [PubMed]
37. Camargo, A.; Rangel-Zúñiga, O.A.; Peña-Orihuela, P.; Marín, C.; Pérez-Martínez, P.; Delgado-Lista, J.; Gutierrez-Mariscal, F.M.; Malagón, M.M.; Roche, H.M.; Tinahones, F.J. Postprandial changes in the proteome are modulated by dietary fat in patients with metabolic syndrome. *J. Nutr. Biochem.* **2013**, *24*, 318–324. [CrossRef] [PubMed]
38. Bonham, M.P.; Linderborg, K.M.; Dordevic, A.; Larsen, A.E.; Nguo, K.; Weir, J.M.; Gran, P.; Luotonen, M.K.; Meikle, P.J.; Cameron-Smith, D. Lipidomic profiling of chylomicron triacylglycerols in response to high fat meals. *Lipids* **2013**, *48*, 39–50. [CrossRef] [PubMed]
39. Pirillo, A.; Norata, G.D.; Catapano, A.L. Postprandial lipemia as a cardiometabolic risk factor. *Curr. Med. Res. Opin.* **2014**, *30*, 1489–1503. [CrossRef] [PubMed]
40. Munsters, M.; Saris, W.H. Body Weight Regulation and Obesity: Dietary Strategies to Improve the Metabolic Profile. *Annu. Rev. Food. Sci. Technol.* **2014**, *5*, 39–51. [CrossRef] [PubMed]
41. Tushuizen, M.E.; Diamant, M.; Heine, R.J. Postprandial dysmetabolism and cardiovascular disease in type 2 diabetes. *Postgrad. Med. J.* **2005**, *81*, 1–6. [CrossRef] [PubMed]
42. Cani, P.D.; Amar, J.; Iglesias, M.A.; Poggi, M.; Knauf, C.; Bastelica, D.; Neyrinck, A.M.; Fava, F.; Tuohy, K.M.; Chabo, C.; *et al.* Metabolic endotoxemia initiates obesity and insulin resistance. *Diabetes* **2007**, *56*, 1761–1772. [CrossRef] [PubMed]
43. Alssema, M.; Schindhelm, R.K.; Dekker, J.M.; Diamant, M.; Nijpels, G.; Teerlink, T.; Scheffer, P.G.; Kostense, P.J.; Heine, R.J. Determinants of postprandial triglyceride and glucose responses after two consecutive fat-rich or carbohydrate-rich meals in normoglycemic women and in women with type 2 diabetes mellitus: The Hoorn Prandial Study. *Metabolism* **2008**, *57*, 1262–1269. [CrossRef] [PubMed]
44. Schindhelm, R.K.; Alssema, M.; Scheffer, P.G.; Diamant, M.; Dekker, J.M.; Barto, R.; Nijpels, G.; Kostense, P.J.; Heine, R.J.; Schalkwijk, C.G.; *et al.* Fasting and Postprandial Glycoxidative and Lipoxidative Stress Are Increased in Women with Type 2 Diabetes. *Diabetes Care* **2007**, *30*, 1789–1794. [CrossRef] [PubMed]
45. Umpaichitra, V.; Banerji, M.A.; Castells, S. Postprandial hyperlipidemia after a fat loading test in minority adolescents with type 2 diabetes mellitus and obesity. *J. Pediatr. Endocrinol. Metab.* **2004**, *7*, 853–864. [CrossRef]
46. Charpentier, G.; Riveline, J.P.; Dardari, D.; Varroud-Vial, M. Should postprandial hyperglycaemia in prediabetic and type 2 diabetic patients be treated? *Drugs* **2006**, *66*, 273–286. [CrossRef] [PubMed]
47. Leiter, L.A.; Ceriello, A.; Davidson, J.A.; Hanefeld, M.; Monnier, L.; Owens, D.R.; Tajima, N.; Tuomilehto, J. Postprandial glucose regulation: New data and new implications. *Clin. Ther.* **2005**, *27*, S42–S56. [CrossRef] [PubMed]
48. Guerci, B.; Verges, B.; Durlach, V.; Hadjadi, S.; Drouin, P.; Paul, J.L. Relationship between altered postprandial lipemia and insulin resistance in normolipidemic and normoglucose tolerant obese patients. *Int. J. Obes. Relat. Metab. Disord.* **2000**, *24*, 468–478. [CrossRef] [PubMed]

7

Efficacy of Aloe Vera Supplementation on Prediabetes and Early Non-Treated Diabetic Patients

Yiyi Zhang [1,†], Wen Liu [2,†], Dan Liu [1], Tieyun Zhao [1] and Haoming Tian [1,*]

[1] Department of Endocrinology and Metabolism, West China Hospital, Sichuan University, Chengdu 610041, China; tibby5211@gmail.com (Y.Z.); danliu565@sina.com (D.L.); zty112356@gmail.com (T.Z.)

[2] Phase I Clinical Research Unit, West China Hospital, Sichuan University, Chengdu 610041, China; wenliu112@126.com

* Correspondence: hmtian999@126.com

† These authors contributed equally to this work.

Abstract: The aim of this study was to evaluate evidence for the efficacy of aloe vera on managing prediabetes and early non-treated diabetes mellitus. We performed a systematic search of PubMed, Embase, and Cochrane Central Register of Controlled Trials until 28 January 2016. A total of five randomized controlled trials (RCTs) involving 415 participants were included. Compared with the controls, aloe vera supplementation significantly reduced the concentrations of fasting blood glucose (FBG) ($p = 0.02$; weighed mean difference [WMD]: −30.05 mg/dL; 95% confidence interval [CI]: −54.87 to −5.23 mg/dL), glycosylated hemoglobin A1c (HbA1c) ($p < 0.00001$; WMD: −0.41%; 95% CI: −0.55% to −0.27%), triglyceride ($p = 0.0001$), total cholesterol (TC) ($p < 0.00001$), and low density lipoprotein-cholesterol (LDL-C) ($p < 0.00001$). Aloe vera was superior to placebo in increasing serum high density lipoprotein-cholesterol (HDL-C) levels ($p = 0.04$). Only one adverse event was reported. The evidence from RCTs showed that aloe vera might effectively reduce the levels of FBG, HbA1c, triglyceride, TC and LDL-C, and increase the levels of HDL-C on prediabetes and early non-treated diabetic patients. Limited evidence exists about the safety of aloe vera. Given the small number and poor quality of RCTs included in the meta-analysis, these results are inconclusive. A large-scale, well-designed RCT is needed to further address this issue.

Keywords: aloe vera; prediabetes; randomized controlled trials; meta-analysis

1. Introduction

Diabetes mellitus is a group of metabolic disorders that is one of the major global health threats to humans due to its increasing prevalence, disabling complications, and chronic course [1]. Both impaired glucose tolerance and impaired fasting glucose are called "prediabetes", which does not reach the diagnostic cutoff values that would precipitate a diagnosis of type 2 diabetes mellitus (T2DM) [2]. It is predicated that approximately 5%–10% of the prediabetic population would suffer from diabetes after approximately a year, and the number of prediabetes patients could reach up to 470 million globally by 2030 [3]. Thus, preventing or delaying the onset of clinical T2DM in prediabetic subjects is a reasonable way to combat the diabetes epidemic and to lessen healthcare costs. Current medications to control blood glucose may have dangerous side effects over time, such as increased risk of liver toxicity, weight gain, and cardiovascular diseases [4]. Therefore, it is not surprising that complementary medicines and natural products, such as oats, are gaining increasing popularity among patients with hyperglycemia, due to affordability and fewer side effects [5]. Many traditional remedies for diabetes mellitus use plant sources, and over 400 species were reported to display hypoglycemic effects, although few of them have been evaluated [6,7].

Aloe is a succulent plant belonging to the Liliaceal family, of which there are more than 200 species found worldwide [8]. Aloe vera is a common name for *Aloe barbadensis*, which is the most widely-used species of aloe. Aloe vera has had applications in health and cosmetic products for many centuries, as well as anti-tumor, antioxidant, anti-inflammatory, and laxative properties [9,10]. It includes over 75 active ingredients that contain enzymes, vitamins, sugars, minerals, lignin, amino acids, and salicylic acid, and most of the constituents appear to be of biological importance in curing diseases [11].

The hypoglycemic effects of aloe vera have been investigated by various researchers. However, there is no consensus on the beneficial effects of aloe vera supplementation in the preventing or improvment of metabolic-syndrome-related disorders [12]. Some studies with rodents have demonstrated the hypoglycemic effect of aloe vera, whereas other studies have shown no significant effects [13,14]. Similarly, there is growing evidence that aloe vera derived extracts showed a preventive effect against insulin resistance and a lipid-lowering effect; however, there is still a great deal of controversy about these data, which have made it difficult to draw any definitive conclusions [14,15]. Therefore, we conducted a meta-analysis to quantitatively summarize and critically evaluate the evidence from randomized clinical trials (RCTs) involving the use of aloe vera as a hypoglycemic supplement.

2. Materials and Methods

2.1. Search Strategy

We searched the following three electronic databases from their inception until 28 January 2016 for the identification of studies: PubMed, Embase and Cochrane Central Register of Controlled Trials. Keywords for databases searching were: ("prediabetes" OR "pre-diabetes" OR "prediabetic state" OR "hyperglycemia" OR "borderline diabetes" OR "impaired glucose tolerance" OR "impaired fasting glucose" OR "diabetes prevention" OR "prevention of diabetes" OR "diabetes mellitus" OR "diabetes mellitus type 2" OR "non-insulin dependent diabetes mellitus") AND ("Aloe" OR "Aloe vera" OR "Aloe barbadensis" OR "Aloe barbadensis extract" OR "Aloe vera extract"). All of the indexed studies were retrieved, and the reference lists of the identified publications were reviewed for additional pertinent studies. No language restriction was applied for searching. The literature search and study selection were carried out independently by two reviewers (Y.Z. and W.L.) with a standardized approach. Any inconsistencies were resolved by consultation with a third reviewer (D.L.).

2.2. Inclusion Criteria

The diagnostic of prediabetes or T2DM was based on the definitions described by the World Health Organization [16] or the American Diabetes Association [4]. Patients were not limited by age, sex, race, or body size. The inclusion criteria were as follows: (1) randomized controlled trials; (2) studies were included irrespective of whether or not they incorporated lifestyle changes into their trial regimen; (3) studies involving the use of aloe vera as part of a combination product or treatment package were excluded from the systematic review; (4) no history of any hypoglycemic medication use; (5) no history of other diseases like coronary heart disease, stroke, cancer, hepatic disorder, a chronic inflammatory condition, or psychiatric disorders; and (6) primary outcomes reported included at least glucose and/or lipid profile.

2.3. Data Extraction and Quality Assessment

One reviewer screened the titles and abstracts of the RCTs that we identified. Full text articles were obtained for those trials that fulfilled the inclusion criteria or for which sufficient information was given. Two reviewers (Y.Z. and W.L.) independently extracted data from trials that met the inclusion criteria on an Excel spreadsheet; any discrepancies in extracted data were resolved by a group discussion and consensus and final arbitration by the Cochrane editorial base. Attempts were made to seek further information from the authors of the original studies if data were unclear or incomplete. The methodologic quality criteria of randomization, allocation concealed, blinding, and intention-to-treat (ITT) analyses were graded as adequate, inadequate, and unclear. Studies were categorized as double blinding, single blinding, or unclear.

2.4. Statistical Analysis

In our meta-analysis, glucose metabolism, such as fasting blood glucose (FBG), insulin, and glycosylated hemoglobin A1c (HbA1c), were considered primary outcomes. Because diabetes was strongly associated with an increased risk of cardiovascular disease, and often coexists with dyslipidemia, other secondary outcomes included lipid profile, such as triglyceride, total cholesterol (TC), low density lipoprotein-cholesterol (LDL-C), and high density lipoprotein-cholesterol (HDL-C). All outcomes extracted from the literature were continuous data.

Review Manager soft-ware 5.2 provided by the Cochrane Collaboration was used for the meta-analysis. For continuous data, weighted mean differences (WMDs) or standardized mean differences (SMDs) with their 95% confidence intervals (95% CIs) were calculated. Analyses were separately performed for each outcome. Heterogeneity across studies was assessed by the Cochrane's Q-test. The fixed-effects model was used to calculate the total effect size where Cochrane's Q-test $p > 0.10$ and the I^2 statistic $I^2 < 50\%$ indicated statistical homogeneity. If heterogeneity of $p < 0.10$ or $I^2 > 50\%$ was found among the trials, a random-effects model was chosen. Two-tailed p-values $\leqslant 0.05$ or 95% CIs not containing 0 (WMD) were considered statistically significant. Publication bias was not assessed because the number of the included trials was less than 10.

3. Results

3.1. Eligible Studies and Baseline Characteristics

We identified 282 records on aloe vera after searching the three databases mentioned above. Finally, a total of five randomized controlled trials [17–21] from 1996 to 2016 containing 415 participants were included (Figure 1). The key characteristics of these studies are outlined in Table 1.

Most of the included RCTs had flaws in the reporting of their methodology. Although randomization was declared in all studies, only two trials reported how the randomization was conducted [19,21], and none of the studies reported adequate allocation concealment. Three of five studies turned out to be double-blinded [18,19,21], and information relating to withdrawal/dropout was reported adequately in three trials [17,19,21]. ITT analysis was conducted in only one study [19].

All included RCTs involved overweight and/or obese participants, except for one study that did not report [17]. Only one adverse event was reported [19]. Participants in two RCTs [18,21] were allowed to continue their normal lifestyle, whereas the remaining studies did not report this information. The duration of follow-up ranged from 6 to 12 weeks. According to comparators used in these studies, our meta-analysis was divided into two parts.

Table 1. Characteristics of studies included in the meta-analysis.

Study	Main Diagnoses of Study Participants	Mean FBG (mg/dL)	Mean HbA1c (%)	Mean BMI (kg/m^2)	Gender (Male/Female)	Randomized/Analyzed	Daily Dosage (Formulation)	Treatment Duration (Weeks)	Main Outcomes	Adverse Events	Control for Lifestyle Factors	Randomization Appropriate	Allocation Concealed	Sample Size Determined	Groups Similar at Baseline	Blinding	ITT Analysis
Yongchaiyudha, 1996 [17]	Early untreated diabetes	250.7	Unclear	Unclear	50/22	72/70	Two tablespoonful (juice)	6	Glucose and lipid profile	Unclear	Unclear	Unclear	Unclear	Unclear	Yes	Single blinding	Unclear
Devaraj, 2013 [18]	Prediabetes	109	5.9	34.7	15/29	45/44	1.0 g (capsules)	8	Glucose and lipid profile	Unclear	Normal diet and exercise at least 100 min per week	Unclear	Unclear	Unclear	Yes	Double blinding	Unclear
Choi, 2013 [19]	Prediabetes and early untreated diabetes	116.2	6.2	27.4	96/40	136/122	2.8 g (capsules)	8	Glucose, lipid profile and obesity-related biomarkers	One adverse event	Unclear	With the randomization code generated by software	Unclear	Unclear	Yes	Double blinding	Inadequate
Choudhary, 2014 [20]	Untreated diabetes	130.8	Unclear	Unclear	90/0	90/90	0.2 g (powder)	12	Glucose, lipid profile and blood pressure	Unclear	Unclear	Unclear	Unclear	Unclear	Yes	Unclear	Unclear
Alinejad-Mofrad, 2015 [21]	Prediabetes	111.1	6	28.2	21/49	72/70	1.0 g (capsules)	8	Glucose and lipid profile	Unclear	Normal diet and exercise	Blocking randomization	Unclear	Unclear	Yes	Double blinding	Unclear

BMI: body mass index; FBG: fasting blood glucose; HbA1c: hemoglobin A1c; ITT: intention to treat.

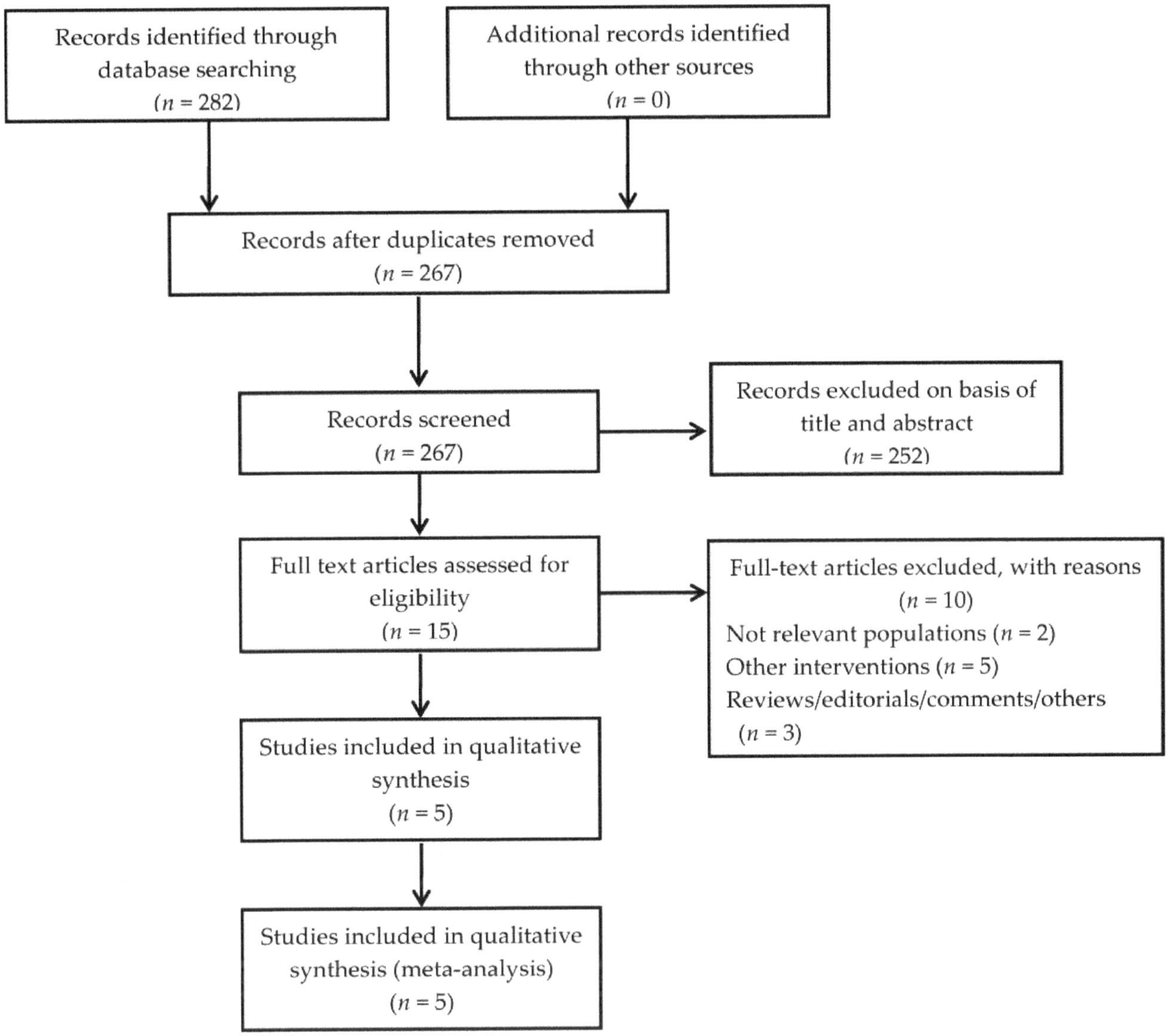

Figure 1. Flow diagram for study identification.

3.2. Meta-Analyses of Primary Outcomes

The changes in FBG were evaluated in the five studies [17–21], which included 328 cases. However, significant heterogeneity was observed among these studies ($p < 0.00001$, $I^2 = 100\%$). The random effects model of meta-analysis was used to combine the effect size. Aloe vera was superior to placebo in reducing FBG levels ($p = 0.02$; WMD: −30.05 mg/dL; 95% CI: −54.87 to −5.23 mg/dL). Two studies compared the effects of aloe vera and placebo on insulin [18,19]. There were no significant changes in the concentration of insulin ($p = 0.15$; SMD: −1.71; 95% CI: −4.07 to 0.64), with heterogeneity existing among these studies ($p < 0.00001$, $I^2 = 96\%$). The changes in HbA1c were evaluated in the two studies [18,21]. Analysis of aggregated data showed a significant reduction in HbA1c ($p < 0.00001$; WMD: −0.41%; 95% CI: −0.55 to −0.27%), without evidence of heterogeneity ($p = 0.61$, $I^2 = 0\%$; Figure 2).

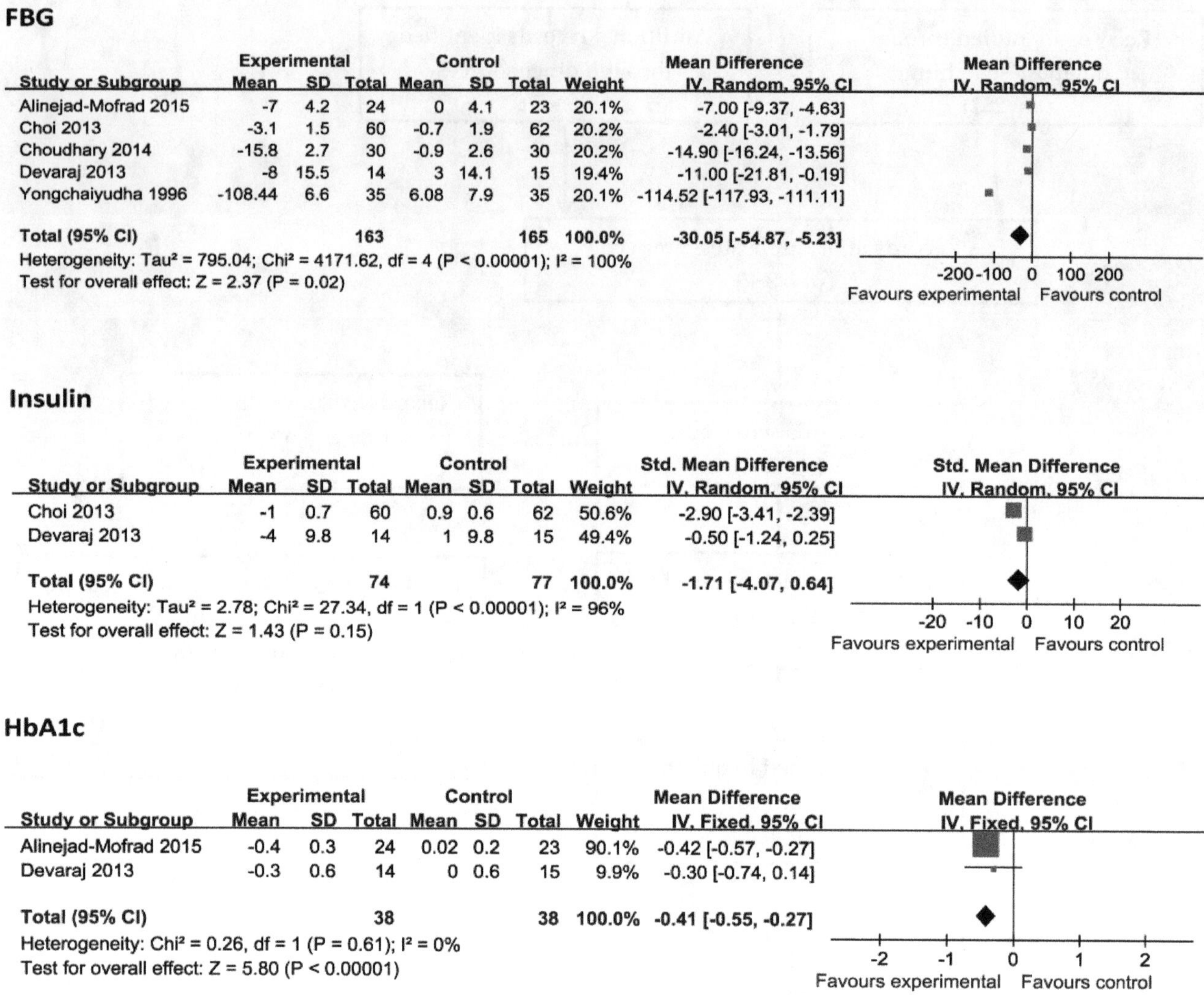

FBG

Study or Subgroup	Experimental Mean	SD	Total	Control Mean	SD	Total	Weight	Mean Difference IV, Random, 95% CI
Alinejad-Mofrad 2015	-7	4.2	24	0	4.1	23	20.1%	-7.00 [-9.37, -4.63]
Choi 2013	-3.1	1.5	60	-0.7	1.9	62	20.2%	-2.40 [-3.01, -1.79]
Choudhary 2014	-15.8	2.7	30	-0.9	2.6	30	20.2%	-14.90 [-16.24, -13.56]
Devaraj 2013	-8	15.5	14	3	14.1	15	19.4%	-11.00 [-21.81, -0.19]
Yongchaiyudha 1996	-108.44	6.6	35	6.08	7.9	35	20.1%	-114.52 [-117.93, -111.11]
Total (95% CI)			**163**			**165**	**100.0%**	**-30.05 [-54.87, -5.23]**

Heterogeneity: Tau² = 795.04; Chi² = 4171.62, df = 4 (P < 0.00001); I² = 100%
Test for overall effect: Z = 2.37 (P = 0.02)

Insulin

Study or Subgroup	Experimental Mean	SD	Total	Control Mean	SD	Total	Weight	Std. Mean Difference IV, Random, 95% CI
Choi 2013	-1	0.7	60	0.9	0.6	62	50.6%	-2.90 [-3.41, -2.39]
Devaraj 2013	-4	9.8	14	1	9.8	15	49.4%	-0.50 [-1.24, 0.25]
Total (95% CI)			**74**			**77**	**100.0%**	**-1.71 [-4.07, 0.64]**

Heterogeneity: Tau² = 2.78; Chi² = 27.34, df = 1 (P < 0.00001); I² = 96%
Test for overall effect: Z = 1.43 (P = 0.15)

HbA1c

Study or Subgroup	Experimental Mean	SD	Total	Control Mean	SD	Total	Weight	Mean Difference IV, Fixed, 95% CI
Alinejad-Mofrad 2015	-0.4	0.3	24	0.02	0.2	23	90.1%	-0.42 [-0.57, -0.27]
Devaraj 2013	-0.3	0.6	14	0	0.6	15	9.9%	-0.30 [-0.74, 0.14]
Total (95% CI)			**38**			**38**	**100.0%**	**-0.41 [-0.55, -0.27]**

Heterogeneity: Chi² = 0.26, df = 1 (P = 0.61); I² = 0%
Test for overall effect: Z = 5.80 (P < 0.00001)

Figure 2. Forest plot of studies that evaluated the effect of aloe vera on primary outcomes compared with placebo. Each block represents a study. Size of square is proportional to the precision of the estimate. Each square represents the weighted mean difference (WMD) or standardized mean difference (SMD) for each study with 95% confidence interval (CI) indicated by horizontal line. FBG, fasting blood glucose; HbA1c, hemoglobin A1c.

3.3. Meta-Analyses of Secondary Outcomes

Four studies [17,18,20,21], which included 206 cases, compared the effects of aloe vera and placebo on triglyceride and TC levels. After analysis of the aggregated results, we found that aloe vera was superior to placebo in reducing serum triglyceride and TC levels ($p = 0.0001$; WMD: −43.92 mg/dL; 95% CI: −66.33 to −21.51 mg/dL and $p < 0.00001$; WMD: −16.94 mg/dL; 95% CI: −23.39 to −10.50 mg/dL, respectively), although heterogeneity existed among these studies ($p < 0.00001$, $I^2 = 100\%$ and $p < 0.00001$, $I^2 = 91\%$, respectively). The changes in HDL-C and LDL-C levels were evaluated in the three studies [18,20,21]. Aloe vera was superior to placebo in increasing serum HDL-C levels ($p = 0.04$; WMD: 2.67 mg/dL; 95% CI: 0.11 to 5.23 mg/dL), and reducing serum LDL-C levels ($p < 0.00001$; WMD: −13.30 mg/dL; 95% CI: −17.19 to −9.41 mg/dL). High heterogeneity was detected with HDL-C and LDL-C variables ($p = 0.0008$, $I^2 = 86\%$ and $p < 0.00001$, $I^2 = 96\%$, respectively; Figure 3).

Triglyceride

Study or Subgroup	Experimental Mean	SD	Total	Control Mean	SD	Total	Weight	Mean Difference IV, Random, 95% CI
Alinejad-Mofrad 2015	-10.4	2.6	24	0.6	1.4	23	30.1%	-11.00 [-12.19, -9.81]
Choudhary 2014	-13.6	1.7	30	-1.8	1.1	30	30.1%	-11.80 [-12.52, -11.08]
Devaraj 2013	-8	83.7	14	18.6	72.4	15	10.2%	-26.60 [-83.74, 30.54]
Yongchaiyudha 1996	-97.59	9.9	35	18.13	10.2	35	29.7%	-115.72 [-120.43, -111.01]
Total (95% CI)			**103**			**103**	**100.0%**	**-43.92 [-66.33, -21.51]**

Heterogeneity: Tau² = 434.47; Chi² = 1848.16, df = 3 (P < 0.00001); I² = 100%
Test for overall effect: Z = 3.84 (P = 0.0001)

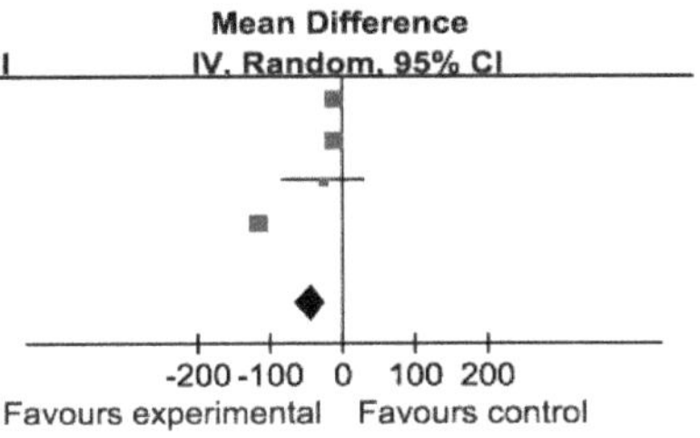

TC

Study or Subgroup	Experimental Mean	SD	Total	Control Mean	SD	Total	Weight	Mean Difference IV, Random, 95% CI
Alinejad-Mofrad 2015	-25	11.2	24	1	3.3	23	28.5%	-26.00 [-30.68, -21.32]
Choudhary 2014	-13.4	2.5	30	-1.8	2.4	30	33.2%	-11.60 [-12.84, -10.36]
Devaraj 2013	-20	29	14	4	29.6	15	7.2%	-24.00 [-45.33, -2.67]
Yongchaiyudha 1996	0.69	6.5	35	13.41	6.7	35	31.2%	-12.72 [-15.81, -9.63]
Total (95% CI)			**103**			**103**	**100.0%**	**-16.94 [-23.39, -10.50]**

Heterogeneity: Tau² = 32.18; Chi² = 35.10, df = 3 (P < 0.00001); I² = 91%
Test for overall effect: Z = 5.16 (P < 0.00001)

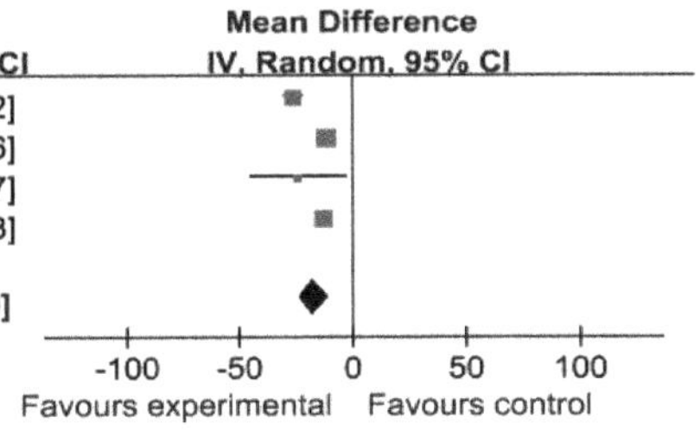

HDL-C

Study or Subgroup	Experimental Mean	SD	Total	Control Mean	SD	Total	Weight	Mean Difference IV, Random, 95% CI
Alinejad-Mofrad 2015	4.2	3.2	24	-0.26	1.4	23	43.9%	4.46 [3.06, 5.86]
Choudhary 2014	2.3	0.9	30	0.6	0.9	30	49.8%	1.70 [1.24, 2.16]
Devaraj 2013	-2	10	14	0.1	15.6	15	6.4%	-2.10 [-11.57, 7.37]
Total (95% CI)			**68**			**68**	**100.0%**	**2.67 [0.11, 5.23]**

Heterogeneity: Tau² = 3.37; Chi² = 14.17, df = 2 (P = 0.0008); I² = 86%
Test for overall effect: Z = 2.05 (P = 0.04)

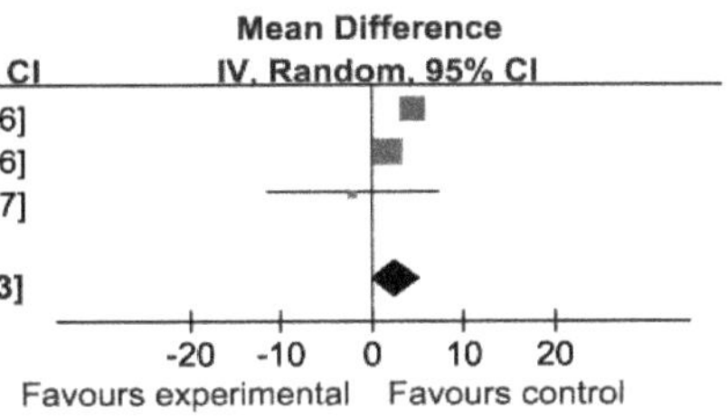

LDL-C

Study or Subgroup	Experimental Mean	SD	Total	Control Mean	SD	Total	Weight	Mean Difference IV, Random, 95% CI
Alinejad-Mofrad 2015	-14.1	1.3	24	1	1.1	23	47.8%	-15.10 [-15.79, -14.41]
Choudhary 2014	-13	1.9	30	-2	1.5	30	47.4%	-11.00 [-11.87, -10.13]
Devaraj 2013	-17	25.1	14	1.1	21	15	4.8%	-18.10 [-35.01, -1.19]
Total (95% CI)			**68**			**68**	**100.0%**	**-13.30 [-17.19, -9.41]**

Heterogeneity: Tau² = 8.11; Chi² = 53.08, df = 2 (P < 0.00001); I² = 96%
Test for overall effect: Z = 6.70 (P < 0.00001)

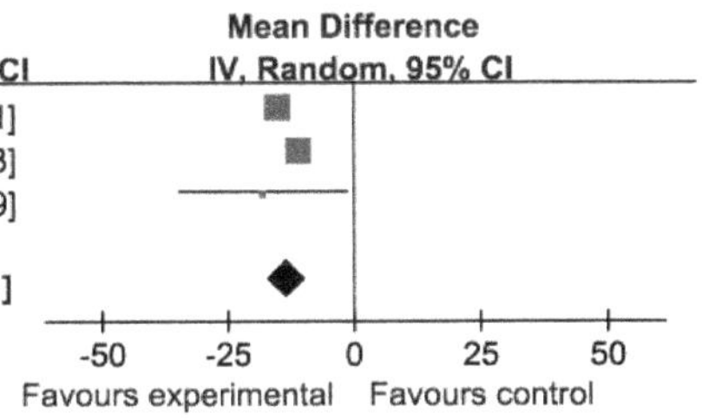

Figure 3. Forest plot of studies that evaluated the effect of aloe vera on secondary outcomes compared with placebo. See Figure 2 for the legend of symbols used. TC, total cholesterol; HDL-C, high density lipoprotein-cholesterol; LDL-C, low density lipoprotein-cholesterol.

4. Discussion

This study is the first meta-analysis regarding the effects of aloe vera for prediabetes and non-treated diabetic patients that has been conducted to synthesize the results from independent randomized controlled studies to draw an overall conclusion. Although significant differences between groups were found for most parameters, the limited evidence reveal a statistically significant difference in reducing serum FBG and HbA1c levels favoring aloe vera over placebo. In addition, aloe vera has also been shown to reduce the levels of triglyceride, TC and LDL-C, and increase the levels of HDL-C.

Our findings are consistent with some animal studies [13,14]. Several mechanisms may be involved in the association between glucose-lipid metabolism and aloe vera. It could be due to the efficacy of high molecular weight polysaccharides or phytosterols isolated from aloe vera gel in enhancing glucose transport by modulating the proximal and distal markers involved in glucose uptake and reducing serum concentrations of cholesterol by reducing the absorptions of cholesterol from the gut. Another theory is that the aloe vera extract can lower the level of blood glucose and lipid in diabetic rats by reducing toxic effects of fat in the liver to improve sensitivity of cells to insulin [14,22,23]. It has also been hypothesized that normalization of plasma lipid status by aloe vera may be explained by its ability to suppress adipogenic gene expression, increased clearance and decreased production of the major transporters of endogenously synthesized cholesterol and triglycerides [14]. Additionally, some researchers believe that aloe vera reduce body fat and improve insulin sensitivity by activating adenosine monophosphate-activated muscle protein kinase, which is important in the regulation of glucose and lipid metabolism [24].

Although some reviews have recently been published about the hypoglycemic effects of aloe vera, the quality of these reviews was limited, and they did not present specific methods on data extraction or assessment of heterogeneity. The following factors have strengthened this meta-analysis. First, studies were included or excluded according to strict criteria. Next, the meta-analysis offered an up-to-date and complete overview of all RCTs involving the efficacy of aloe vera supplementation in managing prediabetes and early non-treated diabetic patients, because it was the result of an extensive search, including gray literature and unpublished studies.

There are several limitations should be considered before recommending the findings of this review to clinicians. First, our analysis was based on small number of trials and the backgrounds of patients varied, which would result in low statistical power and the publication bias could not be excluded. Second, insufficient data were available. Insulin or glycosylated HbA1c was not available in the majority of studies, thereby limiting the reliable results. Next, some studies [17,18,20] did not examine or report whether or not blinding requirements were fully met and allocation concealments were fully achieved. ITT analysis was performed in only one study [19]. Hence, selective bias and measurement bias may have existed in the trails. Finally, significant between-study heterogeneity was detected for most of the variables assessed. Three different aloe vera-based preparations were manufactured in five different regions, Thailand, United States, South Korea, India and Iran. Furthermore, these discrepancies in pharmacological effects of various aloe vera preparations may be due to several other factors, including a lack of consistency among studies in relation to standardization of aloe vera manufacturing process, dosage, duration of treatment, units of laboratory tests and races of the selected patients. Such heterogeneity confounds interpretation of statistical findings. We had initially planned to conduct subgroup analyses, however, there were not a sufficient number of trials to perform this analysis. Therefore, the random-effects model was adopted, although it cannot completely eliminate heterogeneity.

Despite these limitations, the present findings could provide useful information on the future research. First, insulin resistance is thought to be a key factor in the development of diabetes; unfortunately, insulin did not appear in a large number of studies outcomes. Second, lifestyle factors, such as food intake and physical exercise, are very important aspects of blood glucose control. However, the difference in the average daily caloric intake and level of physical activity undertaken by study participants was unclear. Most studies lacked objective outcome measures to estimate the extent to which these variations influenced the outcome of the study result. Therefore, focusing on these supplementary clues may be useful in future research studies on the topic. Third, not all of these included aloe vera preparations were assumed to be identical in the composition and biological activity they possessed, which might lead to the discrepancies in the glucose-lowering effect. The variation in daily dosages makes it difficult to determine the minimum effective dose of aloe vera that can cause a blood glucose reduction. Future studies should focus on the effects of aloe preparations, dosage, and the part of the plant used. Finally, the common adverse effects of aloe vera supplementation are abdominal pain, cramping, and muscle weakness [8,9]. However, only one study briefly described the adverse reactions of subjects in the aloe vera group [19]. The selected trials administered aloe vera for 6–12 weeks. Considering the fact that these studies were of short duration, the safety of long-term aloe vera intake seems uncertain. Thus, it is essential for investigators of future trials to incorporate surveillance time frames into the clinical trials to monitor any medium- and long-term adverse events associated with the use of aloe vera.

5. Conclusions

In conclusion, the currently available data showed that aloe vera might reduce the levels of FBG, HbA1c, triglyceride, TC and LDL-C, and increase the levels of HDL-C in prediabetes and early non-treated diabetic patients; however, limited evidence exists about the safety of aloe vera, given the small RCTs, poor quality of RCTs included, and the considerable heterogeneity seen in the study results, the magnitude of this effect is small and the clinical relevance is uncertain. Large-scale, multi-center and placebo-controlled long-term trials should be rigorously designed to substantiate the current findings and to investigate the long-term effects of aloe vera supplementation on managing prediabetes and T2DM.

Author Contributions: Y.Z. and W.L. contributed equally to this work; Y.Z. and H.T. conceived and designed the study; Y.Z. and W.L. performed data extraction and drafted the paper; Y.Z., W.L., D.L. and T.Z. performed the meta-analysis and discussed study findings; Y.Z., W.L. and H.T. revised the paper for submission for publication.

Abbreviations

The following abbreviations are used in this manuscript:

CI	Confidence interval
FBG	Fasting blood glucose
HbA1c	Hemoglobin A1c
HDL-C	High density lipoprotein-cholesterol
ITT	Intention to treat
LDL-C	Low density lipoprotein-cholesterol
RCT	Randomized clinical trial
SMD	Standardized mean difference
T2DM	Type 2 diabetes mellitus
TC	Total cholesterol
WMD	Weighed mean difference

References

1. Wild, S.; Roglic, G.; Green, A.; Sicree, R.; King, H. Global prevalence of diabetes: Estimates for the year 2000 and projections for 2030. *Diabetes Care* **2004**, *27*, 1047–1053. [CrossRef] [PubMed]
2. American Diabetes Association. Standards of medical care in diabetes-2014. *Diabetes Care* **2015**, *38* (Suppl. S1), S31–S33.
3. Tabák, A.G.; Herder, C.; Rathmann, W.; Brunner, E.J.; Kivimäki, M. Prediabetes: A high-risk state for diabetes development. *Lancet* **2012**, *379*, 2279–2290. [CrossRef]
4. American Diabetes Association. Economic costs of diabetes in the U.S. in 2007. *Diabetes Care* **2008**, *31*, 596–615.
5. Hou, Q.; Li, Y.; Li, L.; Cheng, G.; Sun, X.; Li, S.; Tian, H. The Metabolic Effects of Oats Intake in Patients with Type 2 Diabetes: A Systematic Review and Meta-Analysis. *Nutrients* **2015**, *7*, 10369–10387. [CrossRef] [PubMed]
6. Rizvi, S.I.; Mishra, N. Traditional Indian medicines used for the management of diabetes mellitus. *J. Diabetes Res.* **2013**, *2013*, 712092. [CrossRef] [PubMed]
7. Modak, M.; Dixit, P.; Londhe, J.; Ghaskadbi, S.; Devasagayam, T.P. Indian herbs and herbal drugs used for the treatment of diabetes. *J. Clin. Biochem. Nutr.* **2007**, *40*, 163–173. [CrossRef] [PubMed]
8. Surjushe, A.; Vasani, R.; Saple, D.G. Aloe vera: A short review. *Indian J. Dermatol.* **2008**, *53*, 163–166. [CrossRef] [PubMed]

9. Shelton, R.M. Aloe vera. Its chemical and therapeutic properties. *Int. J. Dermatol.* **1991**, *30*, 679–683. [CrossRef] [PubMed]
10. Hamman, J.H. Composition and applications of Aloe vera leaf gel. *Molecules* **2008**, *13*, 1599–1616. [CrossRef] [PubMed]
11. Radha, M.H.; Laxmipriya, N.P. Evaluation of biological properties and clinical effectiveness of Aloe vera: A systematic review. *J. Tradit. Complement. Med.* **2014**, *5*, 21–26. [CrossRef] [PubMed]
12. Ulbricht, C.; Armstrong, J.; Basch, E.; Basch, S.; Bent, S.; Dacey, C.; Dalton, S.; Foppa, I.; Giese, N.; Hammerness, P.; et al. An evidence-based systematic review of Aloe vera by the natural standard research collaboration. *J. Herb. Pharmacother.* **2007**, *7*, 279–323. [CrossRef] [PubMed]
13. Rajasekaran, S.; Ravi, K.; Sivagnanam, K.; Subramanian, S. Beneficial effects of aloe vera leaf gel extract on lipid profile status in rats with streptozotocin diabetes. *Clin. Exp. Pharmacol. Physiol.* **2006**, *33*, 232–237. [CrossRef] [PubMed]
14. Kim, K.; Kim, H.; Kwon, J.; Lee, S.; Kong, H.; Im, S.A.; Lee, Y.H.; Lee, Y.R.; Oh, S.T.; Jo, T.H.; et al. Hypoglycemic and hypolipidemic effects of processed Aloe vera gel in a mouse model of non-insulin-dependent diabetes mellitus. *Phytomedicine* **2009**, *16*, 856–863. [CrossRef] [PubMed]
15. Yagi, A.; Hegazy, S.; Kabbash, A.; Wahab, E.A. Possible hypoglycemic effect of Aloe vera L. high molecular weight fractions on type 2 diabetic patients. *Saudi Pharm. J.* **2009**, *17*, 209–215. [CrossRef] [PubMed]
16. World Health Organization (WHO). *Definition, Diagnosis and Classification of Diabetes Mellitus and Its Complications. Report of a WHO Consultation. Part 1: Diagnosis and Classification of Diabetes Mellitus*; World Health Organization: Geneva, Switzerland, 1999.
17. Yongchaiyudha, S.; Rungpitarangsi, V.; Bunyapraphatsara, N.; Chokechaijaroenporn, O. Antidiabetic activity of Aloe vera L. juice. I. Clinical trial in new cases of diabetes mellitus. *Phytomedicine* **1996**, *3*, 241–243. [CrossRef]
18. Devaraj, S.; Yimam, M.; Brownell, L.A.; Jialal, I.; Singh, S.; Jia, Q. Effects of Aloe vera supplementation in subjects with prediabetes/metabolic syndrome. *Metab. Syndr. Relat. Disord.* **2013**, *11*, 35–40. [CrossRef] [PubMed]
19. Choi, H.C.; Kim, S.J.; Son, K.Y.; Oh, B.J.; Cho, B.L. Metabolic effects of aloe vera gel complex in obese prediabetes and early non-treated diabetic patients: Randomized controlled trial. *Nutrition* **2013**, *29*, 1110–1114. [CrossRef] [PubMed]
20. Choudhary, M.; Kochhar, A.; Sangha, J. Hypoglycemic and hypolipidemic effect of Aloe vera L. in non-insulin dependent diabetics. *J. Food Sci. Technol.* **2014**, *51*, 90–96. [CrossRef] [PubMed]
21. Alinejad-Mofrad, S.; Foadoddini, M.; Saadatjoo, S.A.; Shayesteh, M. Improvement of glucose and lipid profile status with Aloe vera in pre-diabetic subjects: A randomized controlled-trial. *J. Diabetes Metab. Disord.* **2015**, *14*, 22. [CrossRef] [PubMed]
22. Anand, S.; Muthusamy, V.S.; Sujatha, S.; Sangeetha, K.N.; Bharathi Raja, R.; Sudhagar, S.; Poornima Devi, N.; Lakshmi, B.S. Aloe emodin glycosides stimulates glucose transport and glycogen storage through PI3K dependent mechanism in L6 myotubes and inhibits adipocyte differentiation in 3T3L1 adipocytes. *FEBS Lett.* **2010**, *584*, 3170–3178. [CrossRef] [PubMed]
23. Beppu, H.; Shimpo, K.; Chihara, T.; Kaneko, T.; Tamai, I.; Yamaji, S.; Ozaki, S.; Kuzuya, H.; Sonoda, S. Antidiabetic effects of dietary administration of Aloe arborescens Miller components on multiple low-dose streptozotocin-induced diabetes in mice: Investigation on hypoglycemic action and systemic absorption dynamics of aloe components. *J. Ethnopharmacol.* **2006**, *103*, 468–477. [CrossRef] [PubMed]
24. Shin, E.; Shin, S.; Kong, H.; Lee, S.; Do, S.G.; Jo, T.H.; Park, Y.I.; Lee, C.K.; Hwang, I.K.; Kim, K. Dietary Aloe Reduces Adipogenesis via the Activation of AMPK and Suppresses Obesity-related Inflammation in Obese Mice. *Immune Netw.* **2011**, *11*, 107–113. [CrossRef] [PubMed]

8

Homocysteine Metabolism Gene Polymorphisms (MTHFR C677T, MTHFR A1298C, MTR A2756G and MTRR A66G) Jointly Elevate the Risk of Folate Deficiency

Wen-Xing Li [1,2,†], Shao-Xing Dai [2,†], Jun-Juan Zheng [2], Jia-Qian Liu [2] and Jing-Fei Huang [2,3,4,*]

1 Institute of Health Sciences, Anhui University, Hefei 230601, Anhui, China; liwenxin@mail.kiz.ac.cn
2 State Key Laboratory of Genetic Resources and Evolution, Kunming Institute of Zoology, Chinese Academy of Sciences, Kunming 650223, Yunnan, China; daishaoxing@mail.kiz.ac.cn (S.-X.D.); zhengjunjuan@mail.kiz.ac.cn (J.-J.Z.); liujiaqian@mail.kiz.ac.cn (J.-Q.L.)
3 KIZ-SU Joint Laboratory of Animal Models and Drug Development, College of Pharmaceutical Sciences, Soochow University, Kunming 650223, Yunnan, China
4 Collaborative Innovation Center for Natural Products and Biological Drugs of Yunnan, Kunming 650223, Yunnan, China
* Correspondence: huangjf@mail.kiz.ac.cn
† These authors contributed equally to this work.

Abstract: Folate deficiency is strongly associated with cardiovascular disease. We aimed to explore the joint effect of the methylenetetrahydrofolate reductase (MTHFR) C677T and A1298C, methionine synthase (MTR) A2756G, and methionine synthase reductase (MTRR) A66G polymorphisms on folate deficiency in a Chinese hypertensive population. A total of 480 subjects aged 28–75 were enrolled in this study from September 2005–December 2005 from six hospitals in different Chinese regions. Known genotypes were detected by PCR-RFLP methods and serum folate was measured by chemiluminescence immunoassay. Our results showed that *MTHFR* 677TT and *MTR* 2756AG + GG were independently associated with a higher risk of folate deficiency (TT *vs.* CC + CT, $p < 0.001$ and AG + GG *vs.* AA $p = 0.030$, respectively). However, the *MTHFR* A1298C mutation may confer protection by elevating the serum folate level ($p = 0.025$). Furthermore, patients carrying two or more risk genotypes showed higher odds of folate deficiency than null risk genotype carriers, especially those carrying four risk genotypes. These findings were verified by generalized multifactor dimensionality reduction ($p = 0.0107$) and a cumulative effects model ($p = 0.001$). The results of this study have shown that interactions among homocysteine metabolism gene polymorphisms lead to dramatic elevations in the folate deficiency risk.

Keywords: *MTHFR* C677T; *MTHFR* A1298C; *MTR* A2756G; *MTRR* A66G; folate deficiency

---

1. Introduction

Recently, a large-scale randomized clinical trial confirmed the benefits of folate therapy on the risk of first stroke [1]. A previous meta-analysis has shown that the effect of the *MTHFR* C677T variant on the homocysteine concentration is modified by folate status [2]. Hyperhomocysteinemia and the *MTHFR* 677TT genotype are considered risk factors for cardiovascular diseases (CVDs) [2–5]. The associations between homocysteine metabolism gene polymorphisms and homocysteine, folate, and other B vitamins have been widely studied [6]. Some mutations may result in an elevation in the plasma homocysteine concentration and a reduction in the folate concentration [6–11], thereby exacerbating the risks of several complicated diseases [6,12]. Other studies have demonstrated that high-dose folate intervention therapy [13] or dietary folate supplementation [8] may increase the serum folate level and simultaneously reduce the prevalence of hyperhomocysteinemia and hypertension.

Folate is a crucial vitamin in homocysteine metabolism. Serum folate enters into tissue cells via folate receptors, and then dihydrofolate reductase (DHFR) converts it into tetrahydrofolate. Next, tetrahydrofolate is transformed into 5, 10-methylenetetrahydrofolate, with vitamin B_6 as a cofactor [14]. Then, methylenetetrahydrofolate reductase (MTHFR) converts 5, 10-methylenetetrahydrofolate into 5-methyltetrahydrofolate, providing a methyl group for conversion of homocysteine into methionine in a reaction catalyzed by methionine synthase (MTR) [15,16]. MTR requires vitamin B_{12} (cobalamin) as a coenzyme. Over time, the cobalamin (I) cofactor of MTR is oxidized to form cobalamin (II), leading to inactivation of MTR. Thus, methionine synthase reductase (MTRR) is required for reversion of oxidized cobalamin (II) to CH_3-cobalamin (III) to maintain the activity of MTR [17].

Some common polymorphisms (*MTHFR* C677T, rs1801133; *MTHFR* A1298C, rs1801131; *MTR* A2756G, rs1805087; and *MTRR* A66G, rs1801394) may influence the serum folate level [6,7,10,18]. Numerous studies have demonstrated that the *MTHFR* C677T mutation significantly lowers the serum folate level [7,10,11,19], whereas a recent study has reported no such correlation [20]. The associations of *MTHFR* A1298C and *MTR* A2767G with the folate level remain controversial [10,18]. In addition, the *MTRR* A66G polymorphism itself may not affect the plasma folate level [7]. Further, these mutations may synergistically promote folate deficiency [21,22]. A low folate level may increase the risk of hyperhomocysteinemia, as has been demonstrated in 77% of hypertensive patients in a previous study [23]. In many developed countries (USA, Canada, UK, France, and other western countries), folic acid fortification has been fully implemented. This measure has been reported to reduce the risk of complex diseases [2,6,8]. However, no folate fortification policy has been established in China, India, Pakistan or other Asian countries and, thus, folate deficiency is more common in Asian populations than in European and American populations [9–11].

The aims of our study were to investigate the associations between homocysteine metabolism gene polymorphisms (*MTHFR* C677T, *MTHFR* A1298C, *MTR* A2756G and *MTRR* A66G) and the serum folate level, as well as to explore the independent and interactive effects of the risk genotypes on the incidence of folate deficiency in the Chinese hypertensive population.

2. Experimental Section

2.1. Participants and Procedures

This study was conducted using data collected in a previous study [24]. This was a multicenter, randomized, double-blind controlled trial in hypertensive Chinese adults (clinicaltrials.gov; identifier: NCT00520247). Details regarding "Study subjects", "Randomization and double blinding", "Data collection procedures", and "Laboratory tests" have been previously described [24]. In total, 480 patients with mild or moderate hypertension were recruited from six hospitals in different Chinese regions (Ha'rbin, Shanghai, Shenyang, Beijing, Xi'an, and Nanjing) from September to December 2005. All six hospitals have been certified as clinical pharmacology centers by the State Food and Drug Administration of China. Demographic and clinical information and serum folate and homocysteine concentrations were obtained at baseline. This study was approved by the Ethics Committee of Peking University First Hospital, Beijing, China. The purpose and procedures of the study were carefully explained to all participants, and written informed consent was obtained from each participant.

2.2. DNA Extraction and Genotyping

All participants were requested to provide 2 mL peripheral whole blood, which was collected in ethylenediaminetetraacetic acid (EDTA) and stored at −20 °C. DNA was extracted by conventional methods. The TaqMan probe technique was used for detecting polymorphisms in Hcy pathway genes at our central laboratory. The polymerase chain reaction-restriction fragment length polymorphism (PCR-RFLP) method was applied to detect the *MTHFR* C677T, *MTHFR* A1298C, *MTR* A2756G, and

MTRR A66G genotypes. Each genotyping reaction mixture contained 4 ng dried DNA, 0.08 mL 40 assay locus-specific probe, and 2.0 mL TaqMan universal polymerase chain reaction (PCR) master mix in a final volume of 4 mL, with addition of 1.92 mL sterile water. The main parameters for PCR-RFLP of the four single nucleotide polymorphisms (SNPs) are shown in Table 1. The amplified PCR products were separated on a 3% agarose gel. To ensure the accuracy of genotyping, genotyping calls were observed by two independent researchers. The genotyping call rate for assessments of all genetic variants was ≥98% in this study.

Table 1. Primer sequences and reaction conditions for PCR-RFLP of gene polymorphisms.

Gene	Primer sequence [1]	T [2] and Cycles	Product Size	Restriction Enzyme
MTHFR C677T	F: 5′-TGAAGGAGAAGGTGTCTGCGGGA-3′ R: 5′-AGGACGGTGCGGTGAGAGTG-3′	58 °C, 35	198bp	*Hinf* I
MTHFR A1298C	F: 5′-CTTTGGGGAGCTGAAGGACTACTAC-3′ R: 5′-CACTTTGTGACCATTCCGGTTTG-3′	52 °C, 38	163bp	*Mbo* II
MTR A2756G	F: 5′-GAACTAGAAGACAGAAATTCTCTA-3′ R: 5′-CATGGAAGAATATCAAGATATTAGA-3′	53 °C, 36	189bp	*Hae* III
MTRR A66G	F: 5′-GCAAAGGCCATCGCAGAAGACAT-3′ R: 5′-GTGAAGATCTGCAGAAAATCCATGTA-3′	60 °C, 35	151bp	*Nsp* I

[1] F: forward primer; R: reverse primer. [2] T: annealing temperature.

2.3. Statistical Analysis

Statistical analyses were conducting using IBM SPSS software package (version 19.0 for windows; IBM, Inc., Armonk, NY, USA). The results for the categorical variables (*i.e.*, the clinical centers and genotypes) are presented as numbers and percentages of cases. The continuous variables (*i.e.*, age, height, weight, body mass index (BMI), systolic blood pressure (SBP), and diastolic blood pressure (DBP)) are presented as the mean ± standard deviation. The means for the continuous variables in the two groups were compared using t tests, and the prevalences of the categorical variables were compared using χ^2 tests. Since the serum folate and homocysteine levels were not normally distributed, the geometric means and quartiles were displayed and were analyzed with the Mann-Whitney U test. Hardy-Weinberg equilibrium was also assessed for the genotypic frequencies of the different genes with the χ^2 test.

The unitary linear regression model was used to assess the associations of the *MTHFR* C677T, *MTHFR* A1298C, *MTR* A2756G, and *MTRR* A66G gene polymorphisms with the logarithmic transformed folate level. Unconditional logistic regression (ULR) was performed to estimate the independent and joint effects of the genotypes on folate deficiency, defined as a serum folate level of less than 10 nmol/L [25]. The trend test with the general linear model (GLM) was used to verify the above results. A two-sided p value of <0.05 was considered significant.

Generalized multifactor dimensionality reduction (GMDR, version 0.9, obtained from http://www.ssg.uab.edu/gmdr/) was applied to analyze high-order gene-gene interactions. Some parameters, such as training balance accuracy, testing balance accuracy, p value, and cross-validation consistency (CVC), were obtained. The model with the maximum CVC score, the best prediction accuracy, and a p value of 0.05 or lower was considered the best model. All analyses were adjusted for potential confounding factors, including sex, age, clinical center, height, and weight.

3. Results

A total of 480 patients were recruited for this study. After exclusion of 12 subjects who lacked data on *MTHFR* A1298C (five patients), *MTR* A2756G (six patients) or folate (one patient), a total of 468 subjects were included in our final analysis. Four polymorphisms (*MTHFR* C677T, *MTHFR* A1298C, *MTR* A2756G and *MTRR* A66G) in this population showed no deviation in genotype distribution from expected Hardy-Weinberg equilibrium (p values of 0.711, 0.380, 0.862 and 0.393, respectively). Since only four subjects had the 2756GG genotype, the 2756AG and 2756GG genotypes were combined for the following statistical analyses.

3.1. Demographic and Clinical Characteristics

There were no significant differences in age, BMI, SBP or the frequencies of the four gene polymorphisms between the males and females (Table 2). However, the females had a higher serum folate level ($p < 0.001$), lower serum homocysteine level ($p < 0.001$), and lower DBP ($p < 0.001$) compared with the males.

Table 2. Clinical and epidemiologic characteristics of the population grouped by sex.

Characteristic	Sex		*p*
	Females (n = 268)	**Males (n = 200)**	
Age, year	56.7 ± 9.4	56.7 ± 10.7	0.990
Height, cm	157.6 ± 5.3	169.6 ± 5.9	<0.001
Weight, kg	64.4 ± 9.5	73.3 ± 10.6	<0.001
Body mass index, kg/m^2	25.9 ± 3.6	25.4 ± 3.1	0.115
Systolic blood pressure, mm Hg	154.6 ± 12.0	153.8 ± 11.5	0.465
Diastolic blood pressure, mm Hg	92.0 ± 8.2	95.0 ± 8.7	<0.001
Folate, nmol/L	13.62 (10.48–16.92)	11.50 (8.90–13.40)	<0.001
Homocysteine, μmol/L	11.34 (9.12–14.23)	15.96 (11.50–19.18)	<0.001
	Clinical center		
Ha'rbin	35 (13.1)	24 (12.0)	<0.001
Shanghai	48 (17.9)	13 (6.5)	
Shenyang	44 (16.4)	34 (17.0)	
Beijing	67 (25.0)	47 (23.5)	
Xi'an	30 (11.2)	47 (23.5)	
Nanjing	44 (16.4)	35 (17.5)	
	MTHFR C677T		
CC	64 (23.9)	50 (25.0)	0.880
CT	139 (51.9)	99 (49.5)	
TT	65 (24.3)	51 (25.5)	
	MTHFR A1298C		
AA	190 (70.9)	136 (68.0)	0.260
AC	72 (26.9)	54 (27.0)	
CC	6 (2.2)	10 (5.0)	
	MTR A2756G		
AA	222 (82.8)	160 (80.0)	0.367
AG	45 (16.8)	37 (18.5)	
GG	1 (0.4)	3 (1.5)	
	MTRR A66G		
AA	77 (28.7)	76 (38.0)	0.089
AG	146 (54.5)	91 (45.5)	
GG	45 (16.8)	33 (16.5)	

3.2. Associations between Genotypes and Folate Level

The associations between the genotypes and the serum folate level are shown in Table 3. The patients with the *MTHFR* 677TT genotype had a lower serum folate level than the 677CC carriers (adjusted β (SE): −0.27 (0.01), $p < 0.001$). However, there was no significant difference in folate levels between the 677CT and 677CC genotypes. When the 677CC and 677CT genotypes were grouped together, we found that the 677TT carriers had a lower serum folate level than the 677CC + CT carriers (adjusted β (SE): −0.19 (0.02), $p < 0.001$). However, the patients with the *MTHFR* 1298AC + CC genotypes had a higher serum folate level than those with the wild-type genotype (adjusted β (SE): 0.10 (0.02), $p = 0.025$). Furthermore, the patients with *MTR* 2756AG + GG had a lower serum folate level than the 66AA carriers (adjusted β (SE): −0.12 (0.02), $p = 0.005$). There was no significant correlation between the *MTRR* A66G polymorphism and serum folate.

Table 3. Associations of gene polymorphisms with serum folate level.

Genotype	Folate [1]	log(Folate) [1]	Crude β (SE)	Crude *p*	Adjusted [2] β (SE)	Adjusted [2] *p*
			MTHFR C677T			
CC ($n = 114$)	14.97 ± 6.23	1.14 ± 0.16	Reference		Reference	
CT ($n = 238$)	14.00 ± 6.16	1.11 ± 0.17	−0.09 (0.02)	0.098	−0.07 (0.02)	0.186
TT ($n = 116$)	11.85 ± 5.22	1.04 ± 0.16	−0.30 (0.01)	<0.001	−0.27 (0.01)	<0.001
CC + CT ($n = 352$)	14.32 ± 6.19	1.12 ± 0.17	Reference		Reference	
TT ($n = 116$)	11.85 ± 5.22	1.04 ± 0.16	−0.21 (0.02)	<0.001	−0.19 (0.02)	<0.001
			MTHFR A1298C			
AA ($n = 326$)	13.35 ± 5.81	1.09 ± 0.16	Reference		Reference	
AC ($n = 126$)	14.62 ± 6.61	1.13 ± 0.17	0.10 (0.02)	0.039	0.10 (0.02)	0.026
CC ($n = 16$)	13.73 ± 6.15	1.10 ± 0.18	0.01 (0.02)	0.818	0.03 (0.02)	0.596
AA ($n = 326$)	13.35 ± 5.81	1.09 ± 0.16	Reference		Reference	
AC + CC ($n = 142$)	14.52 ± 6.54	1.13 ± 0.17	0.09 (0.02)	0.049	0.10 (0.02)	0.025
			MTR A2756G			
AA ($n = 382$)	13.95 ± 6.26	1.11 ± 0.17	Reference		Reference	
AG + GG ($n = 86$)	12.61 ± 4.96	1.07 ± 0.17	−0.10 (0.02)	0.041	−0.12 (0.02)	0.006
			MTRR A66G			
AA ($n = 153$)	13.57 ± 5.78	1.10 ± 0.17	Reference		Reference	
AG ($n = 237$)	13.83 ± 5.60	1.11 ± 0.16	0.04 (0.02)	0.480	0.02 (0.02)	0.731
GG ($n = 78$)	13.61 ± 7.76	1.09 ± 0.19	−0.04 (0.01)	0.600	−0.03 (0.01)	0.665
AA ($n = 153$)	13.57 ± 5.78	1.10 ± 0.17	Reference		Reference	
AG + GG ($n = 315$)	13.77 ± 6.19	1.10 ± 0.17	0.02 (0.02)	0.727	0.01 (0.02)	0.841

[1] Data are presented as the mean ± standard deviation (nmol/L). [2] Adjusted for sex, age, clinical center, height, and weight.

The effects of the four genotypes on folate deficiency are shown in Table 4. Using the *MTHFR* 677CC + CT genotypes as references, the odds ratio of the 677TT carriers was 2.34 (95% CI 1.47–3.71, $p < 0.001$). Additionally, the patients with the *MTR* 2756AG + GG genotypes had a higher risk of folate deficiency than the 2756AA carriers (OR = 1.80, 95% CI 1.06–3.05, $p = 0.030$). However, the patients with *MTHFR* 1298AC + CC showed a lower risk of folate deficiency, although this finding did not reach significance. Additionally, we found no significant effect of the *MTRR* A66G polymorphism on folate deficiency.

3.3. Gene-Gene Interactions on Folate Deficiency

We next examined the joint effects of these four gene polymorphisms on deficiency (Table 5). None of the patients had the 677TT/1298AC + CC genotypes, consistent with some previous reports [21,22]. Haplotypes of these two mutations have been suggested to be in complete linkage disequilibrium (p-value < 0.0001) [26]. Compared with the 677CC + CT/1298AC + CC carriers, the patients with the 677TT/1298AA genotypes had higher odds of folate deficiency (OR = 2.45, 95% CI 1.41–4.28, $p = 0.002$). Furthermore, the patients with 677TT/2756AG + GG had a four-fold increased risk of folate deficiency compared with those carrying 677CC + CT/2756AA (OR = 4.13, 95% CI 1.68–10.13, $p = 0.002$), and the 677TT/66AG + GG carriers had higher odds of folate deficiency than the 677CC + CT/66AA carriers (OR = 2.50, 95% CI 1.33–4.67, $p = 0.004$). Additionally, the 1298AA/2756AG + GG and 2756AG + GG/66AG + GG carriers both had higher risks of folate deficiency compared with the reference group. We further performed the trend test to verify these findings and, except for the *MTHFR* A1298C/*MTRR* A66G combination, the other genotype combinations dramatically increased the folate deficiency risk.

Table 4. Effects of gene polymorphisms on folate deficiency.

Genotype	Low folate [1]	High folate [1]	OR (95%CI)	p [2]
		MTHFR C677T		
CC	26 (19.8)	88 (26.1)	Reference	
CT	57 (43.5)	181 (53.7)	1.01 (0.58–1.74)	0.980
TT	48 (36.6)	68 (20.2)	2.35 (1.29–4.26)	0.005
CC + CT	83 (63.4)	269 (79.8)	Reference	
TT	48 (36.6)	68 (20.2)	2.34 (1.47–3.71)	<0.001
		MTHFR A1298C		
AA	98 (74.8)	228 (67.7)	Reference	
AC	27 (20.6)	99 (29.4)	0.61 (0.37–1.01)	0.055
CC	6 (4.6)	10 (3.0)	1.18 (0.40–3.48)	0.770
AA	98 (74.8)	228 (67.7)	Reference	
AC + CC	33 (25.2)	109 (32.3)	0.67 (0.42–1.07)	0.095
		MTR A2756G		
AA	100 (76.3)	282 (83.7)	Reference	
AG + GG	31 (23.7)	55 (16.3)	1.80 (1.06–3.05)	0.030
		MTRR A66G		
AA	41 (31.3)	112 (33.2)	Reference	
AG	60 (45.8)	177 (52.5)	0.99 (0.61–1.60)	0.966
GG	30 (22.9)	48 (14.2)	1.65 (0.90–3.01)	0.105
AA	41 (31.3)	112 (33.2)	Reference	
AG + GG	90 (68.7)	225 (66.8)	1.14 (0.72–1.79)	0.579

[1] Data are presented as the number of cases (percentage). Low folate: serum folate level < 10 nmol/L; high folate: serum folate level ≥ 10 nmol/L. [2] Adjusted for sex, age, clinical center, height, and weight.

We used the GMDR model to explore the effects of high-order gene-gene interactions on folate deficiency (Table 6). The model with *MTHFR* C677T, *MTHFR* A1298C, *MTR* A2756G, and *MTRR* A66G had the highest training balance accuracy (0.6357), a relatively high testing balance accuracy (0.5717), the maximum cross-validation consistency of 10/10, and a significant p value ($p = 0.0107$). Thus, this model is probably the best model for interpreting the effects of high-order gene-gene interactions on folate deficiency.

3.4. Cumulative Effects of Risk Genotypes on Folate Deficiency

We defined the risk genotypes as 677TT, 1298AA, 2756AG + GG, and 66AG + GG. The cumulative effects of these four polymorphisms on folate deficiency are shown in Table 7. Due to the numbers of patients with all these four risk genotypes being relatively low, we combined the patients carrying three or four risk genotypes for evaluation. Compared with the null risk genotype carriers, the patients carrying three risk genotypes had a higher folate deficiency risk, with an odds ratio of 2.53 (95% CI 1.10–5.85; $p = 0.029$). In addition, the patients with four risk genotypes had a nearly four-fold increased risk of folate deficiency (OR = 3.77, 95% CI 1.07–13.27; $p = 0.039$). When we combined the patients with three or four risk genotypes, the increase in the folate deficiency risk remained significant (OR = 2.68, 95% CI 1.18–6.09; $p = 0.019$). Furthermore, the trend test showed a dramatic increase in folate deficiency with an increase in the number of risk genotypes ($p_{trend} = 0.001$). Plausibly, these results further support the conclusion drawn from the GMDR results that potential interactions among these gene polymorphisms may affect the incidence of folate deficiency.

Table 5. Effects of gene-gene interactions on folate deficiency.

Genotype 1	Genotype 2	N_L/N_H [1]	OR (95%CI)	p [2]	Trend test	p [2]
MTHFR C677T	*MTHFR* A1298C					
CC + CT	AC + CC	33/109	Reference		0.16 (0.02)	<0.001
CC + CT	AA	50/160	1.09 (0.65–1.82)	0.757		
TT	AC + CC	0/0	-	-		
TT	AA	48/68	2.45 (1.41–4.28)	0.002		
MTHFR C677T	*MTR* A2756G					
CC + CT	AA	65/225	Reference		0.19 (0.02)	<0.001
CC + CT	AG + GG	18/44	1.69 (0.88–3.23)	0.116		
TT	AA	35/57	2.22 (1.32–3.74)	0.003		
TT	AG + GG	13/11	4.13 (1.68–10.13)	0.002		
MTHFR C677T	*MTRR* A66G					
CC + CT	AA	29/91	Reference		0.15 (0.02)	0.001
CC + CT	AG + GG	54/178	1.02 (0.60–1.73)	0.954		
TT	AA	12/21	2.03 (0.84–4.87)	0.114		
TT	AG + GG	36/47	2.50 (1.33–4.67)	0.004		
MTHFR A1298C	*MTR* A2756G					
AC + CC	AA	26/92	Reference		0.11 (0.02)	0.019
AC + CC	AG + GG	7/17	2.07 (0.72–5.92)	0.177		
AA	AA	74/190	1.50 (0.89–2.54)	0.131		
AA	AG + GG	24/38	2.54 (1.26–5.15)	0.010		
MTHFR A1298C	*MTRR* A66G					
AC + CC	AA	13/38	Reference		0.08 (0.02)	0.088
AC + CC	AG + GG	20/71	0.87 (0.38–1.99)	0.743		
AA	AA	28/74	1.18 (0.54–2.60)	0.680		
AA	AG + GG	70/154	1.46 (0.72–2.98)	0.297		
MTR A2756G	*MTRR* A66G					
AA	AA	30/93	Reference		0.10 (0.02)	0.032
AA	AG + GG	70/189	1.16 (0.69–1.94)	0.570		
AG + GG	AA	11/19	1.73 (0.70–4.29)	0.240		
AG + GG	AG + GG	20/36	2.09 (1.01–4.29)	0.046		

[1] N_L: number of low folate patients (<10 nmol/L); N_H: number of high folate patients ($\geq$10 nmol/L); [2] Adjusted for sex, age, clinical center, height, and weight.

Table 6. GMDR models of effects of high-order interactions on folate deficiency.

Models [1]	Training balance accuracy	Testing balance accuracy	Sign test (p value)	Cross-validation consistency
C677T	0.5842	0.5825	8 (0.0547)	10/10
C677T, A2756G	0.6047	0.5946	10 (0.0010)	10/10
C677T, A2756G, A66G	0.6236	0.5631	10 (0.0010)	6/10
C677T, A2756G, A1298C, A66G	0.6357	0.5717	9 (0.0107)	10/10

[1] All models adjusted for sex, age, clinical center, height and weight.

Table 7. Cumulative effects of risk genotypes [1] on folate deficiency.

Number of risk genotypes	Low folate [2]	High folate [2]	OR (95%CI)	p [3]	p_{trend} [3]
0	10 (7.6)	33 (9.8)	Reference		
1	32 (24.4)	106 (31.5)	1.01 (0.44–2.32)	0.989	
2	40 (30.5)	132 (39.2)	1.17 (0.52–2.63)	0.710	0.001
3	41 (31.3)	58 (17.2)	2.53 (1.10–5.85)	0.029	
4	8 (6.1)	8 (2.4)	3.77 (1.07–13.27)	0.039	
≥3	49 (37.4)	66 (19.6)	2.68 (1.18–6.09)	0.019	

[1] Risk genotypes were defined as *MTHFR* 677TT, *MTHFR* 1298AA, *MTR* 2756AG + GG, and *MTRR* 66AG + GG. [2] Data are presented as the number of cases (percentage). Low folate: serum folate level <10 nmol/L; high folate: serum folate level ≥10 nmol/L. [3] Adjusted for sex, age, clinical center, height, and weight.

4. Discussion

In the present study, the *MTHFR* C677T and *MTR* A2756G polymorphisms each independently reduced the serum folate level and increased the folate deficiency risk. In addition, compared with the wild-type of *MTHFR* A1298C genotype, patients carried the mutant C allele showed higher folate level. We defined the risk genotypes as *MTHFR* 677TT, *MTHFR* 1298AA, *MTR* 2756AG + GG, and *MTRR* 66AG + GG. Assessment of gene-gene interactions using the ULR and GMDR models revealed significant effects of interactions of these four risk genotypes on folate deficiency.

Folate is a crucial factor in cell division and cell maintenance and also plays an important role in regulating epigenetic gene expression [12]. A recent study has shown that three forms of folate supplementation (natural folate-rich foods, folic acid and 5-MTHF) have similar effects on lowering plasma homocysteine [8]. Pravenec *et al.* have indicated that a reduction in the folate level aggravates evidence of oxidative tissue damage and insulin resistance, and elevates blood pressure in spontaneously hypertensive rats [27]. We found that a low folate level resulted in a significant increase in the plasma homocysteine concentration ($p < 0.001$, data not show) and this negative correlation has been widely confirmed [10,23,25,28]. Furthermore, several studies showed that folate supplementation reduced the plasma homocysteine level, urinary 8-iso-prostaglandin $F_{2\alpha}$ and 11-dehydro-thromboxane B_2 excretion, and increased serum folate level especially in hyperhomocysteinemic carriers [29,30]. These results showed the beneficial of folate supplementation on oxidative stress and platelet activation. In addition, a prospective study has shown that folate deficiency is independently predictive of a 53% increased risk of coronary heart disease mortality in older adults [31]. In an Indian cohort, the *MTHFR* 677T allele and folate deficiency independently increased neonatal hyperbilirubinemia risk by approximately four-fold and three-fold, respectively [32]. These findings indicate that folate deficiency may independently increase the risk of CVDs.

According to the threshold of 10 nmol/L, approximately 28% (131) of the Chinese hypertension patients in our study were folate deficient. Toprak *et al.* reported only 201 (1.1%) subjects with a folate level of $\leq$5 nmol/L and 640 (4.7%) with a level of $\leq$6.8 nmol/L out of a total of 17,713 participants [33], suggesting that use of a higher folate cutoff value may improve sensitivity for detecting a deficiency. The relationship between folate and homocysteine may differ depending on whether the folate level is low or high. Selhub *et al.* have reported that the serum homocysteine concentration increases as the serum folate concentration decreases; however, at a high folate level, this correlation may disappear [25]. In addition, the two-phase regression model suggests that the threshold folate level is approximately 10 nmol/L, which is the level at which the homocysteine concentration approaches flat [25]. Therefore, in this study, we defined folate deficiency as a serum folate level of <10 nmol/L.

We observed that the patients with *MTHFR* 677TT had a lower serum folate level ($p < 0.001$, Table 3) and a higher odds of folate deficiency ($p < 0.001$, Table 4) than the 677CC + CT carriers. This negative correlation between *MTHFR* C677T polymorphisms and the folate level has been widely reported [7,10,11,19,34]. A previous study has reported that *MTHFR* 677TT may cause an approximately 70% decrease and 677CT results in a 35% decrease in the mean MTHFR activity [35]. The *MTHFR* C677T mutation is located in the catalytic domain of the enzyme [35,36] and causes an alanine to valine substitution at position 222, resulting in a thermolabile enzyme [22,35]. The homozygous *MTHFR* C677T mutation decreases enzymatic activity and causes a lower rate of reduction of 5, 10-methylene-THF to 5-methyl-THF, resulting in increased availability of 5, 10-methylene-THF for oxidation to the formylated folate forms and accumulation in red blood cells (RBCs) [37]. However, no formylated folates have been found in RBCs of 677CC genotype carriers. Furthermore, because mature RBCs have almost no ability to transport folate, accumulation of formylated-THF RBCs may lead to lower proportions of 5, 10-methylene-THF and 5-methyl-THF in the serum, which could explain the decreased serum folate level observed in individuals with the 677TT genotype. However, Waskiewicz *et al.* failed to find this association in either adult Polish men or women [38]. Moreover, a low folate level and *MTHFR* 677TT may have a synergistic effect on elevating the plasma homocysteine concentration [10,11]. *MTHFR* A1298C is located in the regulatory domain named NADPH and

S-adenosylmethionine binding site [36]. The A1298C mutation does not result in synthesis of a thermolabile protein [22]. Thus, this mutation may not have a significant effect on the serum folate level (AA *vs.* AC + CC, $p = 0.684$) [7]. Further, Yakub *et al.* have not found an effect of *MTHFR* A1298C on the serum folate level [10]. Our results showed that heterozygous and homozygous A1298C mutations resulted in a higher folate level compared with that resulting from the wild-type genotype (adjusted $p = 0.025$, Table 3). Furthermore, *MTHFR* 1298AC + CC may be a protective factor that reduces the risk of folate deficiency, although this finding was not significant (Table 4). Similar to our results, Biselli *et al.* have found that the mean plasma folate concentration is significantly higher in carriers of the altered allele (1298AC and 1298CC) compared with carriers of 1298AA in coronary artery disease patients [18]. One possible reason for this finding is that S-adenosylmethionine is an allosteric inhibitor of MTHFR [36]. Structural prediction revealed that the S-adenosylmethionine binding site in the mutated structure is distorted compared with that in the normal structure [36] and therefore, it may reduce the inhibitory effect of the enzyme. However, in contrast with the results of our study, subjects carrying the 1298CC genotype have been demonstrated to have a lower serum folate level compared with the levels in 1298AC and 1298CC carriers in a study of male clear cell renal cell carcinoma patients and control individuals [19]. Therefore, the potential impact of *MTHFR* A1298C on the serum folate level needs more investigation.

The physiologically active coenzyme form of folate is tetrahydrofolate (THF). *In vivo*, THF is converted into 5, 10-methylene-THF with the aid of vitamin B_6 and then into 5-methyl-THF. The conversion of 5, 10-methylene-THF into 5-methyl-THF is physiologically irreversible [25]. Therefore, reduced MTR activity may decrease the rate of conversion of 5-methyl-THF to THF, then results in physiological folate deficiency. *MTR* A2756G mutation located at position 919 of the protein results in substitution of glycine for aspartic acid [39]. It is located in a domain of the protein that interacts with S-adenosylmethionine and auxiliary proteins that are required for the reductive methylation and reactivation of the vitamin B_{12} cofactor, which can be inactivated by oxidation during catalysis [17,40]. Therefore, this mutation might impair the binding of SAM and/or auxiliary proteins [40] and reduce catalytic efficiency. In this study, we found that the *MTR* 2756AG + GG genotypes resulted in not only a decreased serum folate level ($p = 0.006$, Table 3) but also an increased folate deficiency risk compared with the wild-type genotype ($p = 0.030$, Table 4). In contrast, studies of the Brazilian [7], Pakistani [10], and Jamaican [20] populations have failed to demonstrate a correlation between the *MTR* A2756G polymorphism and folate level. However, serum folate and the *MTHFR* 677CC+CT and *MTR* 2756AA genotypes have been shown to have significant interactions with total homocysteine in pregnant women [7]. Furthermore, in individuals with low intake of folate, vitamin B_6, and vitamin B_{12}, the *MTHFR* 677T and *MTR* 2756G alleles have been shown to result in a high risk of breast cancer [41].

A common *MTRR* polymorphism is the substitution of A for G at nucleotide 66, which results in the substitution of isoleucine by methionine. This mutation is located in the putative flavin mononucleotide-binding domain of the MTRR enzyme, which interacts with MTR [17] and, thus, disrupts the binding of MTRR to the MTR-cobalamin-complex, decreasing the rate of homocysteine remethylation [39]. Our results showed that *MTRR* 66AG + GG may not affect the serum folate level or the incidence of folate deficiency (Tables 3 and 4). Similarly, Feix *et al.* have reported that the *MTRR* A66G polymorphism has no effects on the total homocysteine, folate or vitamin B_{12} concentrations [42]. Although the *MTRR* A66G polymorphism has no significant influence on the serum folate level, the combination of *MTHFR* C677T and *MTRR* A66G have significant interactive effects on the total homocysteine and serum folate concentrations [7].

Based on these findings, we hypothesized that multiple genetic defects will aggravate folate deficiency. Several studies showed the combination effect of *MTHFR* C677T and A1298C decreased serum folate level [7,19,22]. MTHFR is crucial for maintaining an adequate methionine pool and for ensuring that the homocysteine concentration does not reach a toxic level [43]. The homozygous *MTHFR* C677T mutation causes a decrease in the conversion rate of 5, 10-methylene-THF to 5-methyl-THF resulting in a reduction in the 5-methyl-THF level [35]. Subsequently, the supply of methyl groups is diminished, affecting the synthesis of methionine from homocysteine. *MTR* 2756G allele affects the binding of accessory proteins involved in cofactor reduction [44], potentially resulting in reductions in the synthesis rates of 5-methyl-THF to THF and homocysteine to methionine. A low THF level also affects folate circulation. Furthermore, MTRR restores the activity of MTR [17]. Thus, a mutation in MTRR may result in a decreased recovery rate of the oxidant cobalamin, indirectly affecting the serum folate level. As such, the deleterious effects of homocysteine metabolism gene polymorphisms on serum folate level are biologically plausible. In Brazilian children, the folate level has been shown to be significantly decreased in subjects with the 677CC/1298AA/66AA genotypes compared with those carrying 677CC/1298AA/66AG ($p = 0.03$), 677CC/1298AC/66AG ($p = 0.003$) and 677CT/1298AA/66AG ($p = 0.02$) [21]. In our study, the assessment of high-order gene-gene interactions with our GMDR model revealed that all four gene polymorphisms interactively influenced the prevalence of folate deficiency (Table 6). The results from the evaluation of cumulative effects verified these results (Table 7).

To the best of our knowledge, we are the first to demonstrate that the *MTHFR* C677T, *MTHFR* A1298C, *MTR* A2756G, and *MTRR* A66G gene polymorphisms have significant interactive effects on the risk of folate deficiency in Chinese hypertensive patients. A limitation of our study is that the sample size was relatively small. Therefore, we believe that future studies with large samples could be performed to validate our results in a more expansive population.

5. Conclusions

Folate deficiency is a risk factor for cardiovascular disease that is modified by several gene polymorphisms. This study showed that *MTHFR* 677TT, *MTHFR* 1298AA, and *MTR* 2756AG + GG are independently correlated with a high risk of folate deficiency. Furthermore, we have demonstrated that not only pairwise gene-gene interactions but also higher-order interactions of these gene polymorphisms (*MTHFR* C677T, *MTHFR* A1298C, *MTR* A2756G, and *MTRR* A66G) more strongly influence the incidence of folate deficiency. We suggest that individuals who carry those risk genotypes (especially for multiple risk genotypes carriers) should be monitored for their folate circulating levels, and have folate supplementation in case of deficiency. Whether this intervention may translate into a meaningful reduction of cardiovascular events will be hopefully unraveled in the next years.

Acknowledgments: This work was supported by the National Basic Research Program of China (Grant No. 2013CB835100), and the National Natural Science Foundation of China (Grant No. 31123005 and No. 31401142). We gratefully thank Shanqun Jiang, Ph.D. (School of Life Sciences, Anhui University, Hefei, China; and Institute of Biomedicine, Anhui Medical University, Hefei, China) and Xiping Xu, M.D., Ph.D. (Institute of Biomedicine, Anhui Medical University, Hefei, China) for providing clinical trial data and for their helpful advice on data analysis.

Author Contributions: Wen-Xing Li and Shao-Xing Dai analyzed the data. Wen-Xing Li wrote the manuscript. Shao-Xing Dai, Jun-Juan Zheng and Jia-Qian Liu edited the manuscript. Jing-Fei Huang is the corresponding author, and he also edited the manuscript. All authors read and approved the final manuscript.

References

1. Huo, Y.; Li, J.; Qin, X.; Huang, Y.; Wang, X.; Gottesman, R.F.; Tang, G.; Wang, B.; Chen, D.; He, M.; *et al.* Efficacy of folic acid therapy in primary prevention of stroke among adults with hypertension in China: The CSPPT randomized clinical trial. *JAMA* **2015**, *313*, 1325–1335. [CrossRef]
2. Holmes, M.V.; Newcombe, P.; Hubacek, J.A.; Sofat, R.; Ricketts, S.L.; Cooper, J.; Breteler, M.M.B.; Bautista, L.E.; Sharma, P.; Whittaker, J.C.; *et al.* Effect modification by population dietary folate on the association between MTHFR genotype, homocysteine, and stroke risk: A meta-analysis of genetic studies and randomised trials. *The Lancet* **2011**, *378*, 584–594. [CrossRef]
3. Casas, J.P.; Bautista, L.E.; Smeeth, L.; Sharma, P.; Hingorani, A.D. Homocysteine and stroke: Evidence on a causal link from mendelian randomisation. *The Lancet* **2005**, *365*, 224–232. [CrossRef]
4. Ilhan, N.; Kucuksu, M.; Kaman, D.; Ilhan, N.; Ozbay, Y. The 677 C/T MTHFR polymorphism is associated with essential hypertension, coronary artery disease, and higher homocysteine levels. *Arch. Med. Res.* **2008**, *39*, 125–130. [CrossRef] [PubMed]

5. Wang, Y.; Li, X.; Qin, X.; Cai, Y.; He, M.; Sun, L.; Li, J.; Zhang, Y.; Tang, G.; Wang, B.; *et al.* Prevalence of hyperhomocysteinaemia and its major determinants in rural Chinese hypertensive patients aged 45–75 years. *Br. J. Nutr.* **2013**, *109*, 1284–1293. [CrossRef] [PubMed]
6. Wilson, C.P.; McNulty, H.; Scott, J.M.; Strain, J.J.; Ward, M. Postgraduate Symposium: The MTHFR C677T polymorphism, B-vitamins and blood pressure. *Proc. Nutr. Soc.* **2010**, *69*, 156–165. [CrossRef] [PubMed]
7. Barbosa, P.R.; Stabler, S.P.; Machado, A.L.; Braga, R.C.; Hirata, R.D.; Hirata, M.H.; Sampaio-Neto, L.F.; Allen, R.H.; Guerra-Shinohara, E.M. Association between decreased vitamin levels and MTHFR, MTR and MTRR gene polymorphisms as determinants for elevated total homocysteine concentrations in pregnant women. *Eur. J. Clin. Nutr.* **2008**, *62*, 1010–1021. [CrossRef] [PubMed]
8. Zappacosta, B.; Mastroiacovo, P.; Persichilli, S.; Pounis, G.; Ruggeri, S.; Minucci, A.; Carnovale, E.; Andria, G.; Ricci, R.; Scala, I.; *et al.* Homocysteine lowering by folate-rich diet or pharmacological supplementations in subjects with moderate hyperhomocysteinemia. *Nutrients* **2013**, *5*, 1531–1543. [CrossRef] [PubMed]
9. Sukla, K.K.; Raman, R. Association of MTHFR and RFC1 gene polymorphism with hyperhomocysteinemia and its modulation by vitamin B12 and folic acid in an Indian population. *Eur. J. Clin. Nutr.* **2012**, *66*, 111–118. [CrossRef] [PubMed]
10. Yakub, M.; Moti, N.; Parveen, S.; Chaudhry, B.; Azam, I.; Iqbal, M.P. Polymorphisms in MTHFR, MS and CBS genes and homocysteine levels in a Pakistani population. *PloS ONE* **2012**, *7*, e33222. [CrossRef] [PubMed]
11. Husemoen, L.L.; Skaaby, T.; Jorgensen, T.; Thuesen, B.H.; Fenger, M.; Grarup, N.; Sandholt, C.H.; Hansen, T.; Pedersen, O.; Linneberg, A. MTHFR C677T genotype and cardiovascular risk in a general population without mandatory folic acid fortification. *Eur J. Nutr.* **2014**, *53*, 1549–1559. [CrossRef] [PubMed]
12. Czeizel, A.E.; Dudas, I.; Vereczkey, A.; Banhidy, F. Folate deficiency and folic acid supplementation: The prevention of neural-tube defects and congenital heart defects. *Nutrients* **2013**, *5*, 4760–4775. [CrossRef] [PubMed]
13. Qin, X.; Li, J.; Cui, Y.; Liu, Z.; Zhao, Z.; Ge, J.; Guan, D.; Hu, J.; Wang, Y.; Zhang, F.; *et al.* MTHFR C677T and MTR A2756G polymorphisms and the homocysteine lowering efficacy of different doses of folic acid in hypertensive Chinese adults. *Nutr. J.* **2012**, *11*, 2. [CrossRef] [PubMed]
14. Grarup, N.; Sulem, P.; Sandholt, C.H.; Thorleifsson, G.; Ahluwalia, T.S.; Steinthorsdottir, V.; Bjarnason, H.; Gudbjartsson, D.F.; Magnusson, O.T.; Sparso, T.; *et al.* Genetic architecture of vitamin B12 and folate levels uncovered applying deeply sequenced large datasets. *PLoS Genet.* **2013**, *9*, e1003530. [CrossRef] [PubMed]
15. Martinez-Frias, M.L.; Perez, B.; Desviat, L.R.; Castro, M.; Leal, F.; Rodriguez, L.; Mansilla, E.; Martinez-Fernandez, M.L.; Bermejo, E.; Rodriguez-Pinilla, E.; *et al.* Maternal polymorphisms 677C-T and 1298A-C of MTHFR, and 66A-G MTRR genes: Is there any relationship between polymorphisms of the folate pathway, maternal homocysteine levels, and the risk for having a child with Down syndrome? *Am. J. Med. Genet. A.* **2006**, *140*, 987–997. [CrossRef] [PubMed]
16. Biselli, J.M.; Goloni-Bertollo, E.M.; Haddad, R.; Eberlin, M.N.; Pavarino-Bertelli, E.C. The MTR A2756G polymorphism is associated with an increase of plasma homocysteine concentration in Brazilian individuals with Down syndrome. *Braz. J. Med. Biol. Res.* **2008**, *41*, 34–40. [CrossRef] [PubMed]
17. Leclerc, D.; Wilson, A.; Dumas, R.; Gafuik, C.; Song, D.; Watkins, D.; Heng, H.H.; Rommens, J.M.; Scherer, S.W.; Rosenblatt, D.S.; *et al.* Cloning and mapping of a cDNA for methionine synthase reductase, a flavoprotein defective in patients with homocystinuria. *Proc. Natl. Acad. Sci. USA* **1998**, *95*, 3059–3064. [CrossRef] [PubMed]
18. Biselli, P.M.; Guerzoni, A.R.; de Godoy, M.F.; Eberlin, M.N.; Haddad, R.; Carvalho, V.M.; Vannucchi, H.; Pavarino-Bertelli, E.C.; Goloni-Bertollo, E.M. Genetic polymorphisms involved in folate metabolism and concentrations of methylmalonic acid and folate on plasma homocysteine and risk of coronary artery disease. *J. Thromb. Thrombolysis.* **2010**, *29*, 32–40. [CrossRef] [PubMed]
19. Safarinejad, M.R.; Shafiei, N.; Safarinejad, S. Methylenetetrahydrofolate reductase (MTHFR) gene C677T, A1298C and G1793A polymorphisms: Association with risk for clear cell renal cell carcinoma and tumour behaviour in men. *Clin. Oncol.* **2012**, *24*, 269–281. [CrossRef] [PubMed]
20. Jackson, M.D.; Tulloch-Reid, M.K.; McFarlane-Anderson, N.; Watson, A.; Seers, V.; Bennett, F.I.; Egleston, B.; Ragin, C. Complex interaction between serum folate levels and genetic polymorphisms in folate pathway genes: biomarkers of prostate cancer aggressiveness. *Genes. Nutr.* **2013**, *8*, 199–207. [CrossRef] [PubMed]

21. Alessio, A.C.; Annichino-Bizzacchi, J.M.; Bydlowski, S.P.; Eberlin, M.N.; Vellasco, A.P.; Hoehr, N.F. Polymorphisms in the methylenetetrahydrofolate reductase and methionine synthase reductase genes and homocysteine levels in Brazilian children. *Am. J. Med. Genet. A.* **2004**, *128*, 256–260. [CrossRef] [PubMed]
22. Van der Put, N.M.; Gabreels, F.; Stevens, E.M.; Smeitink, J.A.; Trijbels, F.J.; Eskes, T.K.; van den Heuvel, L.P.; Blom, H.J. A second common mutation in the methylenetetrahydrofolate reductase gene: an additional risk factor for neural-tube defects? *Am. J. Hum. Genet.* **1998**, *62*, 1044–1051. [PubMed]
23. Scazzone, C.; Bono, A.; Tornese, F.; Arsena, R.; Schillaci, R.; Butera, D.; Cottone, S. Correlation between low folate levels and hyperhomocysteinemia, but not with vitamin B12 in hypertensive patients. *Ann. Clin. Lab. Sci.* **2014**, *44*, 286–290. [PubMed]
24. Mao, G.; Hong, X.; Xing, H.; Liu, P.; Liu, H.; Yu, Y.; Zhang, S.; Jiang, S.; Wang, X.; Xu, X. Efficacy of folic acid and enalapril combined therapy on reduction of blood pressure and plasma glucose: A multicenter, randomized, double-blind, parallel-controlled, clinical trial. *Nutrition* **2008**, *24*, 1088–1096. [CrossRef] [PubMed]
25. Selhub, J.; Jacques, P.F.; Dallal, G.; Choumenkovitch, S.; Rogers, G. The use of blood concentrations of vitamins and their respective functional indicators to define folate and vitamin B12 status. *Food. Nutr. Bull.* **2008**, *29*, 67–73.
26. Lajin, B.; Alhaj Sakur, A.; Michati, R.; Alachkar, A. Association between MTHFR C677T and A1298C, and MTRR A66G polymorphisms and susceptibility to schizophrenia in a Syrian study cohort. *Asian. J. Psychiatr.* **2012**, *5*, 144–149. [CrossRef] [PubMed]
27. Pravenec, M.; Kozich, V.; Krijt, J.; Sokolova, J.; Zidek, V.; Landa, V.; Simakova, M.; Mlejnek, P.; Silhavy, J.; Oliyarnyk, O.; *et al.* Folate deficiency is associated with oxidative stress, increased blood pressure, and insulin resistance in spontaneously hypertensive rats. *Am. J. Hypertens.* **2013**, *26*, 135–140. [CrossRef] [PubMed]
28. Chmurzynska, A.; Malinowska, A.M.; Twardowska-Rajewska, J.; Gawecki, J. Elderly women: Homocysteine reduction by short-term folic acid supplementation resulting in increased glucose concentrations and affecting lipid metabolism (C677T MTHFR polymorphism). *Nutrition* **2013**, *29*, 841–844. [CrossRef] [PubMed]
29. Santilli, F.; Davi, G.; Patrono, C. Homocysteine, methylenetetrahydrofolate reductase, folate status and atherothrombosis: A mechanistic and clinical perspective. *Vascul Pharmacol* **2015**. [CrossRef] [PubMed]
30. Dragani, A.; Falco, A.; Santilli, F.; Basili, S.; Rolandi, G.; Cerasa, L.; Lattanzio, S.; Ciabattoni, G.; Patrono, C.; Davi, G. Oxidative stress and platelet activation in subjects with moderate hyperhomocysteinaemia due to MTHFR 677 C–>T polymorphism. *Thromb. Haemost.* **2012**, *108*, 533–542. [CrossRef] [PubMed]
31. Gopinath, B.; Flood, V.M.; Rochtchina, E.; Thiagalingam, A.; Mitchell, P. Serum homocysteine and folate but not vitamin B12 are predictors of CHD mortality in older adults. *Eur. J. Prev. Cardiolog.* **2012**, *19*, 1420–1429. [CrossRef] [PubMed]
32. Sukla, K.K.; Tiwari, P.K.; Kumar, A.; Raman, R. Low birthweight (LBW) and neonatal hyperbilirubinemia (NNH) in an Indian cohort: association of homocysteine, its metabolic pathway genes and micronutrients as risk factors. *PloS ONE* **2013**, *8*, e71587. [CrossRef] [PubMed]
33. Toprak, B.; Yalcin, H.Z.; Colak, A. Vitamin B12 and folate deficiency: should we use a different cutoff value for hematologic disorders? *Int. J. Lab. Hematol.* **2014**, *36*, 409–414. [CrossRef] [PubMed]
34. Chango, A.; Emery-Fillon, N.; de Courcy, G.P.; Lambert, D.; Pfister, M.; Rosenblatt, D.S.; Nicolas, J.P. A polymorphism (80G- > A) in the reduced folate carrier gene and its associations with folate status and homocysteinemia. *Mol. Genet. Metab.* **2000**, *70*, 310–315. [CrossRef] [PubMed]
35. Frosst, P.; Blom, H.J.; Milos, R.; Goyette, P.; Sheppard, C.A.; Matthews, R.G.; Boers, G.J.; den Heijer, M.; Kluijtmans, L.A.; van den Heuvel, L.P.; *et al.* A candidate genetic risk factor for vascular disease: A common mutation in methylenetetrahydrofolate reductase. *Nat. Genet.* **1995**, *10*, 111–113. [CrossRef] [PubMed]
36. Shahzad, K.; Hai, A.; Ahmed, A.; Kizilbash, N.; Alruwaili, J. A structured-based model for the decreased activity of Ala222Val and Glu429Ala methylenetetrahydrofolate reductase (MTHFR) mutants. *Bioinformation* **2013**, *9*, 929–936. [CrossRef] [PubMed]
37. Bagley, P.J.; Selhub, J. A common mutation in the methylenetetrahydrofolate reductase gene is associated with an accumulation of formylated tetrahydrofolates in red blood cells. *Proc. Natl. Acad. Sci. USA* **1998**, *95*, 13217–13220. [CrossRef] [PubMed]

38. Waskiewicz, A.; Piotrowski, W.; Broda, G.; Sobczyk-Kopciol, A.; Ploski, R. Impact of MTHFR C677T gene polymorphism and vitamins intake on homocysteine concentration in the Polish adult population. *Kardiologia. Polska.* **2011**, *69*, 1259–1264. [PubMed]
39. Olteanu, H.; Munson, T.; Banerjee, R. Differences in the efficiency of reductive activation of methionine synthase and exogenous electron acceptors between the common polymorphic variants of human methionine synthase reductase. *Biochemistry* **2002**, *41*, 13378–13385. [CrossRef] [PubMed]
40. Harmon, D.L.; Shields, D.C.; Woodside, J.V.; McMaster, D.; Yarnell, J.W.; Young, I.S.; Peng, K.; Shane, B.; Evans, A.E.; Whitehead, A.S. Methionine synthase D919G polymorphism is a significant but modest determinant of circulating homocysteine concentrations. *Genet. Epidemiol.* **1999**, *17*, 298–309. [CrossRef]
41. Qiao, J.H.; Jiao, D.C.; Lu, Z.D.; Cui, S.D.; Liu, Z.Z. Association of methylenetetrahydrofolate reductase and methionine synthase polymorphisms with breast cancer risk and interaction with folate, vitamin B6, and vitamin B12 intakes. *Tumour. Biol.* **2014**, *35*, 11895–11901. [CrossRef] [PubMed]
42. Feix, A.; Winkelmayer, W.C.; Eberle, C.; Sunder-Plassmann, G.; Födinger, M. Methionine synthase reductase MTRR 66A > G has no effect on total homocysteine, folate, and Vitamin B12 concentrations in renal transplant patients. *Atherosclerosis* **2004**, *174*, 43–48. [CrossRef] [PubMed]
43. Goyette, P.; Sumner, J.S.; Milos, R.; Duncan, A.M.; Rosenblatt, D.S.; Matthews, R.G.; Rozen, R. Human methylenetetrahydrofolate reductase: Isolation of cDNA, mapping and mutation identification. *Nat. Genet.* **1994**, *7*, 195–200. [CrossRef] [PubMed]
44. Chen, L.H.; Liu, M.L.; Hwang, H.Y.; Chen, L.S.; Korenberg, J.; Shane, B. Human methionine synthase. cDNA cloning, gene localization, and expression. *J. Biol. Chem.* **1997**, *272*, 3628–3634. [CrossRef] [PubMed]

9

A Moderate Low-Carbohydrate Low-Calorie Diet Improves Lipid Profile, Insulin Sensitivity and Adiponectin Expression in Rats

Jie-Hua Chen [1,†], Caiqun Ouyang [1,†], Qiang Ding [2], Jia Song [1], Wenhong Cao [3] and Limei Mao [1,*]

1 Department of Nutrition and Food Hygiene, School of Public Health and Tropical Medicine, Southern Medical University, Guangzhou 510515, Guangdong, China; siyanpijiehua@gmail.com (J.C.); oycq108729@163.com (C.O.); songj_lin@163.com (J.S.)
2 Department of Nutrition and Food Hygiene, School of Public Health, Tongji Medical College, Huazhong University of Science and Technology, Wuhan 430030, Hubei, China; dq0306@163.com
3 Department of Nutrition, The Gillings School of Global Public Health, The University of North Carolina at Chapel Hill, Chapel Hill, NC 27599, USA; caow@unc.edu
* Correspondence: mlm912@smu.edu.cn
† These authors contributed equally to this work.

Abstract: Calorie restriction (CR) via manipulating dietary carbohydrates has attracted increasing interest in the prevention and treatment of metabolic syndrome. There is little consensus about the extent of carbohydrate restriction to elicit optimal results in controlling metabolic parameters. Our study will identify a better carbohydrate-restricted diet using rat models. Rats were fed with one of the following diets for 12 weeks: Control diet, 80% energy (34% carbohydrate-reduced) and 60% energy (68% carbohydrate-reduced) of the control diet. Changes in metabolic parameters and expressions of adiponectin and peroxisome proliferator activator receptor γ (PPARγ) were identified. Compared to the control diet, 68% carbohydrate-reduced diet led to a decrease in serum triglyceride and increases inlow density lipoprotein-cholesterol (LDL-C), high density lipoprotein-cholesterol (HDL-C) and total cholesterol; a 34% carbohydrate-reduced diet resulted in a decrease in triglycerides and an increase in HDL-cholesterol, no changes however, were shown in LDL-cholesterol and total cholesterol; reductions in HOMA-IR were observed in both CR groups. Gene expressions of adiponectin and PPARγ in adipose tissues were found proportionally elevated with an increased degree of energy restriction. Our study for the first time ever identified that a moderate-carbohydrate restricted diet is not only effective in raising gene expressions of adiponectin and PPARγ which potentially lead to better metabolic conditions but is better at improving lipid profiles than a low-carbohydrate diet in rats.

Keywords: dietary intervention; metabolic syndrome; adiponectin; peroxisome proliferator activator receptor γ; dietary carbohydrate restriction; rats

---

1. Introduction

Metabolic syndrome (MetS) is a collection of medical conditions that can lead to obesity, diabetes, cardiovascular disease and hypertension. The prevalence of MetS is on a rapid rise due to the shifted paradigm of diet and lifestyle and thus has afflicted many people worldwide. It is well known that calorie restriction (CR) improves some markers of MetS [1–3], such as blood pressure, blood glucose and plasma cholesterol, as demonstrated in a number of animal models, and humans [3,4].

Besides functioning as primary energy storage reservoirs, adipose tissue also acts as an endocrine organ secreting numerous protein hormones into the circulation [5]. It was reported that a reduction in White Adipose Tissue (WAT) via CR is likely to change the levels of its secreted hormones. Among all the WAT depots, Visceral Adipose Tissue (VAT) is closely related in particular to MetS and thus is a pathogenic fat depot [6]. The VAT compartment secretes adipokines and cytokines that are predisposed to the development of metabolic traits [7]. Adiponectin is an adipokine and mainly expressed in adipose tissues. Adiponectin has been shown as an insulin-sensitive hormone that participates in the regulation of glucose and lipid metabolism. It was found that adiponectin levels rise during CR [8].

Several elements are capable of modulating adiponectin gene expression, most notably peroxisome proliferator activator receptor γ (PPAR-γ) [9], which is expressed in adipose tissues. A response element of PPARγ was discovered on the promoter of adiponectin gene [10]. Treatment with PPARγ agonists induced adiponectin synthesis during adiponeogenesis [11–13]. PPARγ can also be upregulated by CR through its antioxidative action [14,15].

The beneficial effect of CR on prevention and treatment of MetS has been widely recognized. The optimal CR diet, however, remains to be identified. Among all the CR diets, CR via manipulating dietary carbohydrate content has attracted increasing interest due to its effectiveness on weight loss, glycemic control, insulin sensitivity and the management of cardiovascular risk factors [16]. However, there is little consensus about the extent of dietary carbohydrate restriction to elicit the optimal result in controlling metabolic parameters. In the present study, 12-week CR by varying dietary carbohydrate content (80% or 60% energy (34% or 68% carbohydrate reduction) of the control diet) was employed in Wistar rats to investigate the changes in metabolic parameters and expressions of adiponectin and PPARγ. The results of the study will provide a new perspective and new scientific evidence for the prevention and treatment of MetS.

2. Experimental Section

2.1. Animals and Diets

Thirty-six male Wistar rats (two months old, body weight 240–260 g) were obtained from a local supplier for laboratory animals (Laboratory Animal Center of Hubei Province; Wuhan, China). Rats were housed individually under laboratory conditions (12 h day and night lighting cycle, 22 °C $\pm$ 2 °C, 50% $\pm$ 10% humidity). All experimental protocols were reviewed and approved by Tongji Medical College Council of Animal Care Committee. Rats were randomly assigned into three different groups, *ad libitum* group (AL group; n = 12), calorie restriction group 1 (CR1 group; n = 12) and calorie restriction group 2 (CR2 group; n = 12). All rats had *ad libitum* access to drinking water.

Rat chow diets were prepared based on the Association of Official Analytical Chemists (AOAC) and AIN-93G formulas to meet the nutrient and energy requirements for the growth and development of rats [17]. Rats were fed with these diets for 12 weeks. AL group had *ad libitum* access to the feed whereas CR1 and CR2 group were maintained on a CR regimen with daily access to 80% and 60% of the calorie intake of AL group, respectively (Table 1). Starch was the only nutrient reduced from diets to achieve calorie restriction for CR1 and CR2 groups whereas the amount of other nutrients provided were at the same level as those in the AL group to ensure sufficient nutrients were provided to maintain normal growth of rats. As starch constitutes 58.5% (w/w) of the control diet, 80% and 60% CR correspond to 34% and 68% carbohydrate reduction in CR1 and CR2 group, respectively. The amount of feed consumed by each rat was recorded daily and body weights of rats were monitored weekly. At the end of the 12-week study, rats fasted for 10 h overnight and blood samples were collected. Rats were then sacrificed by decapitation. Serum samples were obtained from all blood samples promptly after blood collection and stored at −80 °C. The peri-epididymal and perirenal adipose tissues were obtained, weighed and frozen immediately in liquid nitrogen prior to storage at −80 °C.

Table 1. Composition of rat chow diet *.

Components	AL Group		CR1 Group [a]		CR2 Group [b]	
	g/kg Diet	**% Energy**	**g/0.8 kg Diet**	**% Energy**	**g/0.6 kg Diet**	**% Energy**
Casein	200.0	20.2	200.0	25.2	200.0	33.8
Vitamin mix **	10.0	-	10.0	-	10.0	-
Mineral mix **	35.0	-	35.0	-	35.0	-
Sucrose	50.0	5.0	50.0	6.3	50.0	8.4
Corn starch	585.0	58.9	385.0	48.6	185.0	31.2
Fiber	50.0	-	50.0	-	50.0	-
Lipid	70.0	15.9	70.0	19.9	70.0	26.6
Total amount (g)	1000.0	100.0	800.0	100.0	600.0	100.0
Total Calorie/kg diet (Kcal)	3970.0		3170.0		2370.0	
Energy ratio (%)						
Protein/Total	20		25		34	
Carbohydrate/Total	64		55		40	
Lipid/Total	16		20		26	

* Abbreviations: AL: *ad libitum*; CR: calorie restriction; ** The composition of vitamin and mineral mix can be referred to AIN-93G; [a] CR1 group was provided with 80% of *ad libitum* intake based on AL group; [b] CR2 group was provided with 60% of *ad libitum* intake based on AL group.

2.2. Biochemical Measurements

Commercial ELISA kit (R & D Systems, Minneapolis, MN, USA) was used to measure serum adiponectin at the baseline and at the end of the study. Fasting blood glucose, fasting serum insulin, serum total cholesterol, fasting triglyceride and serum high density lipoprotein cholesterol (HDL-C) were determined by enzymatic colorimetric analysis using commercialized kits purchased from BioSino Bio-technology and Science Inc., Beijing, China. All the measurements were performed using an automatic enzymatic analyser (BioTek SpectraMax M2, Winooski, VT, USA). Triglyceride level was measured using glycerol-3-phosphate oxidase-p-aminophenazone (GPO-PAP) method. Total cholesterol was determined using cholesterol oxidase-p-aminophenazone (CHOD-PAP) method. After precipitation of very-low-density lipoprotein (VLDL) and low-density lipoprotein cholesterol (LDL-C), HDL-C was measured, as well. Serum LDL-C were then obtained based on Friedewald equation, in which, LDL-C = Total Cholesterol − (Triglyceride/5 + HDL-C) [18]. Blood glucose level was determined by glucose oxidase method. Insulin level was determined with a commercialized radioimmunoassay kit. Homeostasis Model Assessment of Insulin Resistance (HOMA-IR) was calculated based on the relationship between fasting plasma glucose and insulin: HOMA-IR = fasting plasma glucose (mmol/L) × insulin (mIU/L)/22.5 [19].

2.3. Semiquantitative Reverse Transcriptase Polymerase Chain Reaction

Total RNA of the epididymal adipose tissue was extracted using Trizol reagent (Promega, Madison, WI, USA). The concentration of RNA was determined using nucleic acid analyser (Eppendorf, Germany). RNA (3 μg) was reverse transcribed in a 25 μL reaction system into complementary DNA which was then amplified using polymerase chain reaction (PCR). The following primers were used for PCR: 5′-TCCCTCCACCCAAGGAAACT-3′ (sense) and 5′-TTGCCAGTGCTGCCGTGATA-3′ (antisense) for adiponectin; 5′-CATCACTATCGGCAATGAGC-3′ (sense) and 5′-GACAGCACTG TGTTGGCATA-3′ (antisense) for β-actin; 5′-TCCGTGATGGAAGACCACTC-3′ (sense) and 5′-CCCTTGCATCCTTCACAAGC-3′ for PPARγ. β-actin served as a loading control.

All PCR reactions contained 0.2 mmol/L dNTP (deoxyribonucleotide triphosphate), 1.5 μL complementary DNA, 0.25 μmol/L of each primer, 1 × PCR buffer, and 0.8 μL Taq polymerase. The following cycling profile was used for PCR reactions: 5 min of denaturation at 95 °C followed by 30 cycles with 1 min at 94 °C, 45 s at 58 °C and 1 min at 72 °C for adiponectin or 35 cycles with 1 min at 94 °C, 40 s at 56 °C and 1 min at 72 °C for PPARγ or 35 cycles with 1 min at 94 °C, 45 s at 59 °C and 1 min at 72 °C for β-actin and the final extension step of 10 min at 72 °C in a PCR Thermocycler (Biometra, Göttingen, Germany).

PCR products were subjected to electrophoresis in 1.5% agarose gels and the results were analyszed by gel imaging and analysis system (Biometra, Göttingen, Germany). The expression levels of adiponectin mRNA and PPARγ mRNA were shown using the absorbance ratio of target mRNA and β-actin mRNA.

2.4. Statistical Analysis

All the data were analysed using one-way ANOVA followed by Least Significant Difference (LSD)-test with SPSS version 12 software (SPSS Inc., Chicago, IL, USA). Transformation was applied to correct for unequal variances. Pearson correlation coefficient was used to analyze the linear relationship between adiponectin mRNA level and different parameters, *i.e.*, body weight, blood glucose, total cholesterol, triglyceride, HDL-C and insulin. Similar tests were applied to analyze the linear relationship between PPARγ mRNA level and those parameters. In all tests, a value of $p \leq 0.05$ was considered statistically significant.

3. Results

3.1. Calorie Intake and Body Weight

Average calorie intakes of all three groups demonstrated a similar decreasing trend over the 12-week feeding period due to decreased growth rates of rats with maturation (Figure 1). In good agreement with the study design, the ratio of total calorie intake of AL, CR1 and CR2 groups during the feeding period was calculated as 100:81:61.

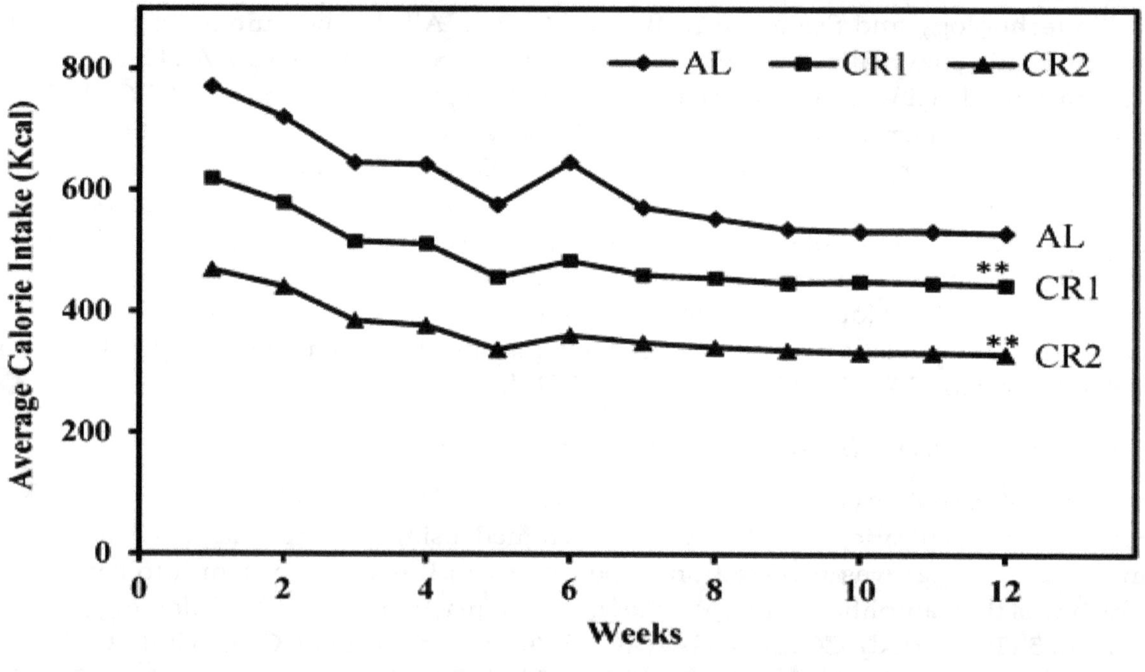

Figure 1. Weekly average calorie intakes of three groups over the 12-week feeding period. Average calorie intake of rats across all groups was shown to be higher at the beginning of the study when rats were fast-growing and then slowly decreased to a plateau with decreasing growth rates of rats. One-way ANOVA followed by LSD-test was used to detect significant differences of the means of the body weights at the end of the study ** $p < 0.001$.

The effect of CR on body weights of rats was found to be significant (Figure 2). Compared to the control group AL, growth rates of rats in CR1 and CR2 group were much slower. Our results indicated that significant differences of body weights of rats among groups were detected in Week 4 ($p < 0.05$) and the differences were greater towards the end of the study ($p < 0.001$).

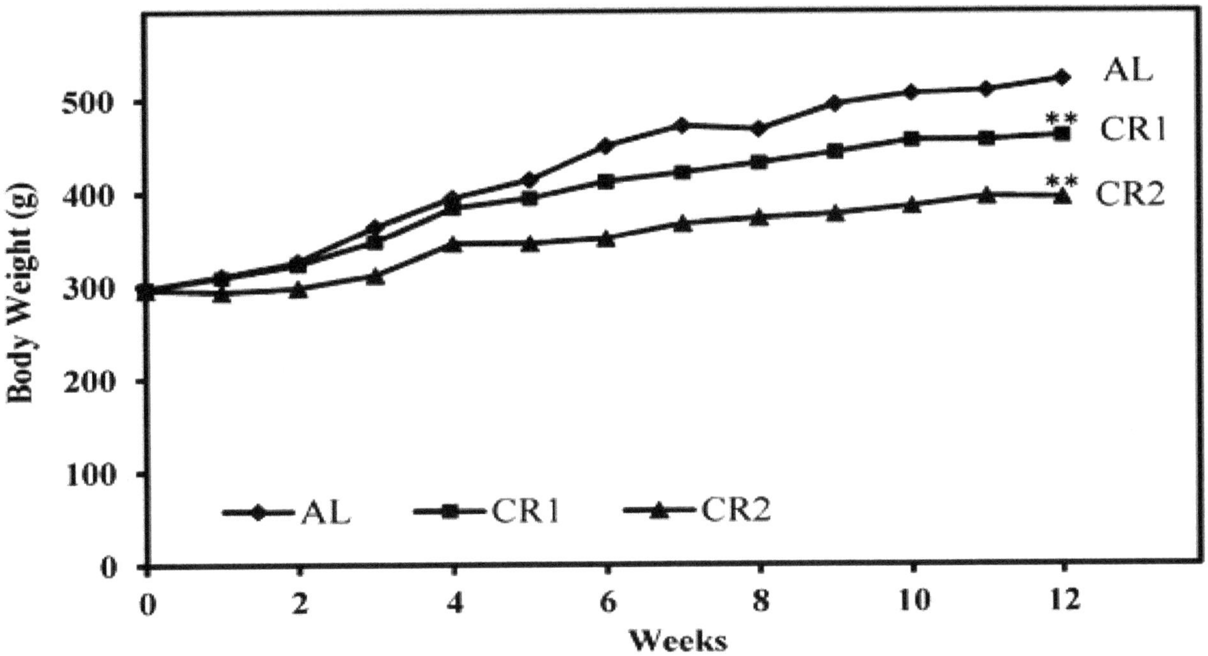

Figure 2. Change of body weights of rats from three groups over the 12-week feeding period. One-way ANOVA followed by LSD-test was used to detect significant differences of the means of the body weights at the end of the study ** $p < 0.001$.

3.2. Changes in Metabolic Parameters

Both 80% (CR1) and 60% (CR2) calorie-restricted diets led to a significant decrease in triglyceride as compared to control diet (AL) ($p < 0.05$; Table 2). However, total cholesterol was found increased in CR2 group ($p < 0.05$) whereas no change was observed in CR1 when compared to AL group ($p > 0.05$; Table 2). Though HDL-C in CR1 and CR2 groups were higher than those in AL group ($p < 0.05$), no significant differences were observed in the ratios of total cholesterol to HDL-C among all the groups ($p > 0.05$). The effect of CR on LDL-C resembled that on total cholesterol which LDL-C increased only in CR2 group ($p < 0.05$).

Table 2. Fasting blood lipid, metabolic and insulin responses in rats of different levels of calorie restriction [†,*].

Group	mmol/L							
	Triglyceride	Total Cholesterol	HDL-C	LDL-C	Total Cholesterol/HDL-C	Glucose	Insulin (IU/mL)	HOMA-IR [#]
AL	1.55 ± 0.59	1.47 ± 0.40	0.69 ± 0.16	0.47±0.39	2.14 ± 0.53	5.54 ± 0.98	23.92 ± 8.76	5.59 ± 0.41
CR1	1.19 ± 0.32 [a]	1.58 ± 0.39	0.82 ± 0.19 [a]	0.52±0.47	1.95 ± 0.39	5.46 ± 0.67	16.02 ± 9.43	3.88 ± 0.63 [a]
CR2	0.92 ± 0.13 [a]	2.09 ± 0.71 [a]	0.92 ± 0.22 [a]	0.99±0.61 [a]	2.25 ± 0.36	5.97 ± 0.98	10.53 ± 7.59 [a]	2.79 ± 0.58 [a,b]

[†] Abbreviations: AL: *ad libitum*; CR: calorie restriction; HDL-C: high density lipoprotein cholesterol; LDL-C: low density lipoprotein cholesterol; * Blood samples were collected at the end of the study; Data was presented as arithmetic mean ± 1 SD ($n = 12$ for each group); [#] HOMA-IR (Homeostasis Model Assessment of Insulin Resistance) = Fasting Blood Glucose (mmol/L) × Fasting Insulin (mIU/L)/22.5 [19]; [a] $p < 0.05$ *versus* AL group; [b] $p < 0.05$ *versus* CR1 group.

No significant difference was detected in blood glucose among all groups (Table 2). Insulin levels decreased by CR which was significant in CR2 compared to AL ($p < 0.05$). Insulin resistance, as presented as HOMA-IR, significantly decreased with increased levels of CR ($p < 0.05$).

All groups demonstrated a similar level of serum adiponectin at the beginning of the study (Figure 3). At the end of the study, serum adiponectin was only significantly increased in CR2 group but not in AL and CR1 groups.

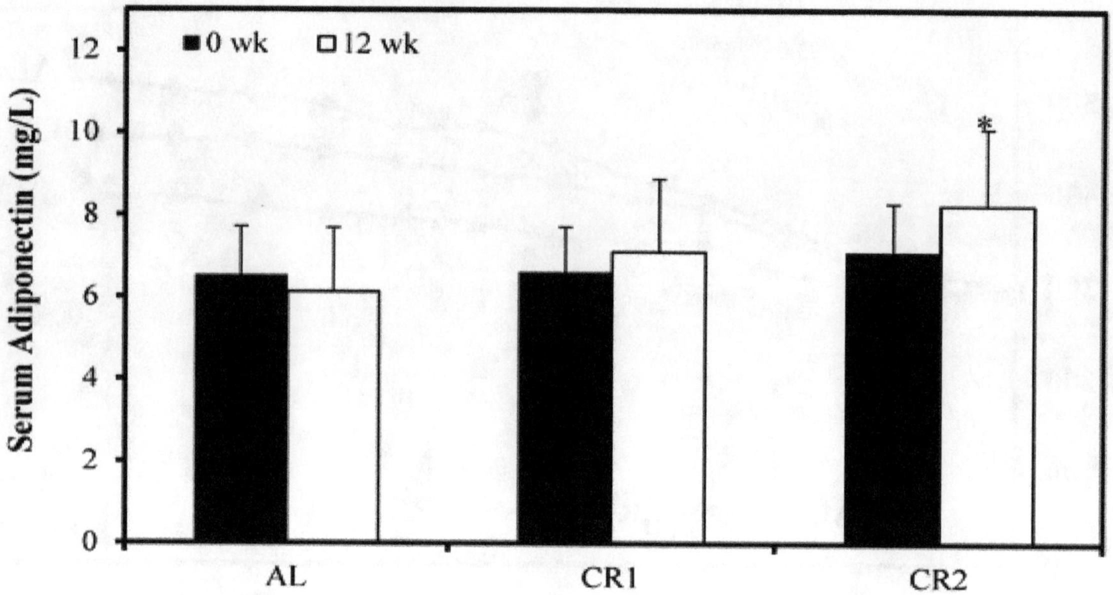

Figure 3. The effect of calorie restriction on serum adiponectin. Serum adiponectin showed no significant difference among all three groups at the beginning of the study. During the 12-week period, only CR2 group demonstrated a significant increase in serum adiponectin level as compared to the baseline. One-way ANOVA followed by LSD-test was used to detect significant differences of the means, * $p < 0.05$.

CR also led to a decrease in mass of visceral adipose tissue (Table 3). At the end of the 12-week study, wet weights of VAT and its percentage to the total body weight in CR groups were significantly lower than those in AL group ($p < 0.05$). As compared to CR1 group, further calorie restriction in CR2 group resulted in a significantly lower visceral fat mass ($p < 0.05$).

Table 3. Effect of calorie restriction on visceral adipose tissue †.

Group	Visceral Fat Mass [g] #,*	Visceral Fat Mass [%] *,Δ
AL	16.47 ± 3.76	3.29 ± 0.48
CR1	12.08 ± 3.71 a	2.51 ± 0.68 a
CR2	6.72 ± 2.61 a,b	1.79 ± 0.69 a,b

† Abbreviations: AL: *ad libitum*; CR: calorie restriction; * Data was presented as arithmetic mean ± 1 S.D. $n = 12$ for each group; # Visceral Fat Mass [g] = total perirenal adipose tissue [g] + total peri-epididymal adipose tissue [g] [20]; Δ Visceral fat mass [%] = Visceral fat mass/Body weight × 100; a $p < 0.05$ *versus* AL group; b $p < 0.05$ *versus* CR1 group.

3.3. Gene Expression

Results obtained from RT-PCR indicated that the expression levels of adiponectin mRNA and PPARγ mRNA in CR groups were significantly higher than those in AL group (Figure 4). Within two CR groups, adiponectin and PPARγ mRNA levels in CR2 group were significantly higher than those in CR1 group (Figure 4(A2,B2)).

3.4. Correlation Analysis

Pearson correlation analysis was performed for mRNA levels of adiponectin, PPARγ with different serum parameters (Table 4). Results showed that no correlation was detected between adiponectin, PPARγ mRNA levels, total cholesterol ($p > 0.05$), and fasting glucose ($p > 0.05$). However, adiponectin, and PPARγ mRNA levels were positively associated with HDL-C ($p < 0.05$) and inversely correlated with body weight ($p < 0.05$), triglyceride ($p < 0.05$) and fasting insulin ($p < 0.05$).

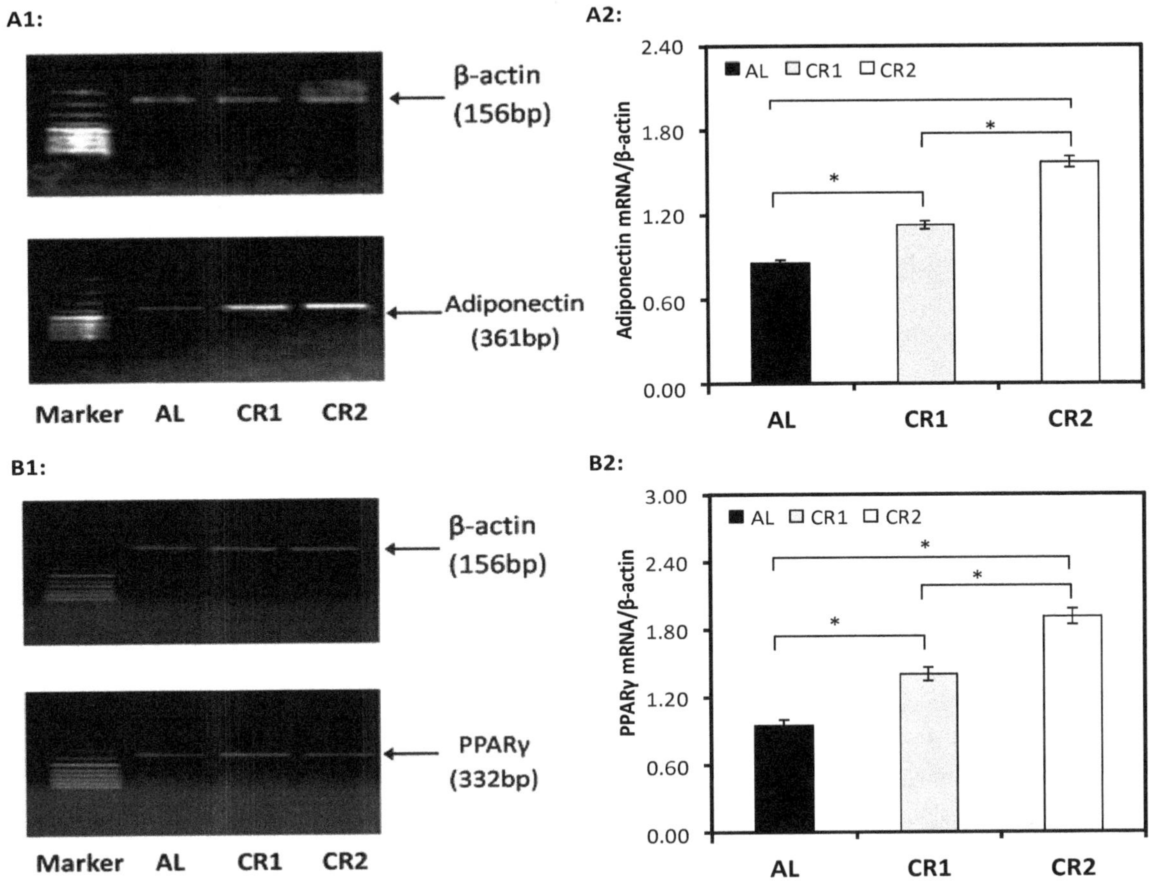

Figure 4. The effect of calorie restriction on the expressions of adiponectin and PPARγ in adipose tissues. (**A1, B1**) demonstrate the expression levels of mRNA of β-actin, adiponectin and PPARγ, respectively, quantified by RT-PCR. The expression levels (absorbance) of mRNA of adiponectin and PPARγ were then normalized against those of β-actin (served as loading control) (**A2, B2**). One-way ANOVA followed by LSD-test was used to detect significant differences of the means, * $p < 0.05$.

Table 4. Correlation analysis of adiponectin mRNA, PPARγ [†] mRNA with different serum parameters.

Independent Variables	Adiponectin		PPARγ	
	r	*p*	*r*	*p*
Body weight	−0.389	0.001	−0.425	0.005
Triglyceride	−0.345	0.042	−0.532	0.032
Total Cholesterol	0.47	0.624	0.673	0.431
HDL-C [†]	0.376	0.026	0.354	0.032
Glucose	0.530	0.231	0.492	0.485
Insulin	−0.411	0.003	−0.537	0.013

[†] Abbreviations: PPAR-γ: peroxisome proliferator activator receptor γ; HDL-C: High density lipoprotein cholesterol.

4. Discussion and Conclusions

MetS represents a cluster of conditions including glucose intolerance, hypertension, dyslipidemia, and insulin resistance. CR via carbohydrate reduction has elicited a great deal of interest among nutritionists because studies have shown that carbohydrate restriction can improve biological markers that define MetS. In the present study, we conducted a 12-week CR with different levels of carbohydrate reduction in healthy Wistar rats to investigate the changes in MetS-associated biomarkers as well as the expressions of insulin-sensitive adiponectin and its regulator PPARγ.

Body weight and peripheral adipose tissues (Table 3) in CR groups were significantly lower than the AL group and the change of these parameters were inversely associated with the degree of CR. VAT is associated with the development of insulin resistance, glucose intolerance, dyslipidemia and hypertension, whereas subcutaneous adipose tissue is not [21–24]. The study conducted by Gerbaix *et al.* has validated that removing perirenal and peri-epididymal adipose tissue in rats appears to be more representative of visceral fat mass as dissection of mesenteric and subcutaneous fat is challenging [20]. Hence, in the present study, visceral fat mass was evaluated as the total weight of perirenal and peri-epididymal adipose tissue (Table 3). Our result indicated that CR via carbohydrate reduction lowered visceral fat mass markedly, even when presented as visceral fat mass %, suggesting the potential beneficial effect of CR via carbohydrate reduction on fat distribution and insulin sensitivity in Wistar rats.

Consistent with the results obtained by previous studies involving carbohydrate restriction [25,26], a 68% carbohydrate reduction in CR2 group led to a significant decrease in serum triglyceride and significant increases in LDL-C, HDL-C and total cholesterol as compared to AL group. Our result suggested that in contrast to traditional carbohydrate restriction diets with a low percentage of carbohydrate or even ketogenic diets, our CR diet with 34% carbohydrate reduction was better at improving lipid profiles, as it not only resulted in an increase in HDL-C and a reduction in triglyceride, but also maintained LDL-C at the same level as those fed with control diets, thereby maintaining the total cholesterol at the same level. Decreases in plasma triglyceride by carbohydrate-restricted diet might be the result of downregulation of hepatic de novo lipogenesis [16,26,27]. In addition, carbohydrate restriction might increase muscle lipoprotein Lipase (LPL), thus enhance triglyceride clearance. Increased tissue expression and activity of LPL may partially explain increases in HDL-C in our experimental groups. Increased LPL-mediated catabolism of triglyceride-rich lipoproteins resulted in transfer of unesterified cholesterol, apoprotein and phospholipid to form mature HDL-C [16,26,27].

It is reported that long-term CR leads to an alteration of glucose homeostasis in humans [16] and rats [15,28,29], resulting in decreased glycemia and insulinemia. Nevertheless, our results demonstrated unchanged plasma glucose in CR groups as compared to the AL group. This finding may be owing to the relatively short experimental period (12-week) and the moderate CR in the present study. When the ingested carbohydrates fail to meet the energy needs of the body, the body starts to mobilize glucose from glycogen storage pools for energy supply, and continues to maintain blood glucose level via gluconeogenesis. The low glycogen storage stimulates insulin action in the body. In good agreement with previous studies [15,28,29], fasting insulin level in the present study demonstrated a decreasing trend with CR but only showed marked reduction in CR2 group. HOMA-IR also manifested a decreasing trend and significant reduction in HOMA-IR was observed in both CR1 and CR2 groups. Maintaining relatively low levels of fasting insulin and HOMA-IR is shown to be beneficial for the prevention and treatment of diabetes.

Adiponectin is considered to have antiatherogenic and antidiabetic effects [30]. In accordance with the findings obtained by Zhu *et al.* [31] and Sung *et al.* [14], our results suggest that though serum adiponectin level was only significantly elevated by 60% calorie-restricted diet, gene expression levels of adiponectin and PPARγ in adipose tissues were proportionally elevated with increased degree of energy restriction (Figures 3 and 4)-lower energy intakes led to higher expression levels. A high level of adiponectin predicts good insulin sensitivity and improves lipid and glucose metabolism [32,33]. Activation of PPARγ can induce the synthesis and secretion of adiponectin as a response element of PPARγ was discovered on the promoter of adiponectin gene [10]. CR might activate PPARγ and thus up-regulate the gene expression of adiponectin. Our result indicated that decreased insulin and HOMA-IR achieved by CR might be a result of increased adiponectin. Consistent with previous findings [7,34], our results demonstrated a significant inverse relationship of VAT adiponectin mRNA level and triglyceride and a significant positive relationship of adiponectin mRNA and HDL-C (Table 4). The present study additionally showed a significant association of PPARγ mRNA with triglyceride and HDL-C. Our correlation analysis suggested that elevated gene expression of adiponectin and PPARγ might lead to elevated level of HDL-C and reduced level of serum triglyceride.

Both low-carbohydrate CR diet [16,35] and low-fat, high-carbohydrate diet [36] have been proposed for the prevention of MetS. Despite the fact that a low-fat, high-carbohydrate diet has been advocated for controlling weight [37], a low-carbohydrate CR diet has gained in popularity. Although the low-fat, high carbohydrate diet was better at reducing total cholesterol and LDL-C [26], it is controversial [38], because it raises plasma triglycerides [39] and may adversely affect LDL composition [40,41]. The greater the amount of carbohydrates that are substituted for fat, the greater the increase in triglycerides [42]. Increasing evidence has pointed to the role of triglycerides in atherogenic risk [43]. Consumption of a low-carbohydrate CR diet, however, as shown in our present study and numerous previous studies, resulted in a reduction in triglycerides due to lack of substrates for triglyceride synthesis in liver. In addition, elevated levels of HDL-C were observed in subjects on low-carbohydrate CR diets [16,44], whereas HDL-C declined in subjects on low fat, high-carbohydrate diets [45]. The elevated HDL-C and reduced triglycerides in plasma are the advantages of a carbohydrate restricted diet over a high carbohydrate diet [24].

The long-term low-carbohydrate CR diet, however, is difficult for patients to comply with. Studies have shown the efficacy of a moderate-carbohydrate CR diet in weight management and improvement of serum lipid profiles [46]. In addition, a moderate-carbohydrate CR diet is more acceptable to people for the prevention and treatment of type 2 diabetes, as a strict carbohydrate restricted diet is not required [47,48]. In the present study, for the first time ever, we identified that a moderate-carbohydrate diet (34% carbohydrate reduction) is not only effective in raising gene expressions of adiponectin and PPARγ that potentially lead to better metabolic conditions but is also better in improving lipid profiles than a low-carbohydrate diet in rats. Our results suggest that a moderate-carbohydrate CR diet can be a new dietary intervention strategy for prevention and treatment of MetS.

There are certainly some limitations in this study. First, the investigation period (12 weeks) may be too short to predict long-term effects of CR on expression of adiponectin, PPARγ and serum parameters. Second, RT-PCR is a semiquantitative technique. Although our conclusions were based on the results of the adiponectin, PPARγ expression and other serum parameters, more quantitative techniques such as real-time PCR for mRNA or Western blotting for protein expression of adiponectin should be used in a future study. Finally, whether the conclusion drawn from rats in the present study can be extrapolated to other organisms, such as humans, remains to be determined.

Acknowledgments: This project was supported by grants from the National Natural Science Foundation of China (Grant No. 81273072, 2012; Grant No.30571561, 2006).

Author Contributions: Jie-Hua Chen and Limei Mao were involved in study design, data collection and analysis and have contributed to manuscript writing. Qiang Ding, Jia Song and Caiqun Ouyang carried out data collection and analysis. Wenhong Cao was involved in data analysis.

References

1. Verdery, R.B.; Walford, R.L. Changes in plasma lipids and lipoproteins in humans during a 2-year period of dietary restriction in biosphere 2. *Arch. Intern. Med.* **1998**, *158*, 900–906. [CrossRef] [PubMed]
2. Walford, R.L.; Mock, D.; Verdery, R.; MacCallum, T. Calorie restriction in biosphere 2: Alterations in physiologic, hematologic, hormonal, and biochemical parameters in humans restricted for a 2-year period. *J. Gerontol. A Biol. Sci. Med. Sci.* **2002**, *57*, B211–B224. [CrossRef] [PubMed]
3. Bordone, L.; Guarente, L. Calorie restriction, sirt1 and metabolism: Understanding longevity. *Nat. Rev. Mol. Cell Biol.* **2005**, *6*, 298–305. [CrossRef] [PubMed]
4. Takahashi, S.; Masuda, J.; Shimagami, H.; Ohta, Y.; Kanda, T.; Saito, K.; Kato, H. Mild caloric restriction up-regulates the expression of prohibitin: A proteome study. *Biochem. Biophys. Res. Commun.* **2011**, *405*, 462–467. [CrossRef] [PubMed]

5. Oana, F.; Takeda, H.; Matsuzawa, A.; Akahane, S.; Isaji, M.; Akahane, M. Adiponectin receptor 2 expression in liver and insulin resistance in db/db mice given a beta3-adrenoceptor agonist. *Eur. J. Pharmacol.* **2005**, *518*, 71–76. [CrossRef] [PubMed]
6. Bjorndal, B.; Burri, L.; Staalesen, V.; Skorve, J.; Berge, R.K. Different adipose depots: Their role in the development of metabolic syndrome and mitochondrial response to hypolipidemic agents. *J. Obes.* **2011**, *2011*, 490650. [CrossRef] [PubMed]
7. Sadashiv; Tiwari, S.; Paul, B.N.; Kumar, S.; Chandra, A.; Dhananjai, S.; Negi, M.P. Adiponectin mrna in adipose tissue and its association with metabolic risk factors in postmenopausal obese women. *Hormones (Athens)* **2013**, *12*, 119–127. [PubMed]
8. Combs, T.P.; Berg, A.H.; Rajala, M.W.; Klebanov, S.; Iyengar, P.; Jimenez-Chillaron, J.C.; Patti, M.E.; Klein, S.L.; Weinstein, R.S.; Scherer, P.E. Sexual differentiation, pregnancy, calorie restriction, and aging affect the adipocyte-specific secretory protein adiponectin. *Diabetes* **2003**, *52*, 268–276. [CrossRef] [PubMed]
9. Vaiopoulos, A.G.; Marinou, K.; Christodoulides, C.; Koutsilieris, M. The role of adiponectin in human vascular physiology. *Int. J. Cardiol.* **2012**, *155*, 188–193. [CrossRef] [PubMed]
10. Iwaki, M.; Matsuda, M.; Maeda, N.; Funahashi, T.; Matsuzawa, Y.; Makishima, M.; Shimomura, I. Induction of adiponectin, a fat-derived antidiabetic and antiatherogenic factor, by nuclear receptors. *Diabetes* **2003**, *52*, 1655–1663. [CrossRef] [PubMed]
11. Combs, T.P.; Wagner, J.A.; Berger, J.; Doebber, T.; Wang, W.J.; Zhang, B.B.; Tanen, M.; Berg, A.H.; O'Rahilly, S.; Savage, D.B.; *et al.* Induction of adipocyte complement-related protein of 30 kilodaltons by ppargamma agonists: A potential mechanism of insulin sensitization. *Endocrinology* **2002**, *143*, 998–1007. [PubMed]
12. Maeda, N.; Takahashi, M.; Funahashi, T.; Kihara, S.; Nishizawa, H.; Kishida, K.; Nagaretani, H.; Matsuda, M.; Komuro, R.; Ouchi, N.; *et al.* Ppargamma ligands increase expression and plasma concentrations of adiponectin, an adipose-derived protein. *Diabetes* **2001**, *50*, 2094–2099. [CrossRef] [PubMed]
13. Yang, W.S.; Jeng, C.Y.; Wu, T.J.; Tanaka, S.; Funahashi, T.; Matsuzawa, Y.; Wang, J.P.; Chen, C.L.; Tai, T.Y.; Chuang, L.M. Synthetic peroxisome proliferator-activated receptor-gamma agonist, rosiglitazone, increases plasma levels of adiponectin in type 2 diabetic patients. *Diabetes Care* **2002**, *25*, 376–380. [CrossRef] [PubMed]
14. Sung, B.; Park, S.; Yu, B.P.; Chung, H.Y. Modulation of ppar in aging, inflammation, and calorie restriction. *J. Gerontol. A Biol. Sci. Med. Sci.* **2004**, *59*, 997–1006. [CrossRef] [PubMed]
15. Zhu, M.; Miura, J.; Lu, L.X.; Bernier, M.; DeCabo, R.; Lane, M.A.; Roth, G.S.; Ingram, D.K. Circulating adiponectin levels increase in rats on caloric restriction: The potential for insulin sensitization. *Exp. Gerontol.* **2004**, *39*, 1049–1059. [CrossRef] [PubMed]
16. Volek, J.S.; Fernandez, M.L.; Feinman, R.D.; Phinney, S.D. Dietary carbohydrate restriction induces a unique metabolic state positively affecting atherogenic dyslipidemia, fatty acid partitioning, and metabolic syndrome. *Prog. Lipid Res.* **2008**, *47*, 307–318. [CrossRef] [PubMed]
17. Reeves, P.G.; Nielsen, F.H.; Fahey, G.C., Jr. AIN-93 purified diets for laboratory rodents: Final report of the american institute of nutrition ad hoc writing committee on the reformulation of the AIN-76A rodent diet. *J. Nutr.* **1993**, *123*, 1939–1951. [PubMed]
18. Tanno, K.; Okamura, T.; Ohsawa, M.; Onoda, T.; Itai, K.; Sakata, K.; Nakamura, M.; Ogawa, A.; Kawamura, K.; Okayama, A. Comparison of low-density lipoprotein cholesterol concentrations measured by a direct homogeneous assay and by the friedewald formula in a large community population. *Clin. Chim. Acta* **2010**, *411*, 1774–1780. [CrossRef] [PubMed]
19. Matthews, D.R.; Hosker, J.P.; Rudenski, A.S.; Naylor, B.A.; Treacher, D.F.; Turner, R.C. Homeostasis model assessment: Insulin resistance and beta-cell function from fasting plasma glucose and insulin concentrations in man. *Diabetologia* **1985**, *28*, 412–419. [CrossRef] [PubMed]
20. Gerbaix, M.; Metz, L.; Ringot, E.; Courteix, D. Visceral fat mass determination in rodent: Validation of dual-energy X-ray absorptiometry and anthropometric techniques in fat and lean rats. *Lipids Health Dis.* **2010**, *9*, 140. [CrossRef] [PubMed]
21. Fox, C.S.; Massaro, J.M.; Hoffmann, U.; Pou, K.M.; Maurovich-Horvat, P.; Liu, C.Y.; Vasan, R.S.; Murabito, J.M.; Meigs, J.B.; Cupples, L.A.; *et al.* Abdominal visceral and subcutaneous adipose tissue compartments: Association with metabolic risk factors in the framingham heart study. *Circulation* **2007**, *116*, 39–48. [CrossRef] [PubMed]

22. Freedland, E.S. Role of a critical visceral adipose tissue threshold (CVATT) in metabolic syndrome: Implications for controlling dietary carbohydrates: A review. *Nutr. Metab. (Lond.)* **2004**, *1*, 12. [CrossRef] [PubMed]
23. Wajchenberg, B.L. Subcutaneous and visceral adipose tissue: Their relation to the metabolic syndrome. *Endocr. Rev.* **2000**, *21*, 697–738. [CrossRef] [PubMed]
24. Sasakabe, T.; Haimoto, H.; Umegaki, H.; Wakai, K. Effects of a moderate low-carbohydrate diet on preferential abdominal fat loss and cardiovascular risk factors in patients with type 2 diabetes. *Diabetes Metab. Syndr. Obes.* **2011**, *4*, 167–174. [CrossRef] [PubMed]
25. Sharman, M.J.; Kraemer, W.J.; Love, D.M.; Avery, N.G.; Gomez, A.L.; Scheett, T.P.; Volek, J.S. A ketogenic diet favorably affects serum biomarkers for cardiovascular disease in normal-weight men. *J. Nutr.* **2002**, *132*, 1879–1885. [PubMed]
26. Volek, J.S.; Sharman, M.J.; Forsythe, C.E. Modification of lipoproteins by very low-carbohydrate diets. *J. Nutr.* **2005**, *135*, 1339–1342. [PubMed]
27. Volek, J.S.; Sharman, M.J.; Gomez, A.L.; Scheett, T.P.; Kraemer, W.J. An isoenergetic very low carbohydrate diet improves serum HDL cholesterol and triacylglycerol concentrations, the total cholesterol to HDL cholesterol ratio and postprandial pipemic responses compared with a low fat diet in normal weight, normolipidemic women. *J. Nutr.* **2003**, *133*, 2756–2761. [PubMed]
28. Masoro, E.J.; McCarter, R.J.; Katz, M.S.; McMahan, C.A. Dietary restriction alters characteristics of glucose fuel use. *J. Gerontol.* **1992**, *47*, B202–B208. [CrossRef] [PubMed]
29. Wetter, T.J.; Gazdag, A.C.; Dean, D.J.; Cartee, G.D. Effect of calorie restriction on *in vivo* glucose metabolism by individual tissues in rats. *Am. J. Physiol.* **1999**, *276*, E728–E738. [PubMed]
30. Yang, X.; Zhang, Y.; Lin, J.; Pen, A.; Ying, C.; Cao, W.; Mao, L. A lower proportion of dietary saturated/monounsaturated/polyunsaturated fatty acids reduces the expression of adiponectin in rats fed a high-fat diet. *Nutr. Res.* **2012**, *32*, 285–291. [CrossRef] [PubMed]
31. Zhu, M.; Lee, G.D.; Ding, L.; Hu, J.; Qiu, G.; de Cabo, R.; Bernier, M.; Ingram, D.K.; Zou, S. Adipogenic signaling in rat white adipose tissue: Modulation by aging and calorie restriction. *Exp. Gerontol.* **2007**, *42*, 733–744. [CrossRef] [PubMed]
32. Saltiel, A.R.; Kahn, C.R. Insulin signalling and the regulation of glucose and lipid metabolism. *Nature* **2001**, *414*, 799–806. [CrossRef] [PubMed]
33. Tschritter, O.; Fritsche, A.; Thamer, C.; Haap, M.; Shirkavand, F.; Rahe, S.; Staiger, H.; Maerker, E.; Haring, H.; Stumvoll, M. Plasma adiponectin concentrations predict insulin sensitivity of both glucose and lipid metabolism. *Diabetes* **2003**, *52*, 239–243. [CrossRef] [PubMed]
34. Yang, W.S.; Chen, M.H.; Lee, W.J.; Lee, K.C.; Chao, C.L.; Huang, K.C.; Chen, C.L.; Tai, T.Y.; Chuang, L.M. Adiponectin mRNA levels in the abdominal adipose depots of nondiabetic women. *Int. J. Obes. Relat. Metab. Disord.* **2003**, *27*, 896–900. [CrossRef] [PubMed]
35. Accurso, A.; Bernstein, R.K.; Dahlqvist, A.; Draznin, B.; Feinman, R.D.; Fine, E.J.; Gleed, A.; Jacobs, D.B.; Larson, G.; Lustig, R.H.; *et al.* Dietary carbohydrate restriction in type 2 diabetes mellitus and metabolic syndrome: Time for a critical appraisal. *Nutr. Metab. (Lond.)* **2008**, *5*, 9. [CrossRef] [PubMed]
36. Krauss, R.M.; Deckelbaum, R.J.; Ernst, N.; Fisher, E.; Howard, B.V.; Knopp, R.H.; Kotchen, T.; Lichtenstein, A.H.; McGill, H.C.; Pearson, T.A.; *et al.* Dietary guidelines for healthy american adults: A statement for health professionals from the nutrition committee, American heart association. *Circulation* **1996**, *94*, 1795–1800. [CrossRef] [PubMed]
37. Halton, T.L.; Willett, W.C.; Liu, S.; Manson, J.E.; Albert, C.M.; Rexrode, K.; Hu, F.B. Low-carbohydrate-diet score and the risk of coronary heart disease in women. *N. Engl. J. Med.* **2006**, *355*, 1991–2002. [CrossRef] [PubMed]
38. Schneeman, B.O. Carbohydrate: Friend or foe? Summary of research needs. *J. Nutr.* **2001**, *131*, 2764S–2765S. [PubMed]
39. Parks, E.J.; Hellerstein, M.K. Carbohydrate-induced hypertriacylglycerolemia: Historical perspective and review of biological mechanisms. *Am. J. Clin. Nutr.* **2000**, *71*, 412–433. [PubMed]
40. Dreon, D.M.; Fernstrom, H.A.; Miller, B.; Krauss, R.M. Low-density lipoprotein subclass patterns and lipoprotein response to a reduced-fat diet in men. *FASEB J.* **1994**, *8*, 121–126. [PubMed]

41. Dreon, D.M.; Fernstrom, H.A.; Williams, P.T.; Krauss, R.M. A very low-fat diet is not associated with improved lipoprotein profiles in men with a predominance of large, low-density lipoproteins. *Am. J. Clin. Nutr.* **1999**, *69*, 411–418. [PubMed]
42. Retzlaff, B.M.; Walden, C.E.; Dowdy, A.A.; McCann, B.S.; Anderson, K.V.; Knopp, R.H. Changes in plasma triacylglycerol concentrations among free-living hyperlipidemic men adopting different carbohydrate intakes over 2 y: The dietary alternatives study. *Am. J. Clin. Nutr.* **1995**, *62*, 988–995. [PubMed]
43. Yuan, G.; Al-Shali, K.Z.; Hegele, R.A. Hypertriglyceridemia: Its etiology, effects and treatment. *CMAJ* **2007**, *176*, 1113–1120. [CrossRef] [PubMed]
44. Fontana, L.; Meyer, T.E.; Klein, S.; Holloszy, J.O. Long-term calorie restriction is highly effective in reducing the risk for atherosclerosis in humans. *Proc. Natl. Acad. Sci. USA* **2004**, *101*, 6659–6663. [CrossRef] [PubMed]
45. Turley, M.L.; Skeaff, C.M.; Mann, J.I.; Cox, B. The effect of a low-fat, high-carbohydrate diet on serum high density lipoprotein cholesterol and triglyceride. *Eur. J. Clin. Nutr.* **1998**, *52*, 728–732. [CrossRef] [PubMed]
46. Johnston, C.S.; Tjonn, S.L.; Swan, P.D.; White, A.; Hutchins, H.; Sears, B. Ketogenic low-carbohydrate diets have no metabolic advantage over nonketogenic low-carbohydrate diets. *Am. J. Clin. Nutr.* **2006**, *83*, 1055–1061. [PubMed]
47. Daly, M.E.; Paisey, R.; Paisey, R.; Millward, B.A.; Eccles, C.; Williams, K.; Hammersley, S.; MacLeod, K.M.; Gale, T.J. Short-term effects of severe dietary carbohydrate-restriction advice in type 2 diabetes—A randomized controlled trial. *Diabet. Med.* **2006**, *23*, 15–20. [CrossRef] [PubMed]
48. Haimoto, H.; Iwata, M.; Wakai, K.; Umegaki, H. Long-term effects of a diet loosely restricting carbohydrates on HbA1c levels, BMI and tapering of sulfonylureas in type 2 diabetes: A 2-year follow-up study. *Diabetes Res. Clin. Pract.* **2008**, *79*, 350–356. [CrossRef] [PubMed]

10

Internal Fat and Cardiometabolic Risk Factors Following a Meal-Replacement Regimen *vs.* Comprehensive Lifestyle Changes in Obese Subjects

Daniel König [1,2,*], Denise Zdzieblik [1], Peter Deibert [2], Aloys Berg [1], Albert Gollhofer [1] and Martin Büchert [3]

[1] Department for Nutrition, Institute for Sports and Sports Science, University of Freiburg, Schwarzwaldstr. 175, 79117 Freiburg, Germany; Daniel.koenig@uniklinik-freiburg.de (D.K.); Denise.Zdzieblik@sport.uni-freiburg.de (D.Z.); berg.aloys@web.de (A.B.); AG@sport.uni-freiburg.de (A.G.)

[2] Department of Exercise and Sports Medicine, Centre for Internal Medicine, University Hospital Freiburg, Hugstetterstr. 175, 79106 Freiburg, Germany; Peter.Deibert@uniklinik-freiburg.de

[3] Department of Radiology—Medical Physics, University Medical Center Freiburg, Breisacher Straße 60a, 79106 Freiburg, Germany; Martin.Buechert@uniklinik-freiburg.de

* Correspondence: Daniel.Koenig@uniklinik-freiburg.de

Abstract: The aim of the present study was to investigate the effect of a meal-replacement regimen *vs.* comprehensive lifestyle changes in overweight or obese subjects on intra-abdominal fat stores (Magnetic Resonance Imaging (MRI) measurements) and cardiometabolic risk factors. Forty-two obese men (n = 18) and women (n = 24) (age 49 ± 8 years; weight 96.3 ± 12.1 kg; BMI 32.7 ± 2.3 kg/m^2) were selected for this randomized parallel-group design investigation. Subjects in the lifestyle group (LS-G; n = 22) received dietary counselling sessions and instructions how to increase physical activity. In the meal replacement group (MR-G; n = 20) meals were replaced by a low-calorie drink high in soy protein. After six months, subjects in the LS-G lost 8.88 ± 6.24 kg and subjects in the MR-G lost 7.1 ± 2.33 kg; $p < 0.01$ for changes within groups; no significant differences were found between the groups. Lean body mass remained constant in both intervention groups. MRI analyses showed that internal fat was significantly reduced in both groups to a comparable amount; the higher fat loss in the LS-G in the abdominal area was due to a higher reduction in subcutaneous fat. Both interventions significantly reduced components of the cardiometabolic risk profile and leptin levels. The decrease in the adipokines fetuin A and resistin was more pronounced in the MR-G. In conclusion, both interventions significantly reduced body weight, total fat mass and internal abdominal fat while preserving lean body mass. The reduction in the adipokines fetuin A and resistin was more pronounced in the meal replacement group suggesting an additional effect of soy protein components.

Keywords: meal replacement; visceral fat; metabolic syndrome; lifestyle intervention

1. Introduction

Hypercaloric diets and sedentary behaviour are cornerstones in the development of obesity, the metabolic syndrome and type 2 diabetes mellitus. Hence, comprehensive lifestyle changes improve both, weight loss and metabolic risk factors.

Several lines of evidence suggest that one of the most important goals for lifestyle interventions is the reduction in fat mass and in particular the reduction in intra-abdominal/internal fat. It has been shown that cardiometabolic risk factors increase as a function of visceral fat accumulation [1]. A higher amount of visceral fat—relative to subcutaneous fat—is related to extra-adipocyte fat storage, reduced insulin sensitivity and increased pro-inflammatory adipokine concentrations. Therefore, the appropriate measurement of the amounts of visceral fat and the ratio of visceral/subcutaneous fat is very important for the evaluation of the pathophysiological impact of total fat stores. Several measures of body composition routinely used in the clinic (e.g., waist circumference, waist/hip ratio or bioimpedance) have failed to predict visceral fat mass accurately [1].

Lifestyle interventions are effective in significantly reducing the amount of visceral fat. However, there is still an ongoing discussion which kind of lifestyle alteration is associated with the highest decrease in visceral fat and thus with the greatest benefit with respect to cardiometabolic risk factors [2–4].

The rational background for the present investigation was that although MR improve body weight and cardiometabolic risk factors [3,5,6], data on the respective effects on different fat stores is not available. MR regimens are criticized as associated with a loss in muscle mass favouring weight regain and that very low calorie diets predominantly reduce visceral fat in the early phase of weight loss interventions [4]. Moreover, little is known if the effects of a comprehensive lifestyle intervention (LSI) including aerobic exercise, psychological coaching and dietary intervention are superior to a MR regimen, particularly with respect to the influence on visceral fat [2].

2. Methods

In the present study, the effects of a six months meal replacement regimen (MR) on body composition and in particular on the amount of visceral and subcutaneous fat were investigated. In addition, body weight, metabolic risk factors and several adipokine concentrations were determined after six weeks and six months in order to document both short and longer term metabolic effects of the intervention. The results were compared to the respective effects of a comprehensive lifestyle intervention (LSI).

2.1. Subjects

Forty-two obese men (n = 18) and women (n = 24) (age 49 ± 8 years; weight 96.3 ± 12.1 kg; BMI 32.7 ± 2.3 kg/m^2) were recruited from the outpatient database of the University Hospital for this randomized parallel-group design investigation. The participants should be between the age of 18 and 65 years (27 $\leqslant$ BMI $\leqslant$ 40) and capable to carry out a six month lifestyle intervention including physical exercise training.

Subjects with type 2 diabetes mellitus, clinically significant illnesses or patients who took anti-diabetic or lipid-lowering drugs were excluded. All subjects completed a comprehensive medical examination and routine blood tests. Written informed consent was provided by all subjects, and the study protocol was approved by the Ethical Committee of the University of Freiburg. Subjects were randomized into two equal groups as described previously using a random list [7]. The data presented here represent the pooled results of two studies that were performed identically in a comparable population group. The randomization process was done for each study separately and the pooling took place after completion of each study.

2.2. Intervention Program

The intervention in the lifestyle group (LS-G) consisted of 10 weekly teaching sessions related to nutrition, physical exercise and motivation. All sessions were held by certified experts in their respective fields. In addition, subjects received a hand-out with dietary advice and recommendations for lifestyle changes that were in accordance with the "German Society of Nutrition" and the "German Society of Sports Medicine and Prevention" [8]. The prescribed diet was a moderate-fat, nutrient-balanced weight reduction diet consisting of 1200 to 1500 kcal per day for women and 1500 to 1800 kcal per day for men, with approximately 50–55 percent of the calories coming from carbohydrates, preferably with a low GI, 25–30 percent from fat, and 15–20 percent from protein. Dietary behaviour was checked using two 24-h dietary recalls that were used for dietary compliance and that were individually discussed at the nutritional teaching sessions.

The subjects in the LS-G were instructed to increase physical activity according to the guidelines of the "German Society of Sports Medicine". They performed three physical activity sessions per week with an intensity ranging between 55% to 75% of VO_2max. In the first six weeks, physical activity was performed as a group session supervised by a physical education teacher two times/week; thereafter, the group sessions took place once a week. Participants were instructed to perform the other physical activity sessions independently.

The subjects assigned to the meal replacement group (MR-G) were instructed to replace two daily meals with a commercially available soy-yoghurt-honey preparation (Almased®) for the first six weeks. During the following 20 weeks, only one daily meal was replaced by the preparation. The dietary intake of fat during this second phase was not to exceed 60 g per day. The first six-week diet contained about 1000 kcal per day for women and 1200 kcal for men, and then, in the following 20 weeks, aimed at a maximum of 1500 kcal for women and 1700 kcal for men.

The data collected at enrolment and after six, and 26 weeks were body weight, waist and abdominal circumference, self-reported medical history, blood pressure, glucose, serum lipids and plasma levels of several adipokines. Leptin, resistin and fetuin A were measured by commercially available ELISA kits (DSL Deutschland GmbH, Sinsheim, Germany). All other laboratory analyses were done in the central laboratory of the University hospital using clinical routine methods. Waist circumference was taken with a non-distensible tape measure according to published guidelines [9]. At baseline and after 26 weeks, body composition analyses using the technique of air displacement plethysmography were performed (Bod Pod®, [10]).

2.3. MRI Measurements

MRI (Magnetic Resonance Imaging) measurements of total abdominal fat and the amount of subcutaneous and internal fat were determined at baseline and after 26 weeks. MRI measurements were performed on a 1.5 T short bore, whole-body MRI system with an inner diameter of 70 cm (Magnetom Espree, Siemens Healthcare, Erlangen, Germany). Data were acquired using a gradient echo based Dixon sequence as described previously [11]. The region of interest was covered by a multi-array spine coil in combination with two multi-array body coils.

Fat/Water MRI data were analysed after a two-point-Dixon fat water image reconstruction using an active contour snake segmentation to separate subcutaneous and internal adipose tissue, including visceral adipose tissue, muscular fat and bone marrow [11]. The classification follows the one used by Shen [12] and was done for the abdominal region ranging from the highest cranial extension of the liver (exhaled position) to the first cranial slice displaying the femoral heads.

2.4. Statistics

Normality of all variables was tested before statistical analyses using the Kolmogorov-Smirnov test procedure. Testing for changes between the examinations within the intervention groups was performed by applying the paired two-sample T-test. Multiple testing was considered using the Holm-Bonferroni method. Testing for changes between groups following the intervention (LS-G *vs.* MR-G) was done by using two-way repeated-measures analysis of variance (ANOVA) for continuous variables. The factors were treatment group (LS-G *vs.* MR-G) and time (levels were pre and post intervention (6 and 26 weeks).

All P values were two-sided and a P value of 0.05 or less was considered to indicate statistical significance. Analysis was conducted with the use of SPSS software (version 20.0.1, IBM, Armonk, NY, USA).

3. Results

As stated before, the data represent the pooled results of two studies that were performed in an absolute identical manner. In total, from the outpatient database of the University Hospital, 117 potentially eligible subjects were contacted and asked concerning exclusion criteria. Seventy-five subjects were invited for screening and 50 subjects were eligible and randomized into the LS-G or MR-G. Forty-two patients completed the study and attended at least 75% of the meetings/training sessions. Eight participants dropped out: One subject changed the residence, five had claustrophobia, one subject was dissatisfied with the randomization outcome and one did not show-up again for follow-up for unknown reason.

For the final analysis, 22 subjects in the lifestyle group (LS-G) and 20 subjects in the meal replacement (MR-G) group were included.

3.1. Anthropometric Parameters

The changes in weight and BMI are shown in Table 1. After six weeks, the decrease in weight and BMI was more distinct in the MR group whereas after six months, weight loss was more pronounced in the LS group. At the end of the study, subjects in the LS-G had lost 8.88 ± 6.24 kg and subjects in the MR-G had lost 7.1 ± 2.33 kg. The changes within each group were highly significant ($p < 0.01$) whereas no significant differences could be observed between the groups. Figure 1 shows the results from the Bod Pod analysis indicating that the higher weight loss in the LS-G was due to a higher decrease in fat mass. Lean body mass did not change in either of the intervention groups. Figure 2 shows the results of the MRI scans. In the abdominal region, subjects in the LS group lost more fat than the MR group (A); however, the differences between the intervention groups were not significant for all MRI measures. Subjects in the MR-G exhibited lower subcutaneous and higher internal abdominal fat in the abdominal region at baseline. The latter findings could be explained by a higher proportion of females in the LS-G compared to the MR-G. However, although the female subjects in this investigation exhibited a higher mean subcutaneous fat mass (11.4 kg) than the male participants (8.6 kg), there were no distinct gender-related changes in the course of the intervention that could explain the different outcome in the LS-G *vs.* MR-G. Both, female and male subjects lost 2.9 kg of total abdominal fat and the surplus amount of subcutaneous fat loss was only 300 g in the female participants. In the LS-G, the surplus in subcutaneous fat loss was 1.4 kg (B) while internal fat loss was almost identical (C).

Table 1. Weight and BMI during the course of the study. Mean ± standard deviation (SD). LS-G, lifestyle intervention group; MR-G, meal replacement group. §, $p < 0.05$ compared to baseline; ◊, $p < 0.01$ compared to baseline (paired *T*-Test). Differences between the intervention groups (ANOVA) were not significant at any point of the investigation.

		Baseline	**6 Weeks**	**6 Months**	**Changes after 6 Weeks**	**Changes after 6 Months**
		Mean (SD)	**Mean (SD)**	**Mean (SD)**	**Mean (SD)**	**Mean (SD)**
Weight (kg)	**LS-G**	95.9 (12.01)	92.1 (11.9) §	87.0 (12.2) ◊	−3.77 (2.85)	−8.88 (6.24)
	MR-G	96.7 (12.6)	91.3 (12.8) ◊	89.7 (13.1) ◊	−5.42 (1.86)	−7.06 (2.33)
BMI (kg/m^2)	**LS-G**	32.5 (2.65)	31.2 (2.62) §	29.4 (2.46) ◊	−1.28 (0.94)	−3.06 (2.13)
	MR-G	32.9 (1.88)	31.0 (2.08) ◊	30.5 (2.43) ◊	−1.85 (0.59)	−2.41 (0.77)

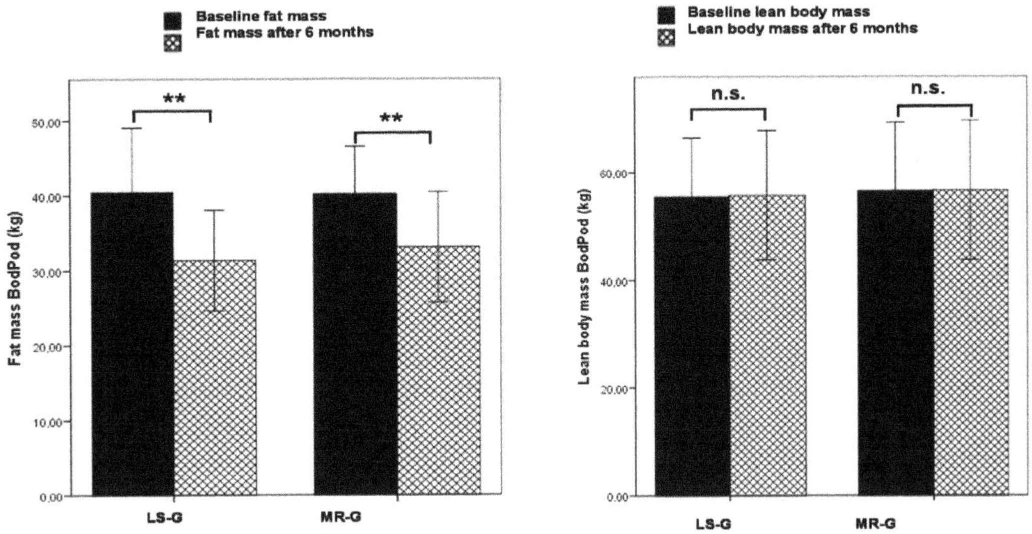

Figure 1. Changes in fat mass (PodBod) and lean body mass (PodBod) after six months by either lifestyle changes (LS-G) or a meal replacement regimen (MR-G); black bar, baseline values; grey hatched bars, post-interventional values after six months. (Error bars: ±1 standard deviation; *, $p < 0.05$; **, $p < 0.01$, n.s., not significant).

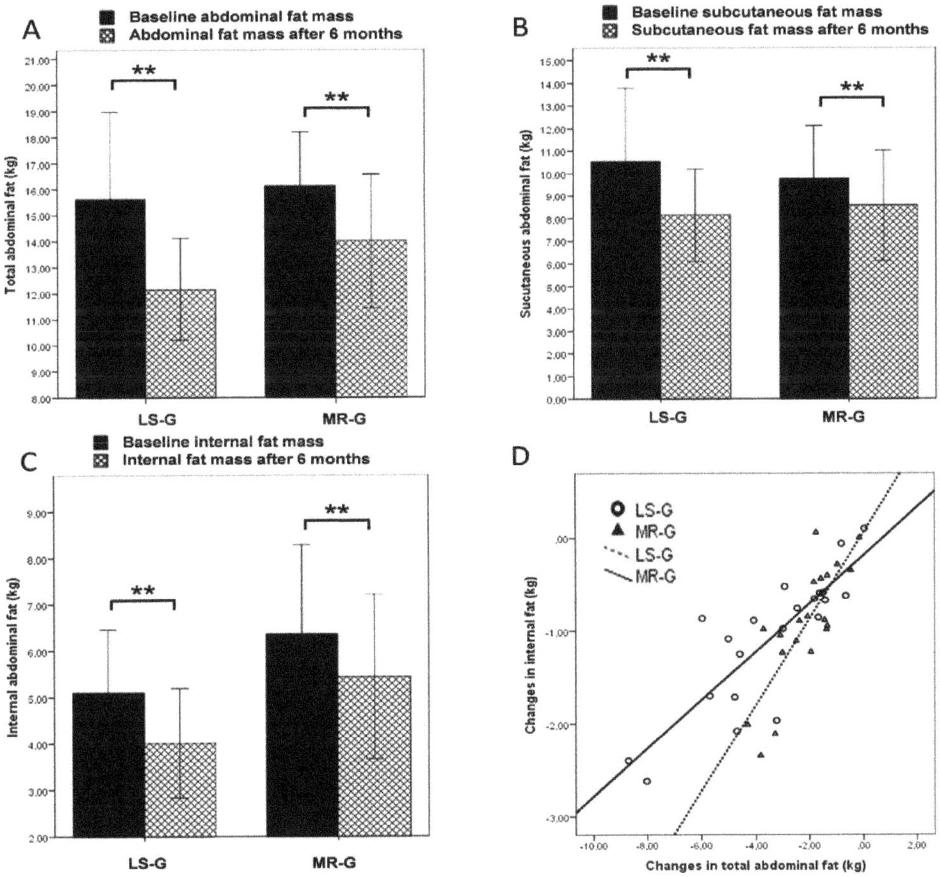

Figure 2. MRI findings: Changes in total abdominal fat mass (**A**); subcutaneous abdominal fat (**B**); internal abdominal fat (**C**) and the correlation between changes in total abdominal fat and internal abdominal fat in dependence of the intervention group (lifestyle changes LS-G or meal replacement regimen MR-G); black bars, baseline values; grey hatched bars, post-interventional values after six months. (Error bars: ±1 standard deviation; *, $p < 0.05$; **, $p < 0.01$).

Per kg fat mass lost during the intervention, participants in the MR-G lost more abdominal fat which is further illustrated by the scatterplot and the linear equation (D).

3.2. Cardiometabolic Risk Factors

Although there were no significant differences between the intervention groups at any time of the study, there were discrepant courses of parameters and differences in the significance levels within the two groups (Table 2). Total cholesterol decreased significantly after six weeks in both groups and rose again to near baseline levels after six months. Triglycerides levels were initially higher in the MR-G and decreased in both groups after six weeks; after six months triglycerides further decreased in the MR-G but rose again in the LS-G. After six month, triglycerides dropped by 51.4 ± 93.1 mg/dL in the MR-G and 19.4 ± 49.2 mg/dL in the LS-G. LDL-Cholesterol dropped significantly in both groups after six weeks with a more pronounced decline in the MR-G. After six months LDL-levels largely returned to baseline in both groups. Initial levels of glucose and HbA1c were higher in subjects in the LS-G. Glucose levels dropped in both groups but the decrease was only significant in the lifestyle group. HbA1c also dropped in both groups and after six months, the changes were significant in both groups. The changes were more distinct in the LS-G, however, comparable to glucose levels, initial HbA1c was also higher in subjects in the lifestyle group.

Table 2. Total cholesterol, triglycerides, LDL- and HDL-cholesterol, glucose and HbA1c levels during the course of the study. Mean ± standard deviation (SD). LS-G, lifestyle intervention group; MR-G, meal replacement group. §, $p < 0.05$ compared to baseline; ◊, $p < 0.01$ compared to baseline (paired *T*-Test). Differences between the intervention groups (ANOVA) were not significant at any point of the investigation.

		Baseline	6 Weeks	6 Months	Changes after 6 Weeks	Changes after 6 Months
		Mean (SD)	Mean (SD)	Mean (SD)	Mean (SD)	Mean (SD)
Cholesterol (mg/dL)	**LS-G**	225 (37.4)	202 (39.9) ◊	215 (33.4)	−23.7 (31.3)	−11.3 (30.1)
	MR-G	228 (38.5)	195 (31.4) ◊	223 (41.4)	−32.3 (24.3)	−4.71 (31.5)
Triglycerides (mg/dL)	**LS-G**	138 (61.4)	103 (37.4) ◊	118 (60.5)	−34.8 (51.1)	−19.4 (49.2)
	MR-G	172 (115)	125 (45.4) ◊	120 (41.9) ◊	−46.9 (88.2)	−51.4 (93.1)
LDL-Cholesterol (mg/dL)	**LS-G**	140.2 (40.4)	131 (34.6) §	139 (31.6)	−8.9 (35.3)	−0.51 (31.3)
	MR-G	147.2 (31.7)	127 (27.5) ◊	150 (36.1)	−20.3 (17.9)	3.27 (24.7)
HDL-Cholesterol (mg/dL)	**LS-G**	53.4 (14.7)	48.8 (8.99) ◊	54.6 (13.2)	−4.53 (10.9)	1.19 (9.17)
	MR-G	50.1 (9.42)	47.4 (7.87) §	52.3 (9.52) ◊	−2.65 (6.76)	2.25 (7.29)
Glucose (mg/dL)	**LS-G**	100.7 (25.1)	91.9 (14) §	92.2 (15.9) ◊	−8.70 (17.3)	−8.48 (15.1)
	MR-G	95.2 (19.9)	93.4 (11.9)	90.2 (10.6) #	−1.35 (10.7)	−4.55 (13.8)
HbA1c (%)	**LS-G**	5.64 (0.52)	5.51 (0.44) ◊	5.51 (0.38) ◊	−0.13 (0.23)	−0.13 (0.26)
	MR-G	5.58 (0.55)	5.52 (0.57)	5.50 (0.42) §	−0.06 (0.18)	−0.07 (0.34)

3.3. Adipokine Levels

None of the adipokines showed significant differences between the groups (Table 3). Plasma leptin levels decreased significantly and to a comparable degree in both groups. The reduction in resistin and fetuin A levels was more pronounced and only significant in the MR-G.

Table 3. Plasma levels of the adipokines Leptin, Resistin and Fetuin A during the course of the study. Mean ± standard deviation (SD). LS-G, lifestyle intervention group; MR-G, meal replacement group. §, $p < 0.05$ compared to baseline; ◊, $p < 0.01$ compared to baseline (paired T-Test).Differences between the intervention groups (ANOVA) were not significant at any point of the investigation.

		Baseline	6 Weeks	6 Months	Changes after 6 Weeks	Changes after 6 Months
		Mean (SD)	Mean (SD)	Mean (SD)	Mean (SD)	Mean (SD)
Leptin (μg(L)	LS-G	19.1 (11.9)	12.7 (8.39) ◊	9.85 (8.02) ◊	−7.91 (10.0)	−10.3 (11.3)
	MR-G	18.7 (19.3)	11.6 (10.9) ◊	9.36 (6.97) ◊	−5.70 (10.7)	−8.47 (13.2)
Resistin (μg/L)	LS-G	4.76 (1.68)	5.03 (1.58)	4.85 (1.88)	0.06 (0.78)	−0.13 (1.12)
	MR-G	5.53 (2.44)	4.67 (1.38) §	4.51 (1.35) ◊	−0.88 (1.64)	−0.88 (1.43)
Fetuin A (μg/mL)	LS-G	0.41 (0.1)	0.41 (0.1)	0.39 (0.09)	0.01 (0.08)	−0.01 (0.08)
	MR-G	0.38 (0.07)	0.36 (0.08) ◊	0.35 (0.08) §	−0.03 (0.06)	−0.03 (0.04)

4. Discussion

The main finding of the present study was that the meal replacement regimen decreased internal abdominal fat stores to the same degree as a comprehensive lifestyle intervention. In addition, total fat loss was not significantly different between the intervention groups, and both groups showed no decrease in fat free mass. The results regarding reductions in body weight and fat mass are in keeping with previous studies investigating the effect of meal replacements or comprehensive lifestyle interventions in overweight or obese subjects [13,14]. This investigation did not confirm the findings of a review by Chaston *et al.* that the preferential loss of internal fat by very low calorie diets disappears when the intervention period is longer than four weeks [4].

Nevertheless, albeit not significant, the lifestyle intervention further reduced total and abdominal fat stores. The results from the MRI-scans suggest that the additional fat loss in the lifestyle group could mainly be attributed to an increased fat loss from subcutaneous fat stores. This could not be explained by the higher proportion of women in the LS-G, since the gender-related differences following the intervention were small compared to the differences between the meal replacement and the lifestyle intervention. Although the evidence cannot be directly deducted from the design of the present investigation, it could be speculated that the greater weight loss is related to the additional training program in the lifestyle group. Previous studies have also shown that additional exercise did not further increase intra-abdominal fat loss when added to a hypocaloric diet [15,16].

However, although the individual amount and the intensity of physical exercise was supervised by the sports instructors, the exact duration and intensity of individual sports activities was not monitored.

Both interventions significantly reduced the metabolic risk profile. From a physician's perspective, the findings after six months had more relevance than the results from six weeks. Regarding changes with clinical significance, the reduction in triglycerides and increase in HDL-cholesterol was more pronounced in the meal replacement group whereas glucose and HbA1c-levels were lower in the lifestyle group. The latter finding could be due to higher baseline levels in the LS-G. Previous investigations have shown that meal replacement regimens induce rapid improvements in metabolic risk factors in subjects with the metabolic syndrome [17,18]. In the present investigation, the metabolic risk profile was relatively low, therefore, the improvements were also relatively small. However, the changes in both groups demonstrated that improvements could be accomplished and that the magnitude of beneficial effects increased as a measure of baseline levels.

Adipokine levels showed no significant differences between the groups during the course of the intervention. These adipokines were selected because they reflect the body's fat stores (leptin) and it has been speculated that they play an important role in the initiation and propagation of the pro-inflammatory state associated with extra-adipocyte fat storage, insulin resistance, internal fat accumulation and atherosclerosis.

Leptin levels were comparably reduced in both groups whereas the reduction in resistin and fetuin A were more pronounced in the subjects in the MR-G. Although the levels of these adipokines were positively correlated with total fat mass and cardiometabolic risk factors (data not shown), the decrease was not directly correlated with a reduction in internal abdominal fat mass. It could be speculated that the higher reduction in fetuin A and resistin could be explained by the specific effects of soy protein. Some, albeit not all investigations have suggested a positive influence of soy protein, and in particular soy isoflavones, on proinflammatory adipokines, insulin resistance and body weight [19–21]. However, it has to be acknowledged that the design of the present investigation was not appropriate to establish a cause-effect relationship.

5. Conclusions

In conclusion, results from the present study have shown that both, lifestyle intervention by increased physical activity/hypocaloric low fat diet and meal replacement using a soy protein formula significantly decreased body weight, total fat mass and internal abdominal fat to a comparable amount while completely preserving lean body mass. Both interventions were associated with an improvement in metabolic risk factors although the effect of the intervention seemed to be dependent on pre-interventional levels. Although the effects in both groups were comparable with respect to internal abdominal fat mass, the reduction in adipokine levels was more pronounced in the meal replacement group suggesting an additional effect of soy protein related compounds e.g., genistein or isoflavones. This, however, needs to be further examined in forthcoming studies. It is important to emphasize that the long-term process of atherosclerosis cannot be influenced by short-term dietary modification. All interventions in obese subjects, particularly in patients with metabolic risk factors and increased atherosclerotic burden, should aim at inducing long-term modifications and not transient alterations in both, weight management and atherosclerotic risk factors.

Acknowledgments: Part of the costs were paid by Almased Wellness Company, Bienenbuettel, Germany. The planning, organisation, monitoring and analysis of the study were performed independently by the investigators.

Author Contributions: Daniel Koenig was the principal investigator of the study. Peter Deibert, Martin Buechert, Denise Zdzieblik and Aloys Berg were involved in the design and execution of the study and performed the statistical analysis. All authors read and approved the final manuscript.

References

1. Fox, C.S.; Massaro, J.M.; Hoffmann, U.; Pou, K.M.; Maurovich-Horvat, P.; Liu, C.Y.; Vasan, R.S.; Murabito, J.M.; Meigs, J.B.; Cupples, L.A.; *et al.* Abdominal visceral and subcutaneous adipose tissue compartments: Association with metabolic risk factors in the Framingham Heart Study. *Circulation* **2007**, *116*, 39–48. [CrossRef] [PubMed]
2. Ross, R.; Janssen, I. Is abdominal fat preferentially reduced in response to exercise-induced weight loss? *Med. Sci. Sports Exerc.* **1999**, *31*, S568–S572. [CrossRef] [PubMed]
3. Xu, D.F.; Sun, J.Q.; Chen, M.; Chen, Y.Q.; Xie, H.; Sun, W.J.; Lin, Y.F.; Jiang, J.J.; Sun, W.; Chen, A.F.; *et al.* Effects of lifestyle intervention and meal replacement on glycaemic and body-weight control in Chinese subjects with impaired glucose regulation: A 1-year randomised controlled trial. *Br. J. Nutr.* **2013**, *109*, 487–492. [CrossRef] [PubMed]
4. Chaston, T.B.; Dixon, J.B. Factors associated with percent change in visceral *versus* subcutaneous abdominal fat during weight loss: Findings from a systematic review. *Int. J. Obes.* **2008**, *32*, 619–628. [CrossRef] [PubMed]
5. Konig, D.; Deibert, P.; Frey, I.; Landmann, U.; Berg, A. Effect of meal replacement on metabolic risk factors in overweight and obese subjects. *Ann. Nutr. Metab.* **2008**, *52*, 74–78. [PubMed]
6. Rothberg, A.E.; McEwen, L.N.; Kraftson, A.T.; Fowler, C.E.; Herman, W.H. Very-low-energy diet for type 2 diabetes: An underutilized therapy? *J. Diabetes Complicat.* **2014**, *28*, 506–510. [CrossRef] [PubMed]

7. Deibert, P.; König, D.; Schmidt-Trucksaess, A.; Zaenker, K.S.; Frey, I.; Landmann, U.; Berg, A. Weight loss without losing muscle mass in pre-obese and obese subjects induced by a high-soy-protein diet. *Int. J. Obes. Relat. Metab. Disord.* **2004**, *28*, 1349–1352. [CrossRef] [PubMed]
8. Halle, M.; Berg, A. Standards der Sportmedizin: Lipidstoffwechsel und körperliche Aktivität. *Deutsch. Z. Sportmed.* **2002**, *53*, 58–59.
9. Lohman, T.C.; Roche, A.F.; Martorell, R. *Anthropometric Standardization Reference Manual*; Human Kinetics Books: Champaign, IL, USA, 1988.
10. McCrory, M.A.; Gomez, T.D.; Bernauer, E.M.; Mole, P.A. Evaluation of a new air displacement plethysmograph for measuring human body composition. *Med. Sci. Sports Exerc.* **1995**, *27*, 1686–1691. [CrossRef] [PubMed]
11. Ludwig, U.A.; Klausmann, F.; Baumann, S.; Honal, M.; Hovener, J.B.; Konig, D.; Deibert, P.; Buchert, M. Whole-body MRI-based fat quantification: A comparison to air displacement plethysmography. *J. Magn. Reson. Imaging* **2014**, *40*, 1437–1444. [CrossRef] [PubMed]
12. Shen, W.; Wang, Z.; Punyanita, M.; Lei, J.; Sinav, A.; Kral, J.G.; Imielinska, C.; Ross, R.; Heymsfield, S.B. Adipose tissue quantification by imaging methods: A proposed classification. *Obes. Res.* **2003**, *11*, 5–16. [CrossRef] [PubMed]
13. Kruschitz, R.; Wallner-Liebmann, S.J.; Lothaller, H.; Luger, M.; Schindler, K.; Hoppichler, F.; Ludvik, B. Evaluation of a meal replacement-based weight management program in primary care settings according to the actual European Clinical Practice Guidelines for the Management of Obesity in Adults. *Wien. Klin. Wochenschr.* **2014**, *126*, 598–603. [CrossRef] [PubMed]
14. Baillot, A.; Romain, A.J.; Boisvert-Vigneault, K.; Audet, M.; Baillargeon, J.P.; Dionne, I.J.; Valiquette, L.; Chakra, C.N.; Avignon, A.; Langlois, M.F. Effects of lifestyle interventions that include a physical activity component in class II and III obese individuals: A systematic review and meta-analysis. *PLoS ONE* **2015**, *10*, e0119017. [CrossRef] [PubMed]
15. Trussardi Fayh, A.P.; Lopes, A.L.; Fernandes, P.R.; Reischak-Oliveira, A.; Friedman, R. Impact of weight loss with or without exercise on abdominal fat and insulin resistance in obese individuals: A randomised clinical trial. *Br. J. Nutr.* **2013**, *110*, 486–492. [CrossRef] [PubMed]
16. Christiansen, T.; Paulsen, S.K.; Bruun, J.M.; Overgaard, K.; Ringgaard, S.; Pedersen, S.B.; Positano, V.; Richelsen, B. Comparable reduction of the visceral adipose tissue depot after a diet-induced weight loss with or without aerobic exercise in obese subjects: A 12-week randomized intervention study. *Eur. J. Endocrinol.* **2009**, *160*, 759–767. [CrossRef] [PubMed]
17. Anderson, J.W.; Luan, J.; Hoie, L.H. Structured weight-loss programs: Meta-analysis of weight loss at 24 weeks and assessment of effects of intervention intensity. *Adv. Ther.* **2004**, *21*, 61–75. [CrossRef] [PubMed]
18. Li, Z.; Hong, K.; Saltsman, P.; DeShields, S.; Bellman, M.; Thames, G.; Liu, Y.; Wang, H.J.; Elashoff, R.; Heber, D. Long-term efficacy of soy-based meal replacements *vs.* an individualized diet plan in obese type II DM patients: Relative effects on weight loss, metabolic parameters, and C-reactive protein. *Eur. J. Clin. Nutr.* **2005**, *59*, 411–418. [CrossRef] [PubMed]
19. Sakamoto, Y.; Naka, A.; Ohara, N.; Kondo, K.; Iida, K. Daidzein regulates proinflammatory adipokines thereby improving obesity-related inflammation through PPARgamma. *Mol. Nutr. Food Res.* **2014**, *58*, 718–726. [CrossRef] [PubMed]
20. Llaneza, P.; Gonzalez, C.; Fernandez-Inarrea, J.; Alonso, A.; Diaz, F.; Arnott, I.; Ferrer-Barriendos, J. Soy isoflavones, diet and physical exercise modify serum cytokines in healthy obese postmenopausal women. *Phytomedicine* **2011**, *18*, 245–250. [CrossRef] [PubMed]
21. Charles, C.; Yuskavage, J.; Carlson, O.; John, M.; Tagalicud, A.S.; Maggio, M.; Muller, D.C.; Egan, J.; Basaria, S. Effects of high-dose isoflavones on metabolic and inflammatory markers in healthy postmenopausal women. *Menopause* **2009**, *16*, 395–400. [CrossRef] [PubMed]

11

Suppression of Endogenous Glucose Production by Isoleucine and Valine and Impact of Diet Composition

Isabel Arrieta-Cruz [1,†], Ya Su [2,†] and Roger Gutiérrez-Juárez [2,*]

1 National Institute of Geriatrics, Ministry of Health, Periférico Sur No. 2767, Col. San Jerónimo Lídice. Del. Magdalena Contreras, Mexico City 10200, Mexico; arrieta777@mail.com

2 Department of Medicine, Albert Einstein College of Medicine, Yeshiva University, 1300 Morris Park Ave, Bronx, NY 10461, USA; ya.su@einstein.yu.edu

* Correspondence: roger.gutierrez@einstein.yu.edu

† These authors contributed equally to this work.

Abstract: Leucine has been shown to acutely inhibit hepatic glucose production in rodents by a mechanism requiring its metabolism to acetyl-CoA in the mediobasal hypothalamus (MBH). In the early stages, all branched-chain amino acids (BCAA) are metabolized by a shared set of enzymes to produce a ketoacid, which is later metabolized to acetyl-CoA. Consequently, isoleucine and valine may also modulate glucose metabolism. To examine this possibility we performed intrahypothalamic infusions of isoleucine or valine in rats and assessed whole body glucose kinetics under basal conditions and during euglycemic pancreatic clamps. Furthermore, because high fat diet (HFD) consumption is known to interfere with central glucoregulation, we also asked whether the action of BCAAs was affected by HFD. We fed rats a lard-rich diet for a short interval and examined their response to central leucine. The results showed that both isoleucine and valine individually lowered blood glucose by decreasing liver glucose production. Furthermore, the action of the BCAA leucine was markedly attenuated by HFD feeding. We conclude that all three BCAAs centrally modulate glucose metabolism in the liver and that their action is disrupted by HFD-induced insulin resistance.

Keywords: branched-chain amino acids; leucine; isoleucine; valine; glucose metabolism; nutrient sensing; hypothalamus; liver

---

1. Introduction

Excessive calorie intake resulting from the consumption of fat-rich diets is the most important environmental factor contributing to the emergence and worsening of the current world pandemic of diabetes and obesity [1,2]. Mammals have developed complex mechanisms for detecting changes in the availability of nutrients and responding to them with metabolic adaptations to maintain homeostasis. Multiple organs and tissues are involved in these physiological adaptive mechanisms of nutrient sensing, but the mediobasal hypothalamus (MBH) of the central nervous system (CNS) has been identified as a key integration center for these nutritional cues [3–6]. Dietary protein and amino acids (AA) exert a powerful influence on insulin action and glucose metabolism. The mechanisms underlying this effect are generally attributed to the metabolic actions of AAs in the liver and skeletal muscle [7–13]. Recently however, a number of metabolic actions of AAs have been localized to the MBH of rodents [14–17]. In particular, we have shown that the metabolism of leucine to acetyl-CoA in the MBH is coupled to the inhibition of endogenous glucose production (EGP) and a consequent decrease of circulating glucose levels [16]. In the brain, leucine is initially metabolized through the consecutive action of five enzymes [18,19]. First, leucine is transaminated to α-KIC by the branched-chain amino transferase (BCAT). Next, α-KIC is oxidatively decarboxylated by the action of the branched-chain α-ketoacid dehyrogenase (BCKDH) to form isovaleryl-CoA, which, after three more reactions, is converted to acetyl-CoA. In our studies [16], interventions that antagonized the activity of the enzyme BCKDH or otherwise prevented the formation of acetyl-CoA in the MBH markedly attenuated the glucoregulatory action of leucine. Thus, the conversion of leucine to acetyl-CoA was required to bring about the glucoregulatory effect. Further experiments also revealed that acetyl-CoA had to be converted to malonyl-CoA. More importantly, we showed that the incapacitation of leucine sensing in the MBH contributes to the development of hyperglycemia [16]. Interestingly, the first two enzymes, BCAT and BCKDH, also catalyze the metabolism of the other two members of the branched-chain amino acids (BCAA) family, isoleucine and valine, to form their respective ketoacid products. Successive enzymatic reactions give rise to various metabolites, including acetyl-CoA, a key intermediate for glucoregulation.

Several studies have shown that acute diet-induced insulin resistance partially obliterates the hypothalamic glucoregulatory response to fatty acids [20–22]. This acquired defect is induced by the consumption of a diet enriched in saturated fat. Furthermore, previous studies indicated that the hypothalamic sensing of glucose and lactate, both of which need to be converted to pyruvate, are attenuated by high-fat diet (HFD) feeding [23]. Importantly, studies in rats revealed that HFD feeding caused a marked decrease in the levels of hypothalamic long-chain fatty acyl CoAs (LCFA-CoA) and that their restoration normalized nutrient-dependent glucoregulation [22]. Based on these findings, we hypothesized that HFD feeding may also perturb the glucoregulatory response to BCAA.

Currently it is not known whether or not isoleucine and valine modulate glucose metabolism; furthermore, the effect of HFD on the central metabolic actions of BCAA has not yet been examined. Here we investigated the possibility that the central metabolism of isoleucine and valine may also be coupled to the regulation of glucose metabolism in the liver. Additionally, to determine whether HFD feeding has an impact on the glucoregulatory action of BCAAs, we infused leucine in the MBH of rats previously fed with a lard-enriched diet. In both cases we assessed glucose metabolism *in vivo* through a combination of pancreatic insulin clamps and measurements of whole body glucose kinetics.

2. Experimental Section

2.1. Animal Studies

The animal studies were approved by the Institutional Animal Care and Use Committee (IACUC) of the Albert Einstein College of Medicine. Ten-week-old Sprague-Dawley male rats (Charles River Laboratories, Wilmington, MA, USA) were used for the studies. The animals were individually housed and subjected to a light–dark cycle (0600–1800/1800–0600) with free access to water and food.

2.1.1. Animal Surgeries

Rats were subjected to stereotaxic surgery for implantation of a stainless steel bilateral cannula in the MBH as previously described [16]. The stereotaxic coordinates for cannula placement were (from bregma): -3.3 mm anterior–posterior axis; 0.4 mm lateral axis; and 9.6 mm vertical axis (depth) [24]. On recovery, the animals underwent a second surgery for the placement of indwelling vascular catheters that were used for infusions and blood sampling during the pancreatic clamp studies [16]. Postoperative recovery was monitored by measuring daily food intake and body weight. Only fully recovered animals were used for the experiments. Proper placement of the cannulas was confirmed histologically in brain slices prepared postmortem.

2.1.2. Diets

In the experiments where we compared leucine, isoleucine, and valine, the rats were fed with a regular chow diet (Cat#5001, Lab Diet, Richmond, IN, USA). In separate experiments designed to test the effect of saturated fat on leucine sensing, the animals were subjected to a 3-day regime of a HFD consisting of regular chow enriched with 10% of lard (Cat#01P5704C-K, Test Diet, Richmond, IN, USA) prior to the clamps.

2.1.3. Intrahypothalamic Infusions

Rats were randomized into three groups and received 6 hr intrahypothalamic (MBH) infusions of the following solutions: (1) Vehicle (artificial cerebrospinal fluid); (2) isoleucine; and (3) valine. For the glucose kinetics experiments, an additional group of animals received leucine at an equimolar dose for comparative purposes. Each AA was dissolved in vehicle and delivered at a total dose of 12 *n*moles over the course of 6 h (0.33 μL/h per side). The protocol and dose was based on our previous *in vivo* studies with leucine [16]. A separate group of rats were subjected to HFD feeding and then similarly infused with leucine during pancreatic clamps.

2.1.4. Pancreatic Clamp Studies and Glucose Kinetics Measurements

All rats on regular chow consumed 60 kcal of food the night prior to the study to ensure comparable nutritional status. Plasma levels of circulating glucose were monitored from the start (t = 0 min) of the central infusion (Figure 1A,B). A primed, continuous infusion of [3-^{3}H] glucose (Perkin Elmer, San Jose, CA, USA; 40 μCi bolus; 0.4 μCi/min) was initiated at t = 120 min and maintained throughout the study to assess glucose kinetics by tracer dilution methodology [25], then a pancreatic clamp with insulin replaced at basal levels was performed (t = 240–360 min). At the end of the study, the animals were euthanized and tissue samples were freeze-clamped *in situ* and stored for subsequent analysis.

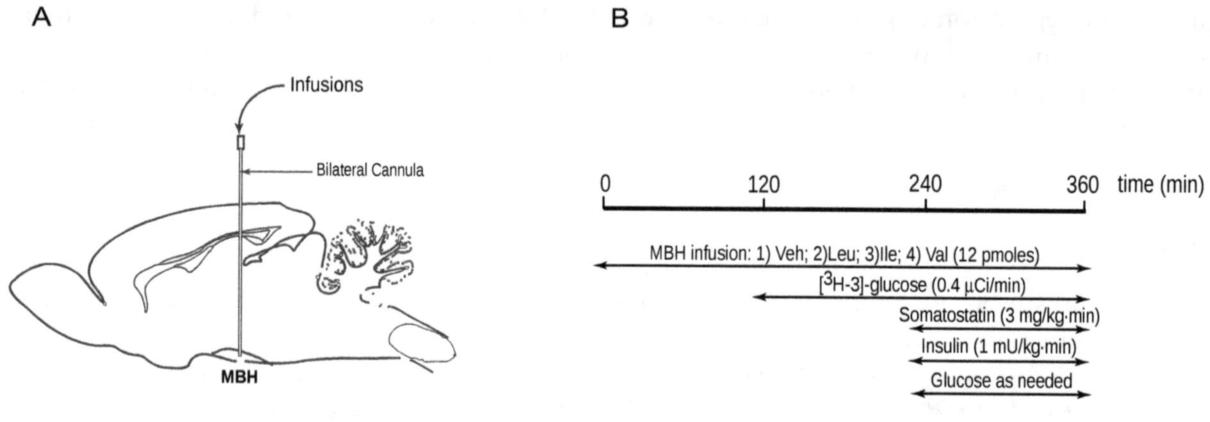

Figure 1. Experimental procedures. (**A**) Schematic of rat brain (sagittal view) with bilateral cannula implanted stereotactically for infusions into the mediobasal hypothalamus (MBH); (**B**) Time-line for *in vivo* central infusions of branched-chain amino acids (BCAAs) during euglycemic pancreatic clamp protocol with isotopic glucose tracer.

2.2. *Analytical Procedures and Calculations*

Plasma glucose was measured using an Analox instrument (Analox Instruments USA Inc., Lunenburg, MA, USA). The radioactivity of [3-^{3}H] glucose in plasma was measured from supernatants of $Ba(OH)_2$ and from $ZnSO_4$ precipitates (Somogyi procedure) of plasma samples after each was evaporated to dryness to remove tritiated water. The rate of glucose uptake and endogenous glucose production were calculated as previously described [26].

2.3. *Statistical Analysis*

All data values are expressed as mean ± S.E.M. of the indicated number of experiments. Statistical comparisons were assessed by unpaired Student's *t* test or analysis of variance (ANOVA) followed by the Tukey HSD test. We used the customary threshold of $p < 0.05$ to declare statistical significance.

3. Results

We first asked if increasing the local levels of isoleucine or valine in the MBH of rats modifies circulating glucose levels. To answer this question we performed intrahypothalamic infusions of these BCAAs under basal conditions and measured blood glucose during the course of the infusion. As predicted, both isoleucine and valine individually decreased the plasma levels of glucose compared to vehicle-infused control animals (Figure 2). Thus isoleucine and valine replicated the glucose-lowering action of leucine.

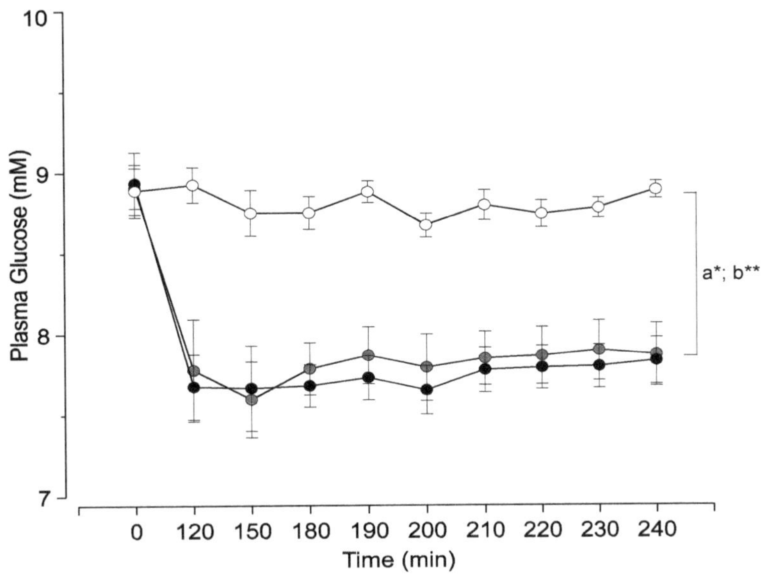

Figure 2. Effect of central isoleucine and valine on circulating glucose levels. Symbols (circles): white, vehicle; black, isoleucine; gray, valine. Each point represents the mean ± s.e.m for 6–8 individual experiments. * a, $p < 0.05$ Isoleucine *vs.* control; ** b, $p < 0.05$ Valine *vs.* control.

To determine if central isoleucine or valine modulates hepatic glucose metabolism, we performed pancreatic insulin clamps and glucose kinetics analysis in the same animals. During the clamps, when glucose and insulin levels in circulation are kept constant, both isoleucine and valine individually produced a marked increase in the glucose infusion rate (GIR) required to maintain euglycemia compared to vehicle (Figure 3A). Kinetic analysis revealed that the increase of GIR was the result of a marked inhibition of EGP (Figure 3B,C), since peripheral glucose utilization (GU) did not change (Figure 3D). The individual effect of isoleucine and valine on all these kinetic parameters was comparable in magnitude to that reported for leucine [16] at the equimolar dose (12 *p*moles) used here. Taken together these results indicate that isoleucine and valine fully replicated the effect of leucine on liver glucose metabolism. On close examination, the individual potency of isoleucine to inhibit EGP was approximately the same as for leucine but somewhat lower than for valine.

Short-term (3-day) feeding of rodents with a diet enriched in saturated fat (HFD) induces insulin resistance in the absence of changes in body weight compared to regular chow (RC) fed animals [27,28]. To examine the consequences of acutely-induced insulin resistance on the ability of BCAAs to inhibit EGP, we subjected rats to three days of HFD feeding and repeated our measurements during central infusions of leucine. We used leucine because its effects on glucose metabolism have been previously characterized in detail by our group [16]. During pancreatic clamps, acute insulin resistance was manifested by decreased GIR (RC = 2.3 ± 0.6 *vs.* HFD = 0.7 ± 0.2 mg/kg·min; $p < 0.05$) due to an increase of EGP (RC = 9.9 ± 0.4 *vs.* HFD = 11.6 ± 0.6 mg/kg·min; $p < 0.05$) without change in GU (RC = 12.3 ± 0.7 *vs.* HFD = 11.9 ± 0.5 mg/kg·min). Next, as shown in Figure 4A, animals treated with HFD required remarkably less glucose infusion to maintain appropriate plasma glucose levels than animals treated with regular chow (not insulin resistant) when infused centrally with leucine.

Analysis of the clamp tracer data revealed that the ability of leucine to reduce EGP was markedly attenuated in these HFD treated animals (Figure 4B,C). Importantly, there was no change in GU (Figure 4D), indicating that all the effect was essentially hepatic. In summary, these results indicate that the short-term consumption of HFD markedly blunts the glucoregulatory action of leucine.

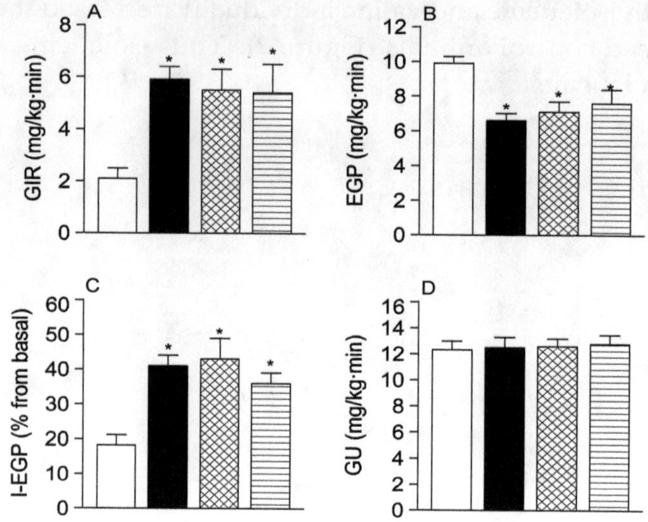

Figure 3. *In vivo* comparison of the central action of isoleucine, valine, and leucine on glucose kinetics during pancreatic insulin clamps. (**A**) Glucose infusion rate (GIR) to maintain euglycemia; (**B**) Endogenous glucose production (EGP); (**C**) Inhibition of EGP by insulin (I-EGP); (**D**) Peripheral glucose utilization (GU). White bars, vehicle; black bars, leucine; check-filled bars, isoleucine; striped bars, valine. Each bar represents the mean ± s.e.m for 6–8 individual experiments. * $p < 0.05$ *vs*. control.

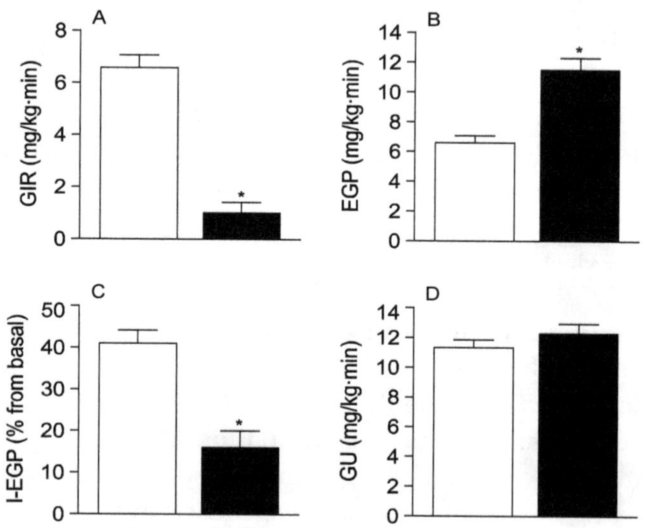

Figure 4. Impact of high-fat diet (HFD) feeding on the central glucoregulatory action of leucine. (**A**) Glucose infusion rate (GIR) to maintain euglycemia; (**B**) Endogenous glucose production (EGP); (**C**) Inhibition of EGP by insulin (I-EGP); (**D**) Peripheral glucose utilization (GU). White bars, regular chow-fed (control) animals; black bars, HFD-fed animals. Each bar represents the mean ± s.e.m for 6 individual experiments. * $p < 0.05$ *vs*. control.

4. Discussion

In the current studies, our measurements of whole body glucose kinetics during pancreatic clamps showed that isoleucine and valine each individually modified the main parameters in a very similar way: increased GIR, decreased EGP, and no change in peripheral GU. At an equimolar dose, the magnitude of their effects were comparable to those of leucine. These findings strongly support our hypothesis that all BCAAs are capable of signalling in the MBH through a common upstream metabolic mechanism. Although the goal of our work was to determine whether or not isoleucine and valine had central glucoregulatory activity rather than studying the mechanisms, it would be appropriate to discuss the possibilities. We think that it is the metabolic fate of these BCAAs that allows them to signal in the MBH. In the case of isoleucine, the explanation seems straightforward because this amino acid is directly converted to acetyl-CoA, which can then be used to generate malonyl-CoA. More intriguing, though, is the effect of valine, since this amino acid is not directly metabolized to acetyl-CoA but rather to propionyl-CoA. This metabolite is converted to succinyl-CoA, which then enters the tricarboxylic acid (TCA) cycle, a feature that makes it a glucogenic amino acid. As a glucogenic AA, valine is the second example of its kind, after proline [17], found to modulate glucose metabolism by acting in the hypothalamus. Interestingly, the glucogenic AA histidine was recently shown to inhibit liver glucose production when delivered in the third ventricle of rats, suggesting that it acts in the hypothalamus [29]. However, in contrast with proline, histidine requires binding to histamine receptors rather than its metabolism in the brain to modify liver glucose fluxes. More importantly, we have shown that physiologically relevant elevations of the circulating levels of leucine or proline modulate hepatic glucose metabolism *in vivo* [16,17]. Similarly, it is possible that physiological elevations of isoleucine and valine also regulate circulating glucose levels, but further studies are required to confirm (or rule out) this idea. Several studies in rodents appear to support a role for BCAAs in the improvement of glucose metabolism reported here. For example, dietary leucine supplementation improves glucose metabolism and prevents obesity in various mouse models [30,31]. Furthermore, mice lacking BCAT in the brain display high circulating levels of leucine in association with a lean phenotype and enhanced insulin sensitivity [32]. Interestingly, recent reports of studies in humans have identified a link between elevated levels of circulating BCAAs and the development of insulin resistance or diabetes [33,34]. However, the details of such an association are not clear, and therefore it is currently unknown how the elevated levels of BCAAs are connected to the development of these disorders of glucose metabolism. Interestingly, in one of these studies [33], the administration of BCAA to HFD-fed rodents induced insulin resistance while the administration of BCAA alone did not. These results not only indicate that BCAAs are not directly involved in the development of insulin resistance, but they also coincide with our report in that HFD feeding modifies the metabolic actions of BCAAs in a detrimental fashion. Thus, our current studies showing a blunting of central glucoregulation by leucine after short-term HFD feeding allows us to add amino acids, or leucine at least, to the list of nutrients whose hypothalamic sensing is nutritionally regulated. In this regard, our previous studies showing that molecular disruption of leucine sensing in the MBH precipitates the development of hyperglycemia in rats fed with a high-protein diet [16] further supports the idea that the faltering of central leucine sensing may contribute to disease development.

5. Conclusions

The MBH responded to a local increase of isoleucine or valine with an inhibition of EGP, which mainly reflects glucose production by the liver. At an equimolar dose, the magnitude of the individual glucoregulatory effect of either isoleucine or valine was similar to that of leucine. Importantly, insulin resistance induced by short-term high fat feeding markedly attenuated the central glucoregulatory effect of leucine. In summary, we conclude that not only leucine but also circulating isoleucine and valine may participate in the acute postprandial regulation of glycemia. Furthermore, consumption of diets rich in saturated fat incapacitates this centrally-mediated glucoregulation.

Acknowledgments: This work was supported by a grant from the National Institutes of Health (DK45024) and an Ajinomoto Amino Acid Research Program grant to R.G.-J. We thank Bing Liu for performing the animal vascular surgeries.

Author Contributions: I.A.-C. performed the experiments, analyzed the data and wrote the manuscript; Y.S. performed the experiments and analyzed the data; R.G.-J. conceived and designed the experiments, analyzed the data and wrote the manuscript.

References

1. Eaton, S.B.; Konner, M. Paleolithic nutrition. A consideration of its nature and current implications. *N. Engl. J. Med.* **1985**, *312*, 283–289.
2. Hill, J.O.; Peters, J.C. Environmental contributions to the obesity epidemic. *Science* **1998**, *280*, 1371–1374.
3. Ukropec, J.; Sebokova, E.; Klimes, I. Nutrient sensing, leptin and insulin action. *Arch. Physiol. Biochem.* **2001**, *109*, 38–51.
4. Obici, S.; Rossetti, L. Minireview: Nutrient sensing and the regulation of insulin action and energy balance. *Endocrinology* **2003**, *144*, 5172–5178.
5. Lindsley, J.E.; Rutter, J. Nutrient sensing and metabolic decisions. *Comp. Biochem. Physiol. B Biochem. Mol. Biol.* **2004**, *139*, 543–559.
6. Schwartz, G.J. Biology of eating behavior in obesity. *Obes. Res.* **2004**, *12* (Suppl. 2), 102S–106S.
7. Rossetti, L.; Rothman, D.L.; DeFronzo, R.A.; Shulman, G.I. Effect of dietary protein on *in vivo* insulin action and liver glycogen repletion. *Am. J. Physiol.* **1989**, *257*, E212–E219.
8. Patti, M.E.; Brambilla, E.; Luzi, L.; Landaker, E.J.; Kahn, C.R. Bidirectional modulation of insulin action by amino acids. *J. Clin. Investig.* **1998**, *101*, 1519–1529.
9. Gannon, M.C.; Nuttall, F.Q.; Saeed, A.; Jordan, K.; Hoover, H. An increase in dietary protein improves the blood glucose response in persons with type 2 diabetes. *Am. J. Clin. Nutr.* **2003**, *78*, 734–741.
10. Nuttall, F.Q.; Gannon, M.C.; Saeed, A.; Jordan, K.; Hoover, H. The metabolic response of subjects with type 2 diabetes to a high-protein, weight-maintenance diet. *J. Clin. Endocrinol. Metab.* **2003**, *88*, 3577–3583.
11. Tremblay, F.; Krebs, M.; Dombrowski, L.; Brehm, A.; Bernroider, E.; Roth, E.; Nowotny, P.; Waldhausl, W.; Marette, A.; Roden, M. Overactivation of S6 kinase 1 as a cause of human insulin resistance during increased amino acid availability. *Diabetes* **2005**, *54*, 2674–2684.
12. Promintzer, M.; Krebs, M. Effects of dietary protein on glucose homeostasis. *Curr. Opin. Clin. Nutr. Metab. Care* **2006**, *9*, 463–468.
13. Tremblay, F.; Lavigne, C.; Jacques, H.; Marette, A. Role of dietary proteins and amino acids in the pathogenesis of insulin resistance. *Annu. Rev. Nutr.* **2007**, *27*, 293–310.
14. Cota, D.; Proulx, K.; Smith, K.A.; Kozma, S.C.; Thomas, G.; Woods, S.C.; Seeley, R.J. Hypothalamic mTOR signaling regulates food intake. *Science* **2006**, *312*, 927–930.
15. Blouet, C.; Jo, Y.H.; Li, X.; Schwartz, G.J. Mediobasal hypothalamic leucine sensing regulates food intake through activation of a hypothalamus-brainstem circuit. *J. Neurosci.* **2009**, *29*, 8302–8311.
16. Su, Y.; Lam, T.K.; He, W.; Pocai, A.; Bryan, J.; Aguilar-Bryan, L.; Gutierrez-Juarez, R. Hypothalamic leucine metabolism regulates liver glucose production. *Diabetes* **2012**, *61*, 85–93.
17. Arrieta-Cruz, I.; Su, Y.; Knight, C.M.; Lam, T.K.T.; Gutiérrez-Juárez, R. Evidence for a role of proline and hypothalamic astrocytes in the regulation of glucose metabolism in rats. *Diabetes* **2013**, *62*, 1152–1158.
18. Suryawan, A.; Hawes, J.W.; Harris, R.A.; Shimomura, Y.; Jenkins, A.E.; Hutson, S.M. A molecular model of human branched-chain amino acid metabolism. *Am. J. Clin. Nutr.* **1998**, *68*, 72–81.
19. Brosnan, J.T.; Brosnan, M.E. Branched-chain amino acids: Enzyme and substrate regulation. *J. Nutr.* **2006**, *136*, 207S–211S.
20. Morgan, K.; Obici, S.; Rossetti, L. Hypothalamic responses to long-chain fatty acids are nutritionally regulated. *J. Biol. Chem.* **2004**, *279*, 31139–31148.
21. Lam, T.K.; Gutierrez-Juarez, R.; Pocai, A.; Rossetti, L. Regulation of blood glucose by hypothalamic pyruvate metabolism. *Science* **2005**, *309*, 943–947.
22. Pocai, A.; Lam, T.K.; Obici, S.; Gutierrez-Juarez, R.; Muse, E.D.; Arduini, A.; Rossetti, L. Restoration of hypothalamic lipid sensing normalizes energy and glucose homeostasis in overfed rats. *J. Clin. Investig.* **2006**, *116*, 1081–1091.
23. Lam, T.K.; Gutierrez-Juarez, R.; Pocai, A.; Bhanot, S.; Tso, P.; Schwartz, G.J.; Rossetti, L. Brain glucose metabolism controls the hepatic secretion of triglyceride-rich lipoproteins. *Nat. Med.* **2007**, *13*, 171–180.
24. Paxinos, G.; Watson, C. *The Rat Brain in Stereotaxic Coordinates*; Elsevier: Amsterdam, The Netherlands, 2007.

25. Gutierrez-Juarez, R.; Obici, S.; Rossetti, L. Melanocortin-independent effects of leptin on hepatic glucose fluxes. *J. Biol. Chem.* **2004**, *279*, 49704–49715.
26. Liu, L.; Karkanias, G.B.; Morales, J.C.; Hawkins, M.; Barzilai, N.; Wang, J.; Rossetti, L. Intracerebroventricular leptin regulates hepatic but not peripheral glucose fluxes. *J. Biol. Chem.* **1998**, *273*, 31160–31167.
27. Kraegen, E.W.; Clark, P.W.; Jenkins, A.B.; Daley, E.A.; Chisholm, D.J.; Storlien, L.H. Development of muscle insulin resistance after liver insulin resistance in high-fat-fed rats. *Diabetes* **1991**, *40*, 1397–1403.
28. Wang, J.; Obici, S.; Morgan, K.; Barzilai, N.; Feng, Z.; Rossetti, L. Overfeeding rapidly induces leptin and insulin resistance. *Diabetes* **2001**, *50*, 2786–2791.
29. Kimura, K.; Nakamura, Y.; Inaba, Y.; Matsumoto, M.; Kido, Y.; Asahara, S.I.; Matsuda, T.; Watanabe, H.; Maeda, A.; Inagaki, F.; *et al.* Histidine augments the suppression of hepatic glucose production by central insulin action. *Diabetes* **2013**, *62*, 2266–2277.
30. Zhang, Y.; Guo, K.; LeBlanc, R.E.; Loh, D.; Schwartz, G.J.; Yu, Y.H. Increasing dietary leucine intake reduces diet-induced obesity and improves glucose and cholesterol metabolism in mice via multimechanisms. *Diabetes* **2007**, *56*, 1647–1654.
31. Guo, K.; Yu, Y.H.; Hou, J.; Zhang, Y. Chronic leucine supplementation improves glycemic control in etiologically distinct mouse models of obesity and diabetes mellitus. *Nutr. Metab. (Lond.)* **2010**, *7*, 57.
32. She, P.; Reid, T.M.; Bronson, S.K.; Vary, T.C.; Hajnal, A.; Lynch, C.J.; Hutson, S.M. Disruption of BCATm in mice leads to increased energy expenditure associated with the activation of a futile protein turnover cycle. *Cell Metab.* **2007**, *6*, 181–194.
33. Newgard, C.B.; An, J.; Bain, J.R.; Muehlbauer, M.J.; Stevens, R.D.; Lien, L.F.; Haqq, A.M.; Shah, S.H.; Arlotto, M.; Slentz, C.A.; *et al.* A branched-chain amino acid-related metabolic signature that differentiates obese and lean humans and contributes to insulin resistance. *Cell Metab.* **2009**, *9*, 311–326.
34. Wang, T.J.; Larson, M.G.; Vasan, R.S.; Cheng, S.; Rhee, E.P.; McCabe, E.; Lewis, G.D.; Fox, C.S.; Jacques, P.F.; Fernandez, C.; *et al.* Metabolite profiles and the risk of developing diabetes. *Nat. Med.* **2011**, *17*, 448–453.

12

The Potential Protective Action of Vitamin D in Hepatic Insulin Resistance and Pancreatic Islet Dysfunction in Type 2 Diabetes Mellitus

Po Sing Leung

School of Biomedical Sciences, Faculty of Medicine, The Chinese University of Hong Kong, Shatin, Hong Kong, China; psleung@cuhk.edu.hk

Abstract: Vitamin D deficiency (*i.e.*, hypovitaminosis D) is associated with increased insulin resistance, impaired insulin secretion, and poorly controlled glucose homeostasis, and thus is correlated with the risk of metabolic diseases, including type 2 diabetes mellitus (T2DM). The liver plays key roles in glucose and lipid metabolism, and its dysregulation leads to abnormalities in hepatic glucose output and triglyceride accumulation. Meanwhile, the pancreatic islets are constituted in large part by insulin-secreting β cells. Consequently, islet dysfunction, such as occurs in T2DM, produces hyperglycemia. In this review, we provide a critical appraisal of the modulatory actions of vitamin D in hepatic insulin sensitivity and islet insulin secretion, and we discuss the potential roles of a local vitamin D signaling in regulating hepatic and pancreatic islet functions. This information provides a scientific basis for establishing the benefits of the maintenance, or dietary manipulation, of adequate vitamin D status in the prevention and management of obesity-induced T2DM and non-alcoholic fatty liver disease.

Keywords: calcitriol; glucose homeostasis; HepG2; hypovitaminosis D; insulin secretion; lipid metabolism

1. Introduction

The liver is a vital organ for metabolic homeostasis, controlling glucose uptake-storage-generation and processing about one third of consumed glucose, and it is a key target for insulin action [1]. Insulin controls lipogenesis (fatty acid and triglycerides biosynthesis) and restrains hepatic gluconeogenesis (glucose production) in the liver. Accordingly, insulin sensitivity has been closely associated with rates of hepatic gluconeogenesis and lipid accumulation [2,3]. Hepatic insulin resistance leads to severely dysregulated glucose homeostasis, resulting in or contributing to hyperglycemia, which then further worsens hepatic insulin insensitivity. This negative cycle progresses toward a pathologic state of hepatic dysfunction and eventually liver disease. Notwithstanding these observations, it is unclear whether hepatic insulin resistance is a cause or consequence of type 2 diabetes mellitus (T2DM), and the underlying mechanism(s) mediating the relationship between hepatic insulin resistance and T2DM remain elusive. In addition to conventional regulatory factors (e.g., genes encoding glycolytic and lipogenic enzymes), changes in life style and nutritional factors have garnered ever increasing attention in the development of preventative and therapeutic approaches to both T2DM and non-alcoholic fatty liver disease (NAFLD). In this context, recent investigations into the interactions of nutritional factors, such as vitamin D, in T2DM-related diseases and their management are of particular interest in terms of both clinical and socio-economic impacts [4–6].

The endocrine pancreas (functionally distinct from the exocrine portions important for production of digestive enzymes) contains insulin-secreting pancreatic islets [7]. Dysfunction or loss of beta cells in pancreatic islets leads to hyperglycemia and hyperlipidemia, two predominant indicators of T2DM [8].

Islet physiology is finely modulated by a myriad of factors, including vitamin D. Vitamin D deficiency, referred to clinically as hypovitaminosis D, impairs insulin secretion and increases insulin resistance, key features of T2DM and related metabolic diseases [9,10]. Interestingly, glucose-stimulated insulin response experiments suggest that early vitamin D supplementation may be protective of insulin secretory function, whereas late supplementation, after vitamin D deficiency and T2DM have been established, may be relatively ineffective [11]. However, the precise modulatory roles of vitamin D in hepatic and islet functions have not been determined.

The purpose of the present review is to provide a critical appraisal of our current knowledge related to the protective effects of vitamin D on hepatic metabolism and islet function, particularly in the context of T2DM and obesity-associated diseases. Such information will be important for informing healthcare providers and patients about the potential benefits of vitamin D supplementation, as a food additive or nutraceutical. In particular, this work focuses on the potential of vitamin D supplementation to oppose the development or worsening of obesity-related diseases, such as T2DM and NAFLD, and thus provide a cost-effective measure for improving hepatic and pancreatic islet functions.

2. Vitamin D Synthesis and Metabolism

The pathophysiology of the insulin-resistant state and islet dysfunction remains enigmatic. Currently, patients with insulin resistance and islet dysfunction are treated with insulin sensitizers and secretagogues, which work mainly by improving glucose disposal via skeletal muscle and suppressing hepatic gluconeogenesis, and by stimulating pancreatic beta-cell insulin secretion, respectively [12]. Mechanism-based studies of the factors that influence insulin secretion and resistance, such as niacin [13,14] and vitamin D (*vide infra*), are needed to identify novel therapeutic targets.

Classically, vitamin D is known for its involvement in the regulation of calcium and bone homeostasis. There are two major forms of vitamin D, namely cholecalciferol (vitamin D_3) and ergocalciferol (vitamin D_2). The primary source of vitamin D in humans is from endogenous biosynthesis in skin cells, a critical step of which hydroxylation of 7-dehydrocholesterol into cholecalciferol is catalyzed by ultraviolet radiation from sunlight [15]. Additionally, cholecalciferol can be found in dietary sources, including fish, egg yolk, beef, and lichen, while ergocalciferol can be found in edible mushrooms and alfalfa. Endogenous and dietary vitamin D molecules, which are biologically inactive themselves, are transported systemically in chylomicrons and converted into the metabolically active 1,25-dihydroxyvitamin D ($1,25(OH)_2D_3$) via a sequence of reactions. In the liver, vitamin D is converted into 25-hydroxyvitamin D ($25(OH)D_3$), the clinically monitored form of plasma vitamin D, by the liver-derived enzyme 25-hydroxylase. Subsequently, $25(OH)D_3$, which is considered a prehormone, is then further hydroxylated to biologically active $1,25(OH)_2D_3$ by kidney-derived 1-α-hydroxylase [16].

The active form of vitamin D, $1,25(OH)_2D_3$, binds vitamin D receptors (VDRs) and activates various transcription factors. For example, activated VDR forms a heterodimer with retinoic X receptor (RXR), and thereby participates in stimulating the RXR nuclear pathway [17]. Indeed, classical vitamin D response elements and other response sites are broadly distributed and critical for pancreatic beta-cell and immune system functions [18–21]. Such findings suggest that manipulations of VDR signaling pathways might be physiologically relevant for the management of diabetes. Figure 1 is a summary of vitamin D synthesis and metabolism, as well as the modulatory action on islet function.

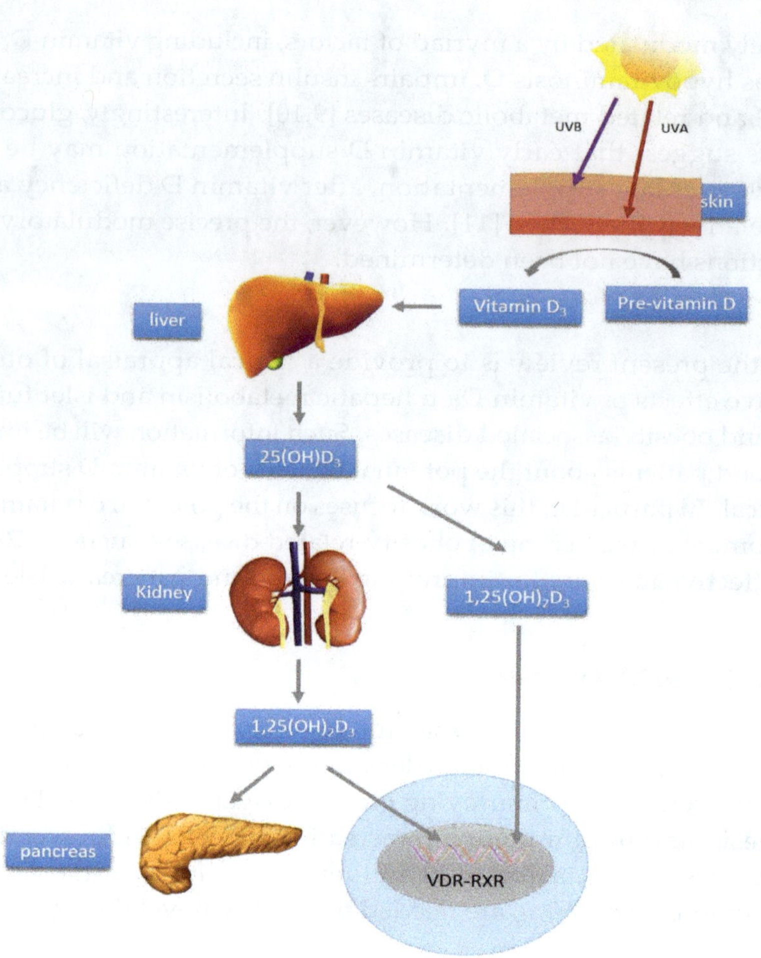

Figure 1. Schematic representation of vitamin D synthesis and metabolism in relation to regulation of pancreatic islet function and survival.

3. Vitamin D and T2DM

Hypovitaminosis D has been correlated with increased risks of a wide variety of chronic diseases. The major causes of hypovitaminosis D are sunlight deprivation (such as by sunscreen, melanin, latitude, and winter), medications and supplements, and malabsorption (such as in Crohn's and celiac diseases, cystic fibrosis, and liver disease). Maintenance of plasma 25(OH)D_3 above 30 ng/mL is recommended for optimal health; some may require dietary supplementation and/or increased exposure to sunlight to attain this level [15]. Of great interest for our present focus, hypovitaminosis D has been reported to impair islet insulin secretion and to increase peripheral insulin resistance, two major risk factors for progression to T2DM; furthermore, hypovitaminosis D is predictive of abnormalities in most of the variables monitored in patients with metabolic syndromes, including T2DM itself [22,23]. It is worthwhile emphasizing that the clinical association between hypovitaminosis and insulin resistance/T2DM might not be a cause-and-effect relationship and that an increase in circulating 25(OH)D_3 concentration might not necessarily reduce the onset of, or progression to, T2DM. In this context, there are considerable randomized clinical trials showing disassociation between plasma levels of active 25(OH)D_3 and the incidence of T2DM, as recently exemplified by a mendelian randomization-derived estimates for glycemic control [24]. In fact, maintenance of adequate vitamin D status and/or its high-dose supplementation have not convincingly displayed long-term glycemic control for human T2DM in several clinical trial studies [25–28]. Such negative studies or discrepancies have yet to be validated by further large-scale clinical studies with large sample sizes, different study designs (cross-sectional and interventional studies, and different populations), as well as by intensive mechanism-driven basic science studies in the future.

T2DM, which is defined as hyperglycemia of sufficient magnitude to cause detrimental effects, results when insulin resistance develops and is followed by dysregulation of insulin secretory responses, with loss of beta-cell mass [29]. Amelioration of both insulin resistance and islet dysfunction are, therefore, both of paramount importance for preventing and treating T2DM. Chronic hyperglycemia and hyperlipidemia are associated with dramatic upregulation of lipid formation and accumulation in the liver and pancreatic islets. Excessive hepatic lipid accumulation causes endoplasmic reticulum (ER) stress and inflammation (lipotoxicity), as well as reduced insulin sensitivity [30,31]. Meanwhile, an increase in intra-islet lipid accumulation impairs glucose-stimulated insulin secretion, and promotes islet inflammation and ER stress, ultimately leading to beta-cell apoptosis and islet failure [32].

Given the importance of vitamin D status for the maintenance of a physiologically healthy liver and pancreas, together with the known involvement of hepatic and pancreatic pathophysiology in T2DM pathogenesis, vitamin D and the VDR represent an area of great therapeutic interest. Identification of agents that can reduce abnormalities of hepatic and islet metabolism simultaneously could yield a substantial advancement in the prevention and treatment of obesity and obesity-related T2DM risk. To this end, there has been a surge of interest in the benefits of maintaining an adequate vitamin D status and the apparent protective mechanism(s) of vitamin D.

4. Vitamin D and Hepatic Metabolism

The liver is a vital organ consisting of functional units called liver lobules, which in turn are composed principally of hepatic cellular plates. The major cell types of the liver are hepatocytes, stellate cells, Kupffer cells, and endothelial cells, with hepatocytes being the functionally predominant cells [1]. As mentioned above, the liver is a major target organ of insulin, wherein insulin regulation helps to maintain glucose homeostasis by making glucose available when it is needed through gluconeogenesis and glycogenolysis, and by storing glucose through glycogenesis when it is present in excess [1]. Gluconeogenesis rate is determined primarily by the transcriptional level of the genes encoding two gluconeogenic enzymes, namely phosphoenolpyruvate carboxykinase (PEPCK) and glucose-6-phosphatase (G6PK) [33]. The opposing process of glycogenesis is mediated by glycogen synthase (GS); GS activity is promoted when glycogen synthase kinase 3 (GSK-3) activity is inhibited [34].

Glucose and lipid metabolism are critical inter-related components of glucose homeostasis. When glucose intake exceeds storage and oxidation capacities, it is converted to fat (*de novo* lipogenesis); however, excessive hepatic lipid causes inflammation and hepatic insulin resistance [35]. Interestingly, numerous studies have suggested that ER stress, which is caused by an imbalance between protein folding stress and the processing capacity of the ER, is closely associated with metabolic disorders. In particular, hepatic ER stress promotes hepatic glucose production, lipogenesis, and insulin resistance in obese and diabetic states [36]. Hence, maintenance of normal hepatic cellular metabolic function appears to be indispensable for preventing the development of hepatic insulin resistance and T2DM.

The metabolic regulating enzyme AMP-activated protein kinase (AMPK) is the therapeutic target of several anti-diabetic agents, such as metformin [37] and adiponectin [38]. It is activated by phosphorylation via either the serine/threonine kinase 11 (a.k.a. liver kinase B1), or the calcium/calmodulin protein kinase kinase beta (CaMKKβ) pathway [39]. The anti-diabetic actions of hepatic AMPK activation are attributed to attenuation of lipogenesis and gluconeogenesis, as well as promotion of lipid oxidation and glycolysis [40]. Additionally, activation of hepatic AMPK has been reported to inhibit Foxo1 activity [41], which results in reduced hepatic ER stress, and to alleviate hepatic steatosis and insulin resistance [42,43]. Furthermore, prior clinical studies have shown that low serum concentrations of $25(OH)D_3$ are independently associated with liver steatosis [44].

Meanwhile, hypovitaminosis D has been proposed to be a causative factor of NAFLD [45]. Although liver steatosis is related to progression of hepatic insulin resistance, no specific lipid has been reported to be both necessary and sufficient for development of liver steatosis. NAFLD appears to involve the accumulation of a variety of lipids, and the levels of multiple lipids can be used as markers of insulin resistance status [46]. Excessive accumulation of certain lipids, such as diacylglycerol and acyl CoA, may interfere with glucose generation and has been linked to risk of hepatic insulin resistance [46–49]. Because hepatic glucose production is tightly regulated by the availability of the enzymes PEPCK and G6PK, and further modulated by the availability of fructose-1,6-bisphosphatase and pyruvate carboxylase [50], down-regulation of these enzymes might reduce abnormal gluconeogenesis in T2DM and ameliorate hepatic insulin resistance.

The research summarized above has led us to propose that vitamin D bioavailability may affect hepatic lipogenesis and gluconeogenesis, and if so, vitamin D supplementation may be used to modulate hepatic insulin resistance and thus reduce T2DM severity. Mechanistically, such effects may be mediated by various vitamin D-regulated pathways, such as AMPK-calmodulin and/or Akt/Notch signaling, as well as through indirect effects on ER stress. In light of the aforementioned negative association between vitamin D status and severity of NAFLD, a well-recognized risk factor for insulin resistance and T2DM, we are now investigating the direct effects of vitamin D on hepatic lipid and glucose production. We obtained preliminary data recently indicating that, at high dosages, calcitriol (the active hormonal metabolite of vitamin D) can ameliorate abnormal hepatic lipid and glucose metabolism in both *in vitro* (1–10 nM in HepG2 cells) and *in vivo* (0.5–2.5 mg/kg for 2 days in db/db mice) models of insulin resistance without any signs of toxicity (unpublished data). Furthermore, we conducted mechanistic experiments showing that increases in cytosolic calcitriol in HepG2 cells activated Ca^{2+}/CaMKKβ/AMPK pathways, and that the activation of these pathways contributed to calcitriol's lipid and glucose regulatory effects.

The involvement of AMPK signaling in calcitriol-mediated metabolic effects is not surprising given that AMPK is the therapeutic target of anti-diabetic medications (e.g., metformin) [37], as well as a target of the obesity regulating endogenous hormone adiponectin, which acts to alleviate insulin resistance [38]. Further study is needed to corroborate these findings, which suggest that calcitriol, when at above-physiological plasma concentrations, can reduce hepatic triglyceride accumulation and glucose output, at least in part, through activation of Ca^{2+}/CaMKKβ/AMPK signaling under insulin-resistant conditions. Importantly, unlike its inactive metabolic precursor cholecalciferol (vitamin D_3), calcitriol does not accumulate in adipose tissue or exert long-lasting effects. Thus, the potential for toxicity that exists with cholecalciferol is much less of a concern with calcitriol, owing to its rapid onset and offset of action. If confirmed, these preliminary data may provide an avenue to supporting the use of vitamin D, at least, as an adjuvant for the management of insulin resistance, NAFLD, and T2DM. Figure 2 is a summary that proposes the direct action of vitamin D in regulating hepatic triglyceride and glucose metabolism.

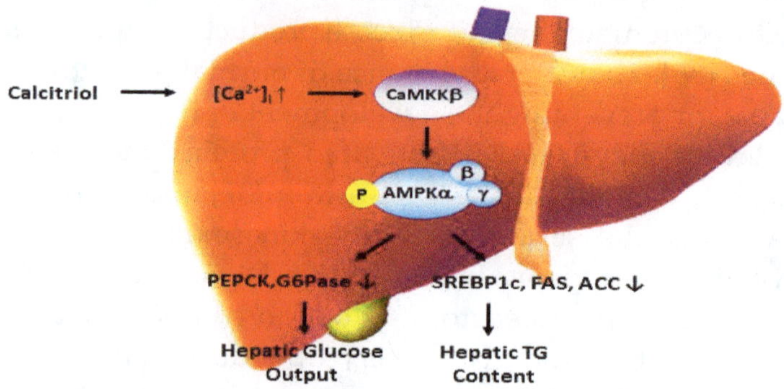

Figure 2. Model of active vitamin D regulation of hepatic triglyceride accumulation and glucose output in a diabetic state.

5. Vitamin D and Pancreatic Islet Function

Emerging data from physiological and genetic studies indicate that islet dysfunction and loss of beta-cell mass are the key determinants of whether an insulin-resistant state will progress to frank hyperglycemia/hyperlipidemia and diabetes; insulin resistance alone is insufficient to predict T2DM [51,52]. High circulating concentrations of glucose and fatty acids in diabetic states are attributed to loss of islet function and mass due to glucolipotoxicity, a process involving oxidative stress, ER stress, and inflammation [53]. Hence, the development of therapeutic agents that can protect islets from glucolipotoxicity could provide a much needed mode of improving the management of T2DM.

Several signaling pathways have been reported to play critical roles in insulin secretion as well as beta-cell growth and survival. For example, activation of Akt is closely associated with beta-cell survival [54–56] and promotes compensatory beta-cell growth in the insulin-resistant state [57]. Akt activation-induced phosphorylation inhibits GSK3 and Foxo1 which, in turn, reverses the toxic effects of glucose and fatty acids on beta-cells [58,59]. In addition, fatty acid-induced ER stress in islets has been linked with decreased Akt activity, and with activation of c-Jun NH_2-terminal kinase (JNK), which, ultimately, contributes to beta-cell apoptosis [60]. These findings lend support to the notion that Akt is a promising target for preservation of islet function and cell mass. In this context, recent studies have demonstrated that angiotensin (1–7), an active component of the renin-angiotensin system (RAS), modulates insulin resistance in skeletal muscle cells by way of Akt signaling pathway activation [61]. Activation of Akt/JNK pathways is also involved in angiotensin (1–7)-mediated modulation of palmitate-induced islet endothelial cell apoptosis [62]. Interestingly, it has been shown that glucagon-like peptide-1 and angiotensin II can prevent glucolipotoxicity-induced apoptosis in pancreatic beta cells additively through the insulin receptor substrate-2/phosphoinostide 3-kinase/Akt/FoxO1 signaling pathways [63]. Hence, it is plausible that other regulators, such as vitamin D (*vide supra*) might, like RAS ligands, exert islet-protective effects through activation of Akt signaling. Further work is needed to examine potential vitamin D-RAS axis interactions in the regulation of islet function and beta-cell survival.

Given the importance of hepatic and pancreatic islet functions in the pathogenesis of insulin resistance and T2DM, we are investigating promising factors and how they, alone or in combination, influence islet function under various pathological and physiological conditions. Of great interest in this context is the local pancreatic RAS and its potential involvement in islet function and survival in T2DM [64]. Previously, we demonstrated that inhibition of islet RAS signaling (*i.e.*, angiotensin II receptor type 1 activation) increased glucose-induced insulin secretion and improved glycemic control [65,66]. Mechanisms proposed for these effects include enhancement of intra-islet blood perfusion [67], reduction of oxidative stress [68], and improvement of the beta-cell proliferation-to-apoptosis balance [69]. Meanwhile, vitamin D is necessary for normal islet insulin secretion [9–11] and it is also a negative endocrine regulator of the RAS, suppressing renal renin secretion [70,71]. Moreover, hypovitaminosis D leads to defective insulin secretion, reduced glucose homeostasis, and increased risk of T2DM in all age bands [72,73], whereas increased pancreatic islet RAS activity in hyperglycemia impairs islet function and survival under hyperglycemic conditions [74]. Given these vitamin D-RAS interactions in islet survival, we set out to examine the potential modulatory action of vitamin D on regulation of islet function and survival through suppression of pancreatic islet RAS [74,75].

Toward this aim, we examined in *ex vivo* experiments how calcitriol (bioactive vitamin D metabolite) affects RAS component expression in islets from normal control, hypovitaminosis D, and VDR knockout mice under physiological and high-glucose conditions. We found that high-glucose–induced upregulation of islet RAS component expression could be prevented and corrected by calcitriol; in corroboration, the VDR knockout mice exhibited overactive islet RAS, compared with that of wild-type mice [76]. On the other hand, the mice with diet-induced hypovitaminosis D developed impaired glucose tolerance and exhibited increased expression RAS components combined with reduced expression of islet function-related genes [76]. Interestingly, we observed in a subsequent study that pharmacological renin inhibition (*i.e.*, aliskiren treatment) without correction of hypovitaminosis D reduced islet RAS hyperactivity, ameliorated islet dysfunction and insulin resistance, and improved glucose tolerance [77].

In summary, treating mice with hypovitaminosis D with RAS inhibitors, without correction of vitamin D deficiency, reduced islet RAS over-activity, ameliorated islet dysfunction and improved glucose tolerance, as predicted. These data indicate that suppression of RAS hyperactivity in a condition of hyperglycemia and hypovitaminosis D is protective against pancreatic islet dysfunction and the development of insulin resistance, thus improving glucose tolerance and glucose homeostasis. If corrected, these findings help to explain the protective role of RAS inhibition against T2DM, as previously reported, and support the use of RAS inhibitors for treating hypertension in people who have, or are at risk of, T2DM. Further work is needed to determine whether alleviation of hypovitaminosis D could work synergistically with RAS inhibition to improve T2DM-related metabolic impairments. In light of these findings, we conclude with Figure 3 that represents a proposed model of how vitamin D regulates pancreatic beta-cell function and survival.

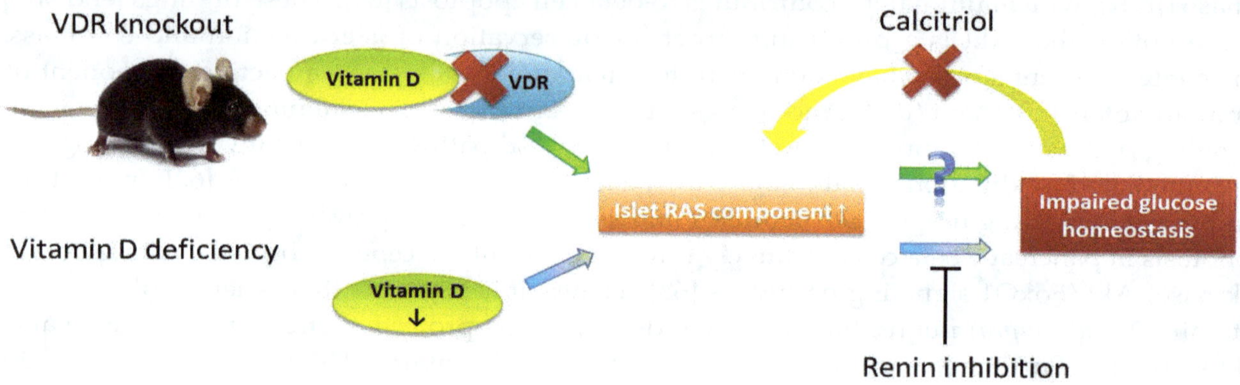

Figure 3. Model of vitamin D in the regulation of pancreatic islet beta-cell function and survival in a diabetic state.

6. Vitamin D and Pancreatic Islet Development

Recent advances in directed differentiation of pancreatic stem cells offer potential for the development of beta-cell replacement therapies for diabetes patients. Unfortunately, however, existing differentiation protocols are complex, time-consuming, and costly; thus there is a desperate need for alternative protocols that can be used to promote beta-cell proliferation, differentiation, and maturation [78]. In this regard, our group has established a system for the isolation and culture of pancreatic progenitor cells (PPCs) derived from human fetal pancreas tissue. These PPCs have a high capacity for proliferation and differentiation when cultured with an appropriate differentiation cocktail; their differentiation can be promoted by morphogens or growth factors related to human pancreatic development, e.g., secreted PDZ domain-containing protein 2 [79,80] and angiotensin II [81], as well as by vitamin A and vitamin D [82]. Vitamin A is a well-established modulator of beta-cell differentiation, and vitamin D is known to affect beta-cell insulin secretion; both vitamin A and vitamin D act through the RXR heterodimerization pathway (*vide supra*) [83–85].

Interestingly, we have demonstrated that the retinoic acid receptor, VDR, and RXR are expressed in first-trimester human fetal PPCs and that all-trans retinoic acid and calcitriol can (each alone) enhance PPC viability [82]. Although further investigations are warranted to elucidate the differentiation properties of PPCs and clarify the roles of vitamin A and vitamin D in islet development and beta-cell differentiation, these data suggest that vitamin A and vitamin D are involved in PPC development and thus should be considered in attempts to develop culture protocols for the development of insulin-secreting islet-like cell clusters (ICC) suitable for clinical transplantation into diabetic patients.

Given the common developmental origins of the liver and pancreas, it is also interesting to note that PPCs can be differentiated in a culture devoid of growth factors by using a microenvironment established by liver stromal cells (LSC) derived from human fetal liver [86]. Specifically, we demonstrated experimentally that a liver stromal cell-induced niche can enhance PPC differentiation into ICCs and enhance ICC functionality. This was the first to report that an LSC-induced niche can enhance ICC differentiation and functionality. Further modifications of the stroma microenvironment may offer an alternative, efficient and cost-effective approach to providing insulin-producing cells for clinical transplantation.

Finally, very recent studies implicated vitamin D in trans-generational risk of metabolic disease. A maternal high-fat diet during pregnancy and lactation was reported to affect hepatic fatty acid metabolism of rat offspring [87]. These animal findings have clinical relevance to obesity-associated diseases in humans and future studies are warranted to examine whether specific plasma fatty acid could be used as an early marker of hepatic dysregulation so as to assist in the identification of offspring that might have a risk of increased adiposity in adulthood. In fact, hypovitaminosis D is closely related to obesity [88] and, in fact, obesity is a causal factor for reduction of serum 25(OH)D levels [89]. These findings suggest that low vitamin D availability due to excessive maternal body fat may contribute to trans-generational impairment of liver fatty acid metabolism [90].

7. Conclusions

Vitamin D might have dual anti-diabetic influences: (1) modulation of hepatic glucose and lipid metabolism; and (2) promotion of pancreatic islet function and survival. Vitamin D could ameliorate hepatic glucose and lipid metabolism abnormalities *in vitro* and *in vivo* through activation of Ca^{2+}/CaMKKβ/AMPK signaling. Furthermore, vitamin D might have a RAS-suppressing influence that may benefit beta-cell function. Taking into consideration some negative data from clinical trial studies, our preliminary results with demonstrated beneficial effects of vitamin D on hepatic and pancreatic functions await to be intensively investigated and validated. In addition, our study findings obtained from cellular and animal models should also be interpreted cautiously since they are not always readily translated into human. However, given the high worldwide prevalence of obesity, T2DM, and related cardio-metabolic sequela that are associated with high healthcare costs and socio-economic implications, the potential protective effects of vitamin D warrants further exploration; if confirmed, vitamin D supplementation may represent a promising, cost-effective preventative and therapeutic agent for the management of obesity-related insulin resistance and diabetes.

Acknowledgments: This work was fully supported by the General Research Fund of the Research Grants Council of the Hong Kong Special Administrative Region, China (Ref. No.: CUHK 14110314), awarded to Po Sing Leung.

References

1. Black, D.D. Hepatobiliary physiology. In *The Gastrointestinal System*; Leung, P.S., Ed.; Springer: Berlin, Germany, 2014; pp. 237–324.
2. Bechmann, L.P.; Hannivoort, R.A.; Gerken, G.; Hotamisligil, G.S.; Trauner, M.; Canbay, A. The interaction of hepatic lipid and glucose metabolism in liver diseases. *J. Hepatol.* **2012**, *56*, 952–964. [CrossRef] [PubMed]
3. Wallace, I.R.; Wallace, H.J.; Mckinley, M.C.; Bell, P.M.; Hunter, S.J. Vitamin D and insulin resistance. *Clin. Endocrinol.* **2015**. [CrossRef] [PubMed]
4. Nwosu, B.U.; Maranda, L. The effects of vitamin D supplementation on hepatic dysfunction, vitamin D status, and glycemic control in children and adolescents with vitamin D deficiency and either type 1 and type 2 diabetes mellitus. *PLoS ONE* **2014**, *9*, e99646. [CrossRef] [PubMed]
5. Minambres, I.; Sanchez-Quesada, J.L.; Vinagre, I.; Sanchez-Hernandez, J.; Urgell, E.; de Leia, A.; Perez, A. Hypovitaminosis D in type 2 diabetes: Relation with features of the metabolic syndrome and glycemic control. *Endocr. Res.* **2015**, *40*, 160–165. [CrossRef] [PubMed]

6. Enciso, P.L.; Wang, L.; Kawahara, Y.; Sakamoto, S.; Shimada, S.; Takeichi, Y.; Takayanagi, R.; Nomura, M. Dietary virtamin D_3 improves postprandial hyperglycemia in aged mice. *Biochem. Biophys. Res. Commun.* **2015**, *461*, 165–171. [CrossRef] [PubMed]
7. Leung, P.S. Physiology of the pancreas. *Adv. Exp. Med. Biol.* **2010**, *690*, 13–27. [PubMed]
8. Leung, P.S. Current research of the RAS in T2DM. *Adv. Exp. Med. Biol.* **2010**, *690*, 131–153. [PubMed]
9. Mathieu, C. Vitamin D and diabetes: Where do we stand? *Diabetes Res. Clin. Pract.* **2015**, *108*, 201–209. [CrossRef] [PubMed]
10. Mezza, T.; Muscogiuri, G.; Sorice, G.P.; Prioletta, A.; Salomone, E.; Pontecorvi, A.; Giaccari, A. Vitamin D deficiency: A new risk factor for type 2 diabetes? *Ann. Nutr. Metab.* **2012**, *61*, 337–348. [CrossRef] [PubMed]
11. Boucher, B.J.; Mannan, N.; Noonan, K.; Hales, C.N.; Evans, S.J.W. Glucose intolerance and impairment of insulin secretion in relation to vitamin D deficiency in East London Asians. *Diabetologia* **1995**, *38*, 1239–1245. [CrossRef] [PubMed]
12. Pajvani, U.B.; Accili, D. The new biology of diabetes. *Diabetologia* **2015**, *58*, 2459–2468. [CrossRef] [PubMed]
13. Wong, T.P.; Chan, L.K.Y.; Leung, P.S. Involvement of the niacin receptor GPR109a in the local control of glucose uptake in small intestine of type 2 diabetic mice. *Nutrients* **2015**, *7*, 7543–7561. [CrossRef] [PubMed]
14. Chen, L.; So, W.Y.; Li, S.Y.T.; Cheng, Q.; Boucher, B.J.; Leung, P.S. Niacin-induced hyperglycemia is partially mediated via niacin receptor GPR109a in pancreatic islets. *Mol. Cell. Endocriol.* **2015**, *404*, 56–66. [CrossRef] [PubMed]
15. Holick, M.F. Sunlight, UV-radiation, vitamin D and skin cancer. *Adv. Exp. Med. Biol.* **2008**, *624*, 1–15. [PubMed]
16. Peechakara, S.V.; Pittas, A.G. Vitamin D as a potential modifier of diabetes risks. *Nat. Clin. Pract. Endocrinol. Metab.* **2008**, *4*, 182–183. [CrossRef] [PubMed]
17. Mathieu, C.; Gysemans, C.; Bouillon, R. Vitamin D and diabetes. *Diabetologia* **2005**, *48*, 1247–1257. [CrossRef] [PubMed]
18. Vidal, M.; Ramana, C.V.; Busso, A.S. Stat1-vitamin D receptor interactions antagonize 1,25-dihyroxyvitamin D transcriptional activity and enhance stat1-mediated transcription. *Mol. Cell. Biol.* **2002**, *22*, 2777–2787. [CrossRef] [PubMed]
19. Maestro, B.; Davila, N.; Carranza, M.C.; Calle, C. Identification of a vitamin D response element in the human insulin receptor gene promoter. *J. Steroid Biochem. Mol. Biol.* **2003**, *84*, 223–230. [CrossRef]
20. Eerligh, P.; Koeleman, B.P.; Dudbridge, F.; Bruining, J.G.; Roep, B.O.; Giphart, M.J. Functional genetic polymorphisms in cytokines and metabolic genes as additional genetic markers for susceptibility to develop type 1 diabetes. *Genes Immun.* **2004**, *5*, 36–40. [CrossRef] [PubMed]
21. Leung, P.S.; Cheng, Q. The novel roles of glucagon-like peptide-1, angiotensin II, and vitamin D in islet function. *Adv. Exp. Med. Biol.* **2010**, *654*, 339–361. [PubMed]
22. Alvarez, J.A.; Ashraf, A. Role of vitamin D in insulin secretion and insulin sensitivity for glucose homeostasis. *Int. J. Endocrinol.* **2010**, *2010*, 351385. [CrossRef] [PubMed]
23. Kayaniyil, S.; Vieth, R.; Retnakaran, R.; Knight, J.A.; Qi, Y.; Gerstein, H.C.; Perkins, B.A.; Harris, S.B.; Zinman, B.; Hanley, A.J. Association of vitamin D with insulin resistance and beta-cell dysfunction in subjects at risk for type 2 diabetes. *Diabetes Care* **2010**, *33*, 1379–1381. [CrossRef] [PubMed]
24. Ye, Z.; Sharp, S.J.; Burgess, S.; Scott, R.A.; Imamura, F.; InterAct Consortium; Langenberg, C.; Wareham, N.J.; Forouhi, N.G. Association between circulating 25-hydroxyvitamin D and incident type 2 diabetes: A mendelian randomization study. *Lancet Diabetes Endocrinol.* **2015**, *3*, 35–42. [CrossRef]
25. Heshmat, R.; Tabatabaei-Malazy, O.; Abbaszadeh-Ahranjiani, S.; Shahbazi, S.; Khooshehchin, G.; Bandarian, F.; Larijani, B. Effect of vitamin D on insulin resistance and anthropometric parameters in type 2 diabetes: A randomized double-blind clinical trial. *DARU* **2012**, *20*, 10. [CrossRef] [PubMed]
26. Ryu, O.H.; Lee, S.; Yu, J.; Choi, M.G.; Yoo, H.J.; Mantero, F. A prospective randomized controlled trial of the effects of vitamin D supplementation on long-term glycemic control in type 2 diabetes mellitus of Korea. *Endocr. J.* **2014**, *61*, 167–176. [CrossRef] [PubMed]
27. Elkassaby, S.; Harrison, L.C.; Mazzitelli, N.; Wentworth, J.M.; Colman, P.G.; Spelman, T.; Fourlanos, S. A randomized controlled trial of high dose vitamin D in recent-onset type 2 diabetes. *Diabetes Res. Clin. Pract.* **2014**, *106*, 576–582. [CrossRef] [PubMed]

28. Krul-Poel, Y.H.; Westra, S.; ten Boekel, E.; ter Wee, M.M.; van Schoor, N.M.; van Wijland, H.; Stam, F.; Lips, P.T.; Simsek, S. Effect of vitamin D supplementation on glycemic control in patients with type 2 diabetes (SUNNY Trial): A randomized placebo-controlled trial. *Diabetes Care* **2015**, *38*, 1420–1426. [CrossRef] [PubMed]
29. Prentki, M.; Nolan, C.J. Islet beta cell failure in type 2 diabetes. *J. Clin. Investig.* **2006**, *116*, 1802–1812. [CrossRef] [PubMed]
30. Kumashiro, N.; Erion, D.M.; Zhang, D.; Kahn, M.; Beddow, S.A.; Chu, X.; Still, C.D.; Gerhard, G.S.; Han, X.; Dziura, J.; *et al.* Cellular mechanism of insulin resistance in nonalcoholic fatty liver disease. *Proc. Natl. Acad. Sci. USA* **2011**, *108*, 16381–16385. [CrossRef] [PubMed]
31. Flamment, M.; Hajduch, E.; Ferré, P.; Foufelle, F. New insights into ER stress-induced insulin resistance. *Trends Endocrinol. Metab.* **2012**, *23*, 381–390. [CrossRef] [PubMed]
32. Del Prato, S. Role of glucotoxicity and lipotoxicity in the pathophysiology of Type 2 diabetes mellitus and emerging treatment strategies. *Diabet. Med.* **2009**, *26*, 1185–1192. [CrossRef] [PubMed]
33. Yabaluri, N.; Bashyam, M.D. Hormonal regulation of gluconeogenic gene transcription in the liver. *J. Biosci.* **2010**, *35*, 473–484. [CrossRef] [PubMed]
34. Roach, P.J.; Cao, Y.; Corbett, C.A.; DePaoli-Roach, A.A.; Farkas, I.; Fiol, C.J.; Flotow, H.; Graves, P.R.; Hardy, T.A.; Hrubey, T.W.; *et al.* Glycogen metabolism and signal transduction in mammals and yeast. *Adv. Enzyme Regul.* **1991**, *31*, 101–120. [CrossRef]
35. Gregor, M.F.; Hotamisligil, G.S. Inflammatory mechanisms in obesity. *Annu. Rev. Immunol.* **2011**, *29*, 415–445. [CrossRef] [PubMed]
36. Hotamisligil, G.S. Endoplasmic reticulum stress and the inflammatory basis of metabolic disease. *Cell* **2010**, *140*, 900–917. [CrossRef] [PubMed]
37. Zhou, G.; Myers, R.; Li, Y.; Chen, Y.; Shen, X.; Fenyk-Melody, J.; Wu, M.; Ventre, J.; Doebber, T.; Fujii, N.; *et al.* Role of AMP-activated protein kinase in mechanism of metformin action. *J. Clin. Investig.* **2001**, *108*, 1167–1174. [CrossRef] [PubMed]
38. Yamauchi, T.; Kamon, J.; Minokoshi, Y.; Ito, Y.; Waki, H.; Uchida, S.; Yamashita, S.; Noda, M.; Kita, S.; Ueki, K.; *et al.* Adiponectin stimulates glucose ultilization and fatty-acid oxidation by activating AMP-activated protein kinase. *Nat. Med.* **2002**, *8*, 1288–1295. [CrossRef] [PubMed]
39. Carling, D.; Sanders, M.J.; Woods, A. The regulation of AMP-activated protein kinase by upstream kinases. *Int. J. Obes. (Lond.)* **2008**, *32*, S55–S59. [CrossRef] [PubMed]
40. Long, Y.C.; Zierath, J.R. AMP-activated protein kinase signaling in metabolic regulation. *J. Clin. Investig.* **2006**, *116*, 1776–1783. [CrossRef] [PubMed]
41. Barthel, A.; Schmoll, D.; Krüger, K.D.; Roth, R.A.; Joost, H.G. Regulation of the forkhead transcription factor FKHR (FOXO1a) by glucose starvation and AICAR, an activator of AMP-activated protein kinase. *Endocrinology* **2002**, *143*, 3183–3186. [CrossRef] [PubMed]
42. Li, Y.; Xu, S.; Giles, A.; Nakamura, K.; Lee, J.W.; Hou, X.; Donmez, G.; Li, J.; Luo, Z.; Walsh, K.; *et al.* Hepatic overexpression of SIRT1 in mice attenuates endoplasmic reticulum stress and insulin resistance in the liver. *FASEB. J.* **2011**, *25*, 1664–1679. [CrossRef] [PubMed]
43. Kamagate, A.; Kim, D.H.; Zhang, T.; Slusher, S.; Gramignoli, R.; Strom, S.C.; Bertera, S.; Ringquist, S.; Dong, H.H. FoxO1 links hepatic insulin action to endoplasmic reticulum stress. *Endocrinology* **2010**, *151*, 3521–3535. [CrossRef] [PubMed]
44. Barchetta, I.; Angelico, F.; Del Ben, M.; Baroni, M.G.; Pozzilli, P.; Morini, S.; Cavallo, M.G. Strong association between non alcoholic fatty liver disease (NAFLD) and low 25(OH) vitamin D levels in an adult population with normal serum liver enzymes. *BMC Med.* **2011**, *9*, 85. [CrossRef] [PubMed]
45. Kwok, R.M.; Torres, D.M.; Harrison, S.A. Vitamin D and nonalcoholic fatty liver disease (NAFLD): Is it more than just an association? *Hepatology* **2013**, *58*, 1166–1174. [CrossRef] [PubMed]
46. Farese, R.V.; Zechner, R.; Newgard, C.B.; Walther, T.C. The problem of establishing relationships between hepatic steatosis and hepatic insulin resistance. *Cell Metab.* **2012**, *15*, 570–573. [CrossRef] [PubMed]
47. Nagle, C.A.; Klett, E.L.; Coleman, R.A. Hepatic triacylglycerol accumulation and insulin resistance. *J. Lipid Res.* **2009**, *50*, S74–S79. [CrossRef] [PubMed]
48. Samuel, V.T.; Petersen, K.F.; Shulman, G.I. Lipid-induced insulin resistance: Unravelling the mechanism. *Lancet* **2010**, *375*, 2267–2277. [CrossRef]

49. Summers, S.A. Sphingolipids and insulin resistance: The five Ws. *Curr. Opin. Lipidol.* **2010**, *21*, 128–135. [CrossRef] [PubMed]
50. Kumashiro, N.; Beddow, S.A.; Vatner, D.F.; Majumdar, S.K.; Cantley, J.L.; Guebre-Egziabher, F.; Fat, I.; Guigni, B.; Jurczak, M.J.; Birkenfeld, A.L.; *et al.* Targeting pyruvate carboxylase reduces gluconeogenesis and adiposity and improves insulin resistance. *Diabetes* **2013**, *62*, 2183–2194. [CrossRef] [PubMed]
51. Bell, G.I.; Polonsky, K.S. Diabetes mellitus and genetically programmed defects in beta-cell function. *Nature* **2001**, *414*, 788–791. [CrossRef] [PubMed]
52. Gerich, J.E. The genetic basis of type 2 diabetes mellitus: Impaired insulin secretion *versus* impaired insulin sensitivity. *Endocr. Rev.* **1998**, *19*, 491–503. [PubMed]
53. Groop, L. Pathogenesis of type 2 diabetes: The relative contribution of insulin resistance and impaired insulin secretion. *Int. J. Clin. Pract. Suppl.* **2000**, *113*, 3–13. [PubMed]
54. Tuttle, R.; Gill, N.S.; Pugh, W.; Lee, J.P.; Koeberlein, B.; Furth, E.E.; Polonsky, K.S.; Naji, A.; Birnbaum, M.J. Regulation of pancreatic β-cell growth and survival by the serine/threonine protein kinase Akt1/PKBalpha. *Nat. Med.* **2001**, *7*, 1133–1137. [CrossRef] [PubMed]
55. Bernal-Mizrachi, E.; Fatrai, S.; Johnson, J.D.; Ohsugi, M.; Otani, K.; Han, Z.; Polonsky, K.S.; Permutt, M.A. Defective insulin secretion and increased susceptibility to experimental diabetes are induced by reduced Akt activity in pancreatic islet β cells. *J. Clin. Investig.* **2004**, *114*, 928–936. [CrossRef] [PubMed]
56. Wrede, C.; Dickson, L.M.; Lingohr, M.K.; Briaud, I.; Rhodes, C.J. Protein kinase B/Akt prevents fatty acid-induced apoptosis in pancreatic β cells (INS-1). *J. Biol. Chem.* **2002**, *277*, 49676–49684. [CrossRef] [PubMed]
57. Jetton, T.L.; Lausier, J.; LaRock, K.; Trotman, W.E.; Larmie, B.; Habibovic, A.; Peshavaria, M.; Leahy, J.L. Mechanisms of compensatory β-cell growth in insulin-resistant rats: Roles of Akt kinase. *Diabetes* **2005**, *54*, 2294–2304. [CrossRef] [PubMed]
58. Martinez, S.; Tanabe, K.; Cras-Méneur, C.; Abumrad, N.A.; Bernal-Mizrachi, E.; Permutt, M.A. Inhibition of Foxo1 protects pancreatic islet beta-cells against fatty acid and endoplasmic reticulum stress-induced apoptosis. *Diabetes* **2008**, *57*, 846–859. [CrossRef] [PubMed]
59. Mussmann, R.; Geese, M.; Harder, F.; Kegel, S.; Andag, U.; Lomow, A.; Burk, U.; Onichtchouk, D.; Dohrmann, C.; Austen, M. Inhibition of GSK3 promotes replication and survival of pancreatic beta cells. *J. Biol. Chem.* **2007**, *282*, 12030–12037. [CrossRef] [PubMed]
60. Srinivasan, S.; Ohsugi, M.; Liu, Z.G.; Fatrai, S.; Mizrachi, E.B.; Permutt, M.A. Endoplasmic reticulum stress-induced apoptosis is partly mediated by reduced insulin signaling through phosphatidylinositol 3-kinase/Akt and increased glycogen synthase kinase-3β in mouse insulinoma cells. *Diabetes* **2005**, *54*, 968–975. [CrossRef] [PubMed]
61. Henriksen, E.J.; Prasannarong, M. The role of the renin-angiotensin system in the development of insulin resistance in skeletal muscle. *Mol. Cell Endocrinol.* **2013**, *378*, 15–22. [CrossRef] [PubMed]
62. Yuan, L.; Lu, C.L.; Wang, Y.; Li, Y.; Li, X.Y. Ang (1–7) protects islet endothelial cells from palmitate-induced apopotosis by AKT, eNOS, p38 MAPK, and JNK pathways. *J. Diabetes Res.* **2014**, *2014*, 391476. [CrossRef] [PubMed]
63. Wang, H.W.; Mizuta, M.; Saitoh, Y.; Noma, K.; Ueno, H.; Nakazato, M. Glucagon-like peptide-1 and candesartan additively improve glucolipotoxicity in pancreatic beta-cells. *Metabolism* **2011**, *60*, 1081–1089. [CrossRef] [PubMed]
64. Leung, P.S. The renin-angiotensin system: Current research progress in the pancreas. In *Advances in Experimental Medicine and Biology*; Springer: Dordrecht, The Netherlands, 2010; Volume 690, p. 207.
65. Lau, T.; Carlsson, P.O.; Leung, P.S. Evidence for a local angiotensin-generating system and dose-dependent inhibition of glucose-stimulated insulin release by angiotensin II in isolated pancreatic islets. *Diabetologia* **2004**, *47*, 240–248. [CrossRef] [PubMed]
66. Chu, K.Y.; Lau, T.; Carlsson, P.O.; Leung, P.S. Angiotensin II type 1 receptor blockade improves beta-cell function and glucose tolerance in a mouse model of type 2 diabetes. *Diabetes* **2006**, *55*, 367–374. [CrossRef] [PubMed]
67. Kampf, C.; Lau, T.; Olsson, R.; Leung, P.S.; Carlsson, P.O. Angiotensin II type 1 receptor inhibition improves the blood perfusion, oxygen tension and first phase of glucose-stimulated insulin secretion in revascularized syngeneic mouse islet grafts. *Diabetologia* **2005**, *48*, 1159–1167. [CrossRef] [PubMed]

68. Chu, K.Y.; Leung, P.S. Angiotensin II Type 1 receptor antagonism mediates uncoupling protein 2-driven oxidative stress and ameliorates pancreatic islet beta-cell function in young Type 2 diabetic mice. *Antioxid. Redox Signal.* **2007**, *9*, 869–878. [CrossRef] [PubMed]
69. Cheng, Q.; Law, P.K.; de Gasparo, M.; Leung, P.S. Combination of the dipeptidyl peptidase IV inhibitor LAF237 with the angiotensin II type 1 receptor antagonist valsartan enhances pancreatic islet morphology and function in a mouse model of type 2 diabetes. *J. Pharmacol. Exp. Ther.* **2008**, *327*, 683–691. [CrossRef] [PubMed]
70. Li, Y.C.; Kong, J.; Wei, M.; Chen, Z.F.; Liu, S.Q.; Cao, L.P. 1,25-Dihydroxyvitamin D_3 is a negiatve endocrine regulator of the renin-angiotensin system. *J. Clin. Investig.* **2002**, *110*, 229–238. [CrossRef] [PubMed]
71. Li, Y.C.; Qiao, G.; Uskokovic, M.; Xiang, W.; Zheng, W.; Kong, J. Vitamin D: A negative endocrine regulator of the renin-angiotensin system and blood pressure. *J. Steroid Biochem. Mol. Biol.* **2004**, *90*, 387–392. [CrossRef] [PubMed]
72. Pittas, A.G.; Lau, J.; Hu, F.B.; Dawson-Gughes, B. The role of vitamin D and calcium in type 2 diabetes: A systemic review and meta-analysis. *J. Clin. Endocrinol. Metab.* **2007**, *92*, 2017–2029. [CrossRef] [PubMed]
73. Pittas, A.G.; Dawson-Gughes, B.; Li, T.; Van Dam, R.M.; Willett, W.C.; Manson, J.E.; Hu, F.B. Vitamin D and calcium intake in relation to type 2 diabetes in women. *Diabetes Care* **2006**, *29*, 650–656. [CrossRef] [PubMed]
74. Cheng, Q.; Leung, P.S. An update on the islet renin-angiotensin system. *Peptides* **2011**, *32*, 1087–1095. [CrossRef] [PubMed]
75. Leung, P.S.; Boucher, B.J. The roles of vitamin D in modulation of the pancreatic renin-angiotensin system. In *Angiotensin Research Progress*; Miura, H., Sasaki, Y., Eds.; Nova Science Publishers: New York, NY, USA, 2008; pp. 201–220.
76. Cheng, Q.; Li, Y.C.; Boucher, B.J.; Leung, P.S. A novel role for vitamin D: Modulation of expression and function of the local renin-angiotensin system in mouse pancreatic islets. *Diabetologia* **2011**, *54*, 2077–2081. [CrossRef] [PubMed]
77. Cheng, Q.; Boucher, B.J.; Leung, P.S. Modulation of hypovitaminosis D-induced islet dysfunction and insulin resistance through direct suppression of the pancreatic islet renin-angiotensin system in mice. *Diabetologia* **2013**, *56*, 553–562. [CrossRef] [PubMed]
78. Leung, P.S.; Ng, K.Y. Current progress in stem cell research and its potential for islet cell transplantation. *Curr. Mol. Med.* **2013**, *13*, 109–125. [CrossRef] [PubMed]
79. Suen, P.M.; Chan, J.C.; Lau, T.K.; Yao, K.M.; Leung, P.S. PDZ-domain-containing 2 (PDZD2) is a novel factor that affects the growth and differentiation of human fetal pancreatic progenitor cells. *Int. J. Biochem. Cell Biol.* **2008**, *40*, 789–803. [CrossRef] [PubMed]
80. Leung, K.K.; Suen, P.M.; Lau, T.K.; Ko, W.H.; Yao, K.M.; Leung, P.S. PDZ-domain containing-2 (PDZD2) drives the maturity of human fetal pancreatic progenitor-derived islet-like cell clusters with functional responsiveness against membrane depolarization. *Stem Cell Dev.* **2009**, *18*, 979–989. [CrossRef] [PubMed]
81. Leung, K.K.; Liang, J.; Ma, M.T.; Leung, P.S. Angiotensin II type 2 receptor is critical for the development of human fetal pancreatic progenitor cells into islet-like cell clusters and their potential for transplantation. *Stem Cells* **2012**, *30*, 525–536. [CrossRef] [PubMed]
82. Ng, K.Y.; Ma, M.T.; Leung, K.K.; Leung, P.S. Vitamin D and vitamin A receptor expression and the proliferative effects of ligand activation of these receptors on the development of pancreatic progenitor cells derived from human fetal pancreas. *Stem Cell Rev.* **2011**, *7*, 53–63. [CrossRef] [PubMed]
83. Niederreither, K.; Dollé, P. Retinoic acid in development: Towards an integrated view. *Nat. Rev. Genet.* **2008**, *9*, 541–553. [CrossRef] [PubMed]
84. Oström, M.; Loffler, K.A.; Edfalk, S. Retinoic acid promotes the generation of pancreatic endocrine progenitor cells and their further differentiation into beta-cells. *PLoS ONE* **2008**, *3*, e2841. [CrossRef] [PubMed]
85. Shi, Y.; Hou, L.; Tang, F. Inducing embryonic stem cells to differentiate into pancreatic beta cells by a novel three-step approach with activin A and all-trans retinoic acid. *Stem Cells* **2005**, *23*, 656–662. [CrossRef] [PubMed]
86. Liang, J.; Ng, K.Y.; Cheng, Q.; Xia, Y.; Wang, C.C.; Leung, P.S. Human fetal liver stromal cells co-culture enhances the differentiation of pancreatic progenitor cells into islet-like cell clusters. *Stem Cell Rev.* **2014**, *10*, 280–294. [CrossRef] [PubMed]
87. Seet, E.L.; Yee, J.K.; Jellyman, J.K.; Hun, G.; Ross, M.G. Maternal high-fat-diet programs rat offspring liver fatty acid metabolism. *Lipids* **2015**, *50*, 565–573. [CrossRef] [PubMed]

88. Fan, H.R.; Lin, L.Q.; Ma, H.; Li, Y.; Sun, C.H. Association between vitamin D receptor gene polymorphism (TaqI) and obesity in Chinese population. *J. Genet.* **2015**, *94*, 473–478. [CrossRef] [PubMed]
89. Wortsman, J.; Matsuoka, L.Y.; Chen, T.C.; Lu, Z.; Holick, M.F. Decreased bioavailability of vitamin D in obesity. *Am. J. Clin. Nutr.* **2000**, *72*, 690–693. [PubMed]
90. Boucher, B.J.; Leung, P.S. "Maternal high-fat-diet programs rat offspring liver fatty acid metabolism": Might reduced vitamin D availability due to increases in maternal body fat contribute to this effect? *Lipids* **2015**, *50*, 837–838. [CrossRef] [PubMed]

13

Protective Effect of Vanillic Acid against Hyperinsulinemia, Hyperglycemia and Hyperlipidemia via Alleviating Hepatic Insulin Resistance and Inflammation in High-Fat Diet (HFD)-Fed Rats

Wen-Chang Chang [1], James Swi-Bea Wu [1], Chen-Wen Chen [1], Po-Ling Kuo [2], Hsu-Min Chien [3], Yuh-Tai Wang [4] and Szu-Chuan Shen [2,*]

1 Graduate Institute of Food Science and Technology, National Taiwan University, P.O. Box 23-14, Taipei 10672, Taiwan; d99641001@ntu.edu.tw (W.-C.C.); jsbwu@ntu.edu.tw (J.S.-B.W.); jenwen0813@hotmail.com (C.-W.C.)

2 Department of Human Development and Family Studies, National Taiwan Normal University, No. 162, Sec. 1, Heping East Road, Taipei 10610, Taiwan; maplebling@gmail.com

3 Department of Nursing, Taipei City Hospital, Renai Branch, No. 10, Sec. 4, Renai Road, Taipei 10629, Taiwan; B1465@tpech.gov.tw

4 Life Science Center, Hsing Wu Institute of Technology, No. 101, Sec. 1, Fen-Liao Road, Lin-Kou District, New Taipei City 244, Taiwan; yuhtai@yahoo.com

* Correspondence: scs@ntnu.edu.tw

Abstract: Excess free fatty acid accumulation from abnormal lipid metabolism results in the insulin resistance in peripheral cells, subsequently causing hyperinsulinemia, hyperglycemia and/or hyperlipidemia in diabetes mellitus (DM) patients. Herein, we investigated the effect of phenolic acids on glucose uptake in an insulin-resistant cell-culture model and on hepatic insulin resistance and inflammation in rats fed a high-fat diet (HFD). The results show that vanillic acid (VA) demonstrated the highest glucose uptake ability among all tested phenolic acids in insulin-resistant FL83B mouse hepatocytes. Furthermore, rats fed HFD for 16 weeks were orally administered with VA daily (30 mg/kg body weight) at weeks 13–16. The results show that levels of serum insulin, glucose, triglyceride, and free fatty acid were significantly decreased in VA-treated HFD rats ($p < 0.05$), indicating the protective effects of VA against hyperinsulinemia, hyperglycemia and hyperlipidemia in HFD rats. Moreover, VA significantly reduced values of area under the curve for glucose ($AUC_{glucose}$) in oral glucose tolerance test and homeostasis model assessment-insulin resistance (HOMA-IR) index, suggesting the improving effect on glucose tolerance and insulin resistance in HFD rats. The Western blot analysis revealed that VA significantly up-regulated expression of hepatic insulin-signaling and lipid metabolism-related protein, including insulin receptor, phosphatidylinositol-3 kinase, glucose transporter 2, and phosphorylated acetyl CoA carboxylase in HFD rats. VA also significantly down-regulated hepatic inflammation-related proteins, including cyclooxygenase-2 and monocyte chemoattractant protein-1 expressions in HFD rats. These results indicate that VA might ameliorate insulin resistance via improving hepatic insulin signaling and alleviating inflammation pathways in HFD rats. These findings also suggest the potential of VA in preventing the progression of DM.

Keywords: vanillic acid; insulin resistance; hyperinsulinemia; hyperglycemia; hyperlipidemia

1. Introduction

As advanced medical technology and improved living standards extend the expectancy of human life, chronic diseases have become a major threat to the health of people. Diabetes mellitus (DM) is one of the fastest-growing chronic diseases. The World Health Organization (WHO) reported that there were more than 347 million people suffering from DM worldwide, and predicted the patient number would double (694 million) by 2030 [1]. The process of DM development involves an initial prediabetes state, and develops into DM if the condition is not appropriately controlled. Therefore, effectively maintaining blood glucose homeostasis has become a crucial issue in DM prevention.

After consuming high-calorie foods, the body is in a hyperglycemic state with an increased insulin secretion, reducing serum glucose to maintain a steady level of serum glucose. Long-term excess intake of high-calorie or high-fat diet (HFD) resulted in increasing blood glucose level and free fatty acid content and induced metabolic related diseases, such as obesity, dyslipidemia, type 2 diabetes mellitus (T2DM), and fatty liver disease [2–4]. The increased blood glucose level caused islet cells to continuously secrete insulin, while the increased free fatty acid content caused an increased lipid synthesis, leading to the accumulation of diacylglycerol in the liver and activation of protein kinase Cε (PKCε). Activated PKCε inhibits the insulin signaling, consequently resulting in hepatic insulin resistance [4]. HFD also tends to be obesity associated. Previous studies indicated that insulin resistance that occurred via obesity is correlated with internal chronic inflammation, which is among the major causes of insulin resistance [5–7]. Increased release of free fatty acids from adipocytes into blood was reported to activate protein kinases, e.g., protein kinase C, which subsequently affected the expression of inhibitor of kappa β kinase, c-Jun N-terminal kinases (JNK), and p38 mitogen-activated protein kinases, stimulating the release of inflammatory factors such as tumor necrosis factor-alpha (TNF-α) and interleukin-6 (IL-6), and causing internal inflammatory responses [8].

Phenolic acids are phytochemicals abundant in various vegetables and fruits. Hydroxybenzoic acid derivatives and hydroxycinnamic acid derivatives are two major categories of phenolic acid [9]. Hydroxycinnamic acid derivative *p*-methoxycinnamic acid promoted glycolysis, reduced gluconeogenesis in the liver of diabetic rats, and increased the secretion of insulin to reduce hyperglycemia in streptozotocin (STZ)-induced diabetic rats [10]. Ferulic acid improved the serum glucose levels and counteracted lipid peroxidation in STZ-induced diabetic mice and KK-Ay spontaneous diabetic mice [11]. Caffeic acid was reported to increase the utilization of glucose by the liver and adipocytes to reduce serum glucose levels in type 2 diabetic mice [12]. Various phenolic acids were found to alleviate the DM and its associated syndromes [9–12]. However, the study of phenolic acids against HFD-induced hyperinsulinemia, hyperglycemia and hyperlipidemia is limited. The aim of the present study is to assess the glucose uptake-enhancing effect *in vitro* and investigate the hypoinsulinemic, hypoglycemic and hypolipidemic effect *in vivo* of phenolic acids. The mechanism of the selected phenolic acid on attenuating insulin resistance in HFD rats is also elucidated.

2. Materials and Methods

2.1. Chemicals

Bovine serum albumin (BSA), caffeic acid, chlorogenic acid, cinnamic acid, D-(+)-glucose, dimethyl sulfoxide (DMSO), disodium hydrogen phosphate (Na_2HPO_4), ferulic acid, 4-(2-hydroxyethyl)-1-piperazineethanesulfonic acid (HEPES), insulin, pioglitazone hydrochloride (Pio), potassium chloride (KCl), potassium dihydrogen phosphate (KH_2PO_4), protocatechuic acid, sinapic acid, sodium chloride (NaCl), sodium phosphate dibasic (Na_2HPO_4), syringic acid, vanillic acid (VA), recombinant mouse tumor necrosis factor (TNF)-α, sulfuric acid (H_2SO_4), Triton X-100, TEMED (*N,N,N,N′*-Tetramethyl-eyhylenediamine), 3-(4,5-dimethylthiazol-2-yl)-2,5-diphenyl-tetrazolium bromide (MTT reagent), and F12 Ham Kaighn's modification (F12K) medium were purchased from Sigma-Aldrich Co. (St. Louis, MO, USA). Fetal bovine serum (FBS) was obtained from Gemini Bio-Products (Woodland, CA, USA). The fluorescent dye 2-(N-(7-nitrobenz-2-oxa-1,3-diazol-4-yl)amino)-2-deoxyglucose (2-NBDG) was purchased from Invitrogen (Camarillo, CA, USA). Bio-Rad protein assay dye reagent was obtained from Bio-Rad Laoboratories (Richmond, VA, USA). All of the chemicals used in this study were of analytical grade.

2.2. Cell Culture

Experiments were performed on a hepatocyte cell line (FL83B) deriving from a fetal mouse (15–17 days). The FL83B cells were incubated in F12K medium containing 10% fetal bovine serum and 1% penicillin and streptomycin (Invitrogen Corporation, Camarillo, CA, USA) in 10 cm Petri dishes at 37 °C and 5% carbon dioxide. Experiments were performed when cells were 80%–90% confluent.

2.3. Tumor Necrosis Factor-Alpha (TNF-α) Induction of Insulin Resistance

The induction of insulin resistance in hepatocytes referred to the method reported by Chang and Shen with minor modifications [13]. FL83B cells were seeded in 10 cm dishes and incubated at 37 °C for 48 h to 80% confluence. Serum-free F12K medium containing 20 ng/mL recombinant mouse TNF-α was then added and incubated for 5 h to induce insulin resistance.

2.4. Uptake of Fluorescent 2-(N-(7-Nitrobenz-2-oxa-1,3-Diazol-4-yl)Amino)-2-Deoxyglucose in FL83B Mouse Hepatocytes

The FL83B cells were detached with trypsin and suspended in 1200 μL of Krebs-Ringer bicarbonate buffer containing 1 μM insulin. Aliquots of the cell suspension (172 μL) were transferred to Eppendorf tubes and co-incubated with 20 μL of 6.25 ng/mL VA and 8 μL of the fluorescent dye 2-NBDG (to a final concentration of 200 μM) in a water bath at 37 °C for 1 h in the dark. The reaction was stopped on ice. The cell suspension was centrifuged at 3000× *g* (4 °C) for 5 min to remove the supernatant. The pellet was washed with phosphate-buffered saline (PBS) and centrifuged 3 times before being suspended in 1 mL of PBS. The fluorescence intensity of the cell suspension was evaluated using flow cytometry (FACScan, Becton Dickinson, Bellport, NY, USA) at an excitation wavelength of 488 nm and an emission wavelength of 542 nm. Fluorescence intensity reflected the cellular uptake of 2-NBDG.

$$\begin{aligned}\text{Amelioration rate (\%)} = {} & ((\text{fluorescence intensity of phenolic acid} - \text{treated group}) - \\ & (\text{fluorescence intensity of TNF} - \alpha - \text{treated group}))/ \\ & (\text{fluorescence intensity of TNF} - \alpha - \text{treated group}) \times 100\ (\%).\end{aligned} \tag{1}$$

2.5. Animals and Diets

Male Sprague-Dawley (SD) rats (5 weeks old) were obtained from the National Laboratory Animal Center, Taipei, Taiwan. The rats were maintained in standard laboratory conditions (22 ± 1 °C and a 12 h light/12 h dark cycle) with free access to food and water. Rats were fed a normal diet for 1 week and had a body weight of approximately 250 g. The rats were divided into 4 groups, with each group containing 6 rats. One group was fed a normal diet for 16 weeks (Control group). A second group was fed an HFD (60% calories from fat) throughout the experimental period (HFD group). A third group was provided an HFD for 16 weeks and daily administered Pio (30 mg/kg body weight) on a daily basis during weeks 13–16 (HFD + Pio group). A final group was provided an HFD for 16 weeks, and orally administered VA (30 mg/kg body weight) on a daily basis during weeks 13–16 (HFD + VA group). The rats were sacrificed at the end of the experiment before the blood samples were collected and the biochemical analysis conducted. The organs such as liver, kidney, perirenal and epididymal adipose tissues were isolated from animals and weighed. The liver was stored at −80 °C for the free fatty acid assay and Western blot analysis.

2.6. Blood Sample Preparation

Blood samples were collected and allowed to clot for 30 min at room temperature and then centrifuged at 3000× *g* for 20 min to obtain the serum, which was stored at −80 °C before use.

2.7. *Biochemical Measurements*

Enzyme-linked immunosorbent assay kits for rat insulin, total bilirubin, blood urea nitrogen, creatinine, total cholesterol, triglyceride, free fatty acid, and leptin were purchased from Randox Laboratories (Crumlin Co., Antrim, UK). Biochemical analyses were performed according to the manufacturer's protocols.

2.8. *Oral Glucose Tolerance Test (OGTT)*

The OGTT was performed on rats in all groups after an overnight fast at week 16. All animals were orally administered 1.5 g of glucose/kg body weight. Blood was sampled from the tail vessels of conscious animals before (t = 0) and 30, 60, 90, and 120 min after glucose administration. The samples were allowed to clot for 30 min and then centrifuged (4 °C, 3000× *g*, 20 min) to obtain the serum. Glucose concentration was determined using a glucose enzymatic kit (Crumlin Co.). The obtained glucose concentration values were plotted against time to provide a curve showing the changes in glucose levels with time, expressed as an integrated area under the curve for glucose ($AUC_{glucose}$).

2.9. *Homeostasis Model Assessment of Insulin Resistance (HOMA-IR) Index [14]*

The HOMA-IR index was calculated using the following equation:

$$\text{HOMA} - \text{IR index} = \text{fasting serum insulin (mU/L)} \times \text{fasting glucose (mmol/L)}/22.5 \quad (2)$$

2.10. *Western Blot Analysis*

Aliquots of supernatants, each containing 50 μg protein, were used to evaluate the expression of insulin receptor (IR), phosphatidylinositol-3 kinase (PI3K), glucose transporter 2 (GLUT-2), cyclooxygenase-2 (COX-2), monocyte chemoattractant protein-1 (MCP-1), and acetyl CoA carboxylase (ACC), phospho-acetyl CoA carboxylase (pACC). The samples were subjected to 10% sodium dodecyl sulfate polyacrylamide gel electrophoresis, and the proteins were electrotransferred to a polyvinylidene difluoride membrane. The membrane was incubated with block buffer (PBS containing 0.05% Tween-20 and 5% *w*/*v* nonfat dry milk) for 1 h, washed with PBS containing 0.05% Tween-20 (PBST) 3 times, and then probed with 1:2000 diluted solutions of anti-IR, anti-PI3K, anti-GLUT-2, anti-COX-2, anti-MCP-1, and anti-ACC, anti-pACC, antibodies (Gene Tex, Irvine, CA, USA) overnight at 4 °C. The intensity of the blot probed with a 1:4000 diluted solution of mouse monoclonal antibody to bind actin (Gene Tex) was used as a control to ensure that a constant amount of protein was loaded into each lane of the gel. The membrane was washed 3 times (5 min each time) in PBST, shaken in a solution of horseradish peroxidase-linked anti-mouse IgG or anti-rabbit IgG secondary antibody, washed 3 more times (5 min each time) in PBST, and then exposed to enhanced chemiluminescence reagent (Millipore) according to the manufacturer's instructions. The films were scanned and analyzed using a UVP Biospectrum image system (Level, Cambridge, UK).

2.11. *Statistical Analysis*

Results presented as mean ± standard deviation (SD) were analyzed using one-way ANOVA and Duncan's new multiple range tests. All comparisons were made relative to controls, and $p < 0.05$ was considered significant.

3. Results and Discussion

3.1. *Effect of Phenolic Acids on Cell Viability and Glucose Uptake Ability in Insulin-Resistant FL83B Mouse Hepatocytes*

The *in vitro* MTT assay is typically used to evaluate the cellular growth inhibition and assess toxicity of drugs or chemicals [15]. Phenolic acids are known to possess antiviral, antioxidative, anticancer, and antihyperglycemic bioactivities [16–18]. However, the effect of phenolic acid on bioactivity and the cytotoxicity in FL83B mouse hepatocytes have not been systematically investigated. Table 1 shows the growth inhibitory of concentration effect of eight naturally occurred phenolic acids on FL83B cells. The results from the cell viability test reveal that the all tested phenolic acids at the concentration of 12.5 μM show above 80%, indicating non-toxicity to FL83B mouse hepatocytes. Therefore, this concentration (12.5 μM) was used to evaluate the glucose uptake-enhancing effect of phenolic acids in insulin resistance cell model.

Table 1. Effects of various concentrations of phenolic acids on cell viability and amelioration rate of glucose uptake in insulin-resistant FL83B cells.

Concentrations / Phenolic Acids	Cell Viability (%) [a]				Amelioration Rate (%) [b]
	12.5 μM	25 μM	50 μM	100 μM	(12.5 μM Phenolic Acid)
Caffeic acid	102.8 ± 15.8	99.4 ± 16.8	82.0 ± 14.3	74.3 ± 8.6	−6.60
Cinnamic acid	86.2 ± 2.1	88.7 ± 2.5	88.6 ± 6.7	89.6 ± 0.1	−11.30
Ferulic acid	92.7 ± 7.3	88.9 ± 9.1	86.7 ± 6.7	77.4 ± 28.2	−22.01
Protocatechuic acid	91.7 ± 10.4	91.8 ± 9.0	75.4 ± 8.1	71.8 ± 9.0	−12.90
Rosmarinic acid	104.3 ± 17.6	97.2 ± 13.1	102.5 ± 16.5	90.7 ± 22.4	−10.28
Sinapic acid	97.2 ± 2.9	102.1 ± 10.1	102.0 ± 10.5	80.0 ± 9.2	−15.37
Syringic acid	90.9 ± 2.2	79.8 ± 17.4	70.2 ± 13.1	64.6 ± 14.5	8.36
Vanillic acid	114.2 ± 26.3	114.8 ± 18.5	109.8 ± 25.5	116.7 ± 17.6	13.66

[a] Cell viability (%) = (A_{570} of sample group)/(A_{570} of control group) × 100 (%); [b] Amelioration rate (%) = ((fluorescence intensity of phenolic acid-treated group) − (fluorescence intensity of TNF-α-treated group))/(fluorescence intensity of TNF-α-treated group) × 100 (%). Data are expressed as percentage relative to control value (100%) or mean ± SD (n = 3).

TNF-α is a cytokine found to interfere with the transmission of insulin signaling and the abilities of liver cells, myofibroblasts, and adipocytes to absorb and metabolize glucose [19–21]. Previously, the 2-NBDG, a modified D-glucose fluorescent derivative, was used to assess the viability of yeast and *Escherichia coli*, and the ability of glucose uptake in FL83B cells treated with TNF-α to induce insulin resistance [13,22,23]. In the present study, fluorescent 2-NBDG was used to evaluate the effect of phenolic acids on glucose uptake ability in insulin-resistant FL83B mouse hepatocytes. As shown in Table 1, VA at concentration of 12.5 μM showed the highest potential for reducing insulin resistance (amelioration rate, 13.66%) among tested phenolic acids. VA was thus used in the subsequent animal experiments.

3.2. Effect of Vanillic Acid on Glucose Tolerance, Serum Insulin and Insulin Resistance Index in High-Fat Diet (HFD)-Fed Rats

HFD is associated with insulin resistance and reduced insulin secretion by β-cells in the pancreas, leading to abnormal glucose tolerance in animal [24–27]. Figure 1a shows the results of OGTT in rats fed HFD for 16 weeks and orally administered with VA daily during the last 4 weeks. The serum glucose levels of rats in the HFD group increased significantly after 30 min, and then decreased slowly. HFD rats treated with Pio or VA exhibited similar changes in serum glucose levels. The $AUC_{glucose}$ for the OGTT, indicating the degree of glucose tolerance in the rats, remained at high levels, thereby indicating low glucose tolerance in the present study. The HFD rats exhibited significantly ($p < 0.05$) lower glucose tolerance than the control rats and VA-treated HFD rats (Figure 1b). In other words, VA can ameliorate the HFD-induced glucose intolerance.

Hyperinsulinemia is likely a marker of insulin resistance, rather than a major, direct contributor to the process [28]. Under hyperglycemic conditions, the pancreas compensates for the decreased insulin response by increasing the insulin secretion; however, the result is hyperinsulinemia to maintain the stable plasma glucose. This process will continue until the reserve capacity is surpassed by metabolic demands and insulin secretion is no longer sufficient; then, blood glucose concentration rises and glucose intolerance and T2DM develop [29–31]. HFD is also reported to be associated with the hyperinsulinemia of rats [32]. In this study, the fasting serum insulin concentration of rats in the HFD group (4.30 ± 1.14 μg/L) was 347.9% higher than that in the control (normal diet) group (0.96 ± 0.33 μg/L) (Figure 1c), indicating the hyperinsulinemia in the HFD rats. However, the serum insulin level of VA-treated HFD rats (2.13 ± 0.64 μg/L) was significantly lower than that in HFD-fed rats, indicating the hypoinsulinemic ability of VA. The rats fed HFD over the long term will develop diabetic symptoms such as insulin resistance [33]. Matthews *et al.* proposed methods using the fasting serum insulin and glucose levels during leisure time to calculate the HOMA-IR index, which is considered a sensitive indicator to assess the degree of insulin resistance [14]. A high HOMA-IR value represents high insulin resistance [14,34]. The advantages of the HOMA-IR are ease of calculation of fasting serum insulin and glucose levels, and potential for extensive use in epidemiological research. As shown in Figure 1d, the HOMA-IR index of VA-treated HFD rats was significantly lower than that of HFD rats, indicating VA may ameliorate the insulin resistance in HFD rats. VA derivative was previously reported to inhibit protein-tyrosine phosphatase 1B (PTP1B) activity, reduce the interference on insulin-signaling proteins, and lead to the alleviation of insulin resistance in T2DM patients [35].

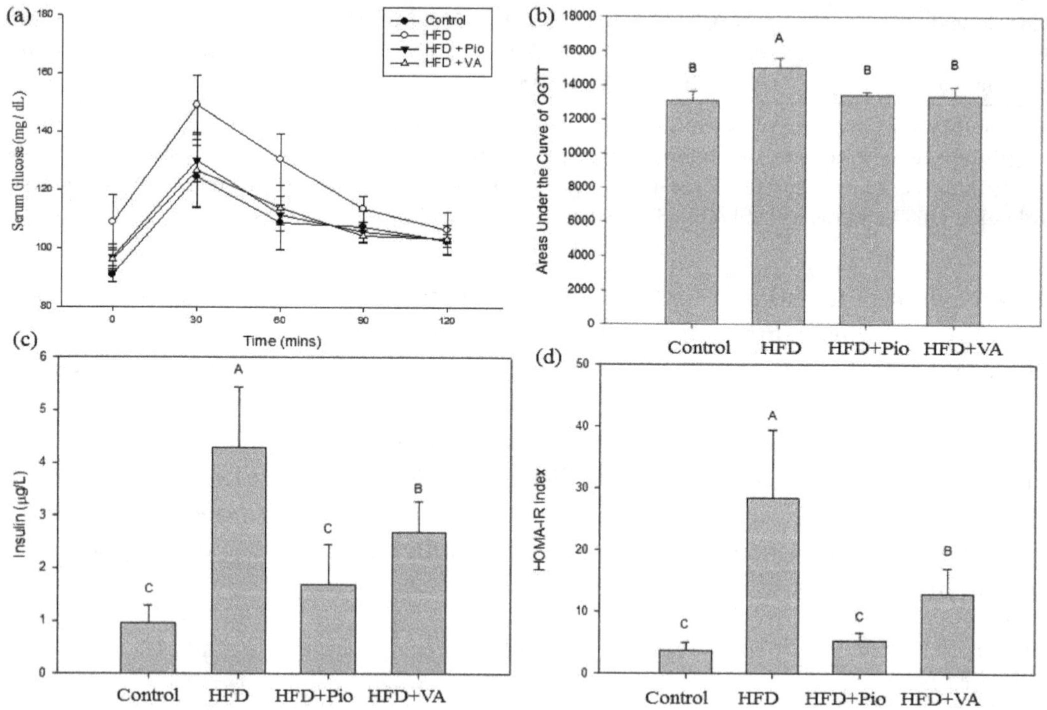

Figure 1. (**a**) Oral glucose tolerance test (OGTT); (**b**) area under the curve for glucose ($AUC_{glucose}$) of OGTT; (**c**) fasting serum insulin, and (**d**) homeostasis model assessment of insulin resistance (HOMA-IR) in rats fed high-fat diet for 16 weeks and orally administered with vanillic acid during the last 4 weeks. Control: normal diet; HFD: high-fat diet (60 kcal % fat); HFD + Pio: HFD (60 kcal % fat) + pioglitazone (30 mg/kg body weight); HFD + VA: HFD (60 kcal % fat) + vanillic acid (30 mg/kg body weight); (A–C) indicate statistically significant differences $p < 0.05$. Data are presented as mean ± SD (6 rats in each group).

3.3. Effect of Vanillic Acid on Energy Intake, Body Weight, and Selected Organ Weight in HFD-Fed Rats

No significant difference ($p > 0.05$) in the energy intakes among tested groups was observed, indicating that orally administered VA exerts no significant effect on energy intake in HFD rats

(Table 2). There was no significant difference in the kidney weights of each group (Table 2). However, after 4 weeks of treatment, the average body, liver and adipose tissue weights of HFD rats were significantly higher than those of Pio and VA-treated HFD rats ($p < 0.05$). HFD was reported to increase serum triglyceride and non-esterified free fatty acid (NEFA) content, thereby resulting in increased lipogenesis in rats [36]. Pio was reported to restrict the increase of adipose tissue and body weight in obese women [37]. Thus, VA was postulated to possess the similar effect as Pio on suppressing accumulation of body fat in HFD-fed rats via the inhibition of lipid synthesis or lipogenesis.

Table 2. The body weight, selected tissue weight, and energy intake in rats fed a high-fat diet for 16 weeks and orally administered with vanillic acid during the last 4 weeks.

Items/Groups	Control	HFD	HFD + Pio	HFD + VA
Body weight (g)	627.1 ± 28.7 C	760.7 ± 63.1 A	686.0 ± 30.4 B	676.9 ± 70.2 B
Diet intake (kcal/rat/day)	104.45 ± 4.43 A	110.04 ± 11.33 A	101.63 ± 5.77 A	104.97 ± 9.91 A
Liver weight (g)	14.6 ± 0.7 B	18.5 ± 2.2 A	13.9 ± 1.4 B	13.9 ± 1.6 B
Kidney weight (g)	1.1 ± 0.4 A	1.4 ± 0.5 A	1.7 ± 0.2 A	0.9 ± 0.6 A
Adipose weight (g)	17.7 ± 4.6 C	56.1 ± 12.7 A	36.7 ± 6.4 B	35.3 ± 12.7 B

Control: normal diet; HFD: high-fat diet (60 kcal % fat); HFD+Pio: HFD (60 kcal % fat) + pioglitazone (30 mg/kg body weight); HFD + VA: HFD (60 kcal % fat) + vanillic acid (30 mg/kg body weight). Adipose weight: total weight of perirenal and epididymal adipose tissues. ($^{A-C}$) indicate statistically significant differences $p < 0.05$. Data are presented as mean ± SD (n = 6/group). Adipose weight includes epididymal fat pad and abdominal adipose tissue weight.

3.4. Effect of Vanillic Acid on Serum Biochemical Parameters in HFD-Fed Rats

Long term consumption HFD resulting in the increment of adipose tissues. The fatty acids from adipocytes are subsequently released into the blood then transported to periphery tissues such as liver and muscle. The process inhibits the utilization of glycogen and glucose and induces insulin resistance in peripheral tissues. HFD was reported to induce dyslipidemia, resulting in elevated serum glucose, triglyceride, NEFA levels and reduced high-density lipoprotein levels in rats [33,38]. After feeding rats for 16 weeks, the fasting serum glucose of the HFD group was 18.1% higher than that of control group (Table 3). The significant difference ($p < 0.05$) between these two groups was consistent to the previous study and revealed that hyperglycemia was induced in HFD-fed rats in the present study [38]. Furthermore, the fasting serum glucose level in VA-treated rats (94.5 ± 1.9 mg/L) was significantly lower than that in the HFD rats ($p < 0.05$) (Table 3), indicating the hypoglycemic ability of VA.

Moreover, the fasting serum triglyceride and free fatty acid concentration of rats in the HFD group are higher than those in the control group by 20.8% and 27.2%, respectively (Table 3), indicating the hyperlipidemia in the HFD rats. However, the fasting serum triglyceride and free fatty acid were significantly reduced in HFD rats supplemented with VA (71.63 ± 13.42 μg/L, 0.76 ± 0.14 mmol/L) compared to the HFD rats ($p < 0.05$), suggesting the hypolipidemic ability of VA.

Leptin is a hormone secreted by adipose tissues and regulates utilization of lipid in human body. The serum leptin concentration of in the HFD rats was significantly ($p < 0.05$) higher than that in control group (Table 3). Comparatively, the serum leptin level was significantly reduced ($p < 0.05$) in HFD rats after 4-weeks VA treatment (Table 3). Previous studies reported a positive correlation between serum leptin concentration and body fat content, and suggested that people with obesity or T2DM have higher serum leptin levels than healthy people do [39,40]. Studies have also indicated that leptin reduces body weight, body fat, energy intake, serum glucose levels, and insulin concentration in mice [41,42]. However, the mechanism underlying such effects was still unidentified. We speculate that HFD promotes leptin production and is involved in the accumulation of hepatic NEFA and the induction of hepatic insulin resistance in rats subsequently.

Table 3. The fasting serum parameters in rats fed high-fat diet for 16 weeks and orally administered with vanillic acid during the last 4 weeks.

Items/Groups	Control	HFD	HFD + Pio	HFD + VA
Glucose (mg/dL)	90.8 ± 1.7 ^{B}	107.2 ± 5.5 ^{A}	97.0 ± 3.7 ^{B}	94.5 ± 1.9 ^{B}
Triglyceride (mg/dL)	74.13 ± 18.20 ^{B}	89.50 ± 11.70 ^{A}	61.50 ± 9.80 ^{B}	71.63 ± 13.42 ^{B}
Free fatty acid (mmol/L)	0.92 ± 0.09 ^{B}	1.17 ± 0.26 ^{A}	0.69 ± 0.16 ^{C}	0.76 ± 0.14 ^{B,C}
Total cholesterol (mg/dL)	62.38 ± 9.71 ^{A}	51.63 ± 14.35 ^{A}	58.13 ± 9.95 ^{A}	40.00 ± 6.41 ^{B}
Leptin (ng/mL)	162.3 ± 32.6 ^{B}	986.3 ± 413.8 ^{A}	429 ± 69.7 ^{B}	303.2 ± 84.2 ^{B}
Bili-total (mg/dL)	0.08 ± 0.01 ^{A}	0.07 ± 0.01 ^{A}	0.05 ± 0.01 ^{B}	0.07 ± 0.02 ^{A}
BUN (mg/dL)	15.33 ± 1.25 ^{A}	9.55 ± 0.91 ^{C}	12.80 ± 1.05 ^{B}	10.96 ± 2.11 ^{C}
Creatinine (mg/dL)	0.35 ± 0.05 ^{AB}	0.38 ± 0.05 ^{A}	0.31 ± 0.04 ^{B}	0.38 ± 0.05 ^{A}

Bili-total: total bilirubin; BUN: blood urea nitrogen. Control: normal diet; HFD: high-fat diet (60 kcal % fat); HFD + Pio: HFD (60 kcal % fat) + pioglitazone (30 mg/kg body weight); HFD + VA: HFD (60 kcal % fat) + vanillic acid (30 mg/kg body weight); (^{A}−−^{C}) indicate statistically significant differences $p < 0.05$. Data are presented as mean ± SD (6 rats in each group).

3.5. *Effect of Vanillic Acid on Hepatic Insulin Signaling, Inflammation and NEFA Formation in HFD-Fed Rats*

Insulin is a hormone with multiple effects. Binding of insulin to the α-subunit of the insulin receptor molecule induces rapid auto-phosphorylation of the β-subunit, which leads to an increase of its tyrosine kinase activity [43]. Tyrosine phosphorylation of insulin receptor proteins induces the cytoplasmic binding activity of insulin receptor substrate-1 (IRS-1) to insulin receptor. IRS-1 plays a pivotal role in transmitting signals from insulin receptors to intracellular PI3K/Akt pathway, which eventually results in the second intracellular step of insulin action, targeting tyrosine-phosphorylated insulin receptor β and IRS-1 [29,43–45]. IR is a condition in which defects in the action of insulin are such that normal levels of insulin do not operate as the signal for glucose uptake [43]. After a 4-week administration of VA, a down-regulation of hepatic insulin signaling-related proteins, such as IR, PI3K, and GLUT-2, was found in HFD group rats as compared with the control group (Figure 2). These results suggested that VA normalizes hepatic insulin signaling and alleviates hepatic insulin resistance in the liver of HFD-fed rats.

The chronic inflammation increases the development of obesity-related insulin resistance [5]. COX-2, an enzyme involved in inflammatory responses, is barely detectable in normal conditions and rapidly up-regulated in the inflammation conditions [28]. MCP-1, an inflammatory cytokine, is up-regulated in the conditions of hyperlipidemia and inflammation [46]. As shown in Figure 3, HFD up-regulated the hepatic COX-2 and MCP-1 protein expressions as compared with the control group. In contrast, the expressions of COX-2 and MCP-1 protein were down-regulated ($p < 0.05$) after a 4-week VA treatment in HFD-fed rats. Diet-induced obesity is a type of inflammatory response, with up-regulated COX-2 and MCP-1 protein expressions observed in the internal tissues of obese rats [47,48].

HFD increases the lipid synthesis in liver and adipose tissues, induces chronic inflammatory responses thus leading to insulin resistance in mice [28,37]. Acetyl CoA carboxylase (ACC), an essential enzyme in fatty acid synthesis, is activated by dephosphorylation and transforms acetyl CoA into malonyl CoA through carboxylation. Enhancing phosphorylation of ACC protein may thus reduce adipose tissue formation and NEFA accumulation in peripheral tissue, including liver [49]. Excess NEFA from adiposity was reported to cause insulin resistance by inhibiting insulin signaling in T2DM [49]. In the present study, the phosphorylated ACC/ACC protein expression of liver significantly decreased, indicating the increment of hepatic lipogenesis in the HFD rats (Figure 4a). The expression of hepatic phosphorylated ACC/ACC protein expression was increased, and the hepatic NEFA level reduced in HFD rats treated with VA for 4 weeks (Figure 4b). The current study suggests that VA may reduce hepatic NEFA accumulation via promoting the phosphorylation of ACC protein expression in liver of HFD rats.

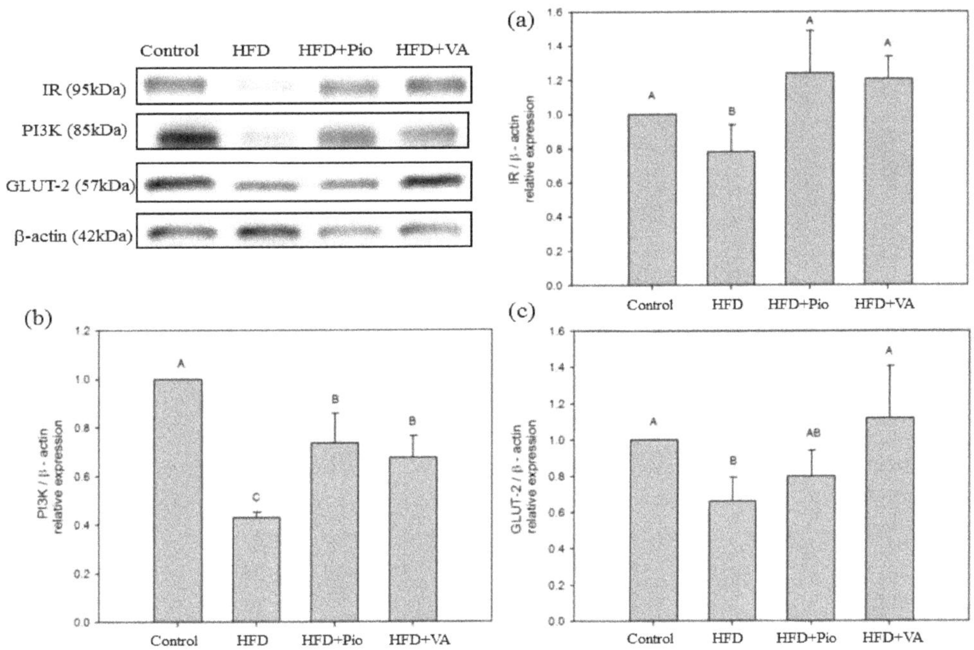

Figure 2. Hepatic (**a**) insulin receptor (IR); (**b**) phosphoinositide 3-kinase (PI3K); and (**c**) glucose transporter 2 (GLUT-2) proteins expression in rat fed high-fat diet for 16 weeks and orally administered vanillic acid during the last 4 weeks. Control: normal diet; HFD: high-fat diet (60 kcal % fat); HFD + Pio: HFD (60 kcal % fat) + pioglitazone (30 mg/kg body weight); HFD + VA: HFD (60 kcal % fat) + vanillic acid (30 mg/kg body weight); (A–C) indicate statistically significant differences $p < 0.05$. Data are presented as mean ± SD (3 rats in each group).

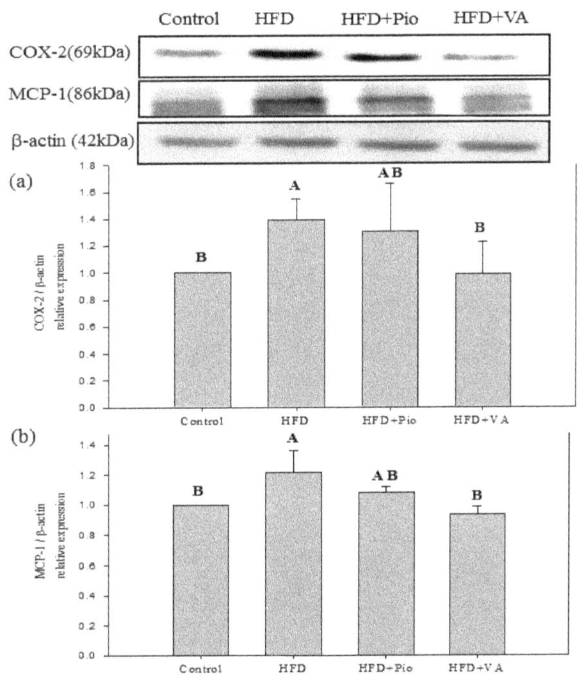

Figure 3. Hepatic (**a**) cyclooxygenase 2 (COX-2) and (**b**) monocyte chemoattractant protein-1 (MCP-1) protein expression in rats fed high-fat diet for 16 weeks and orally administered with vanillic acid during the last 4 weeks. Control: normal diet; HFD: high-fat diet (60 kcal % fat); HFD + Pio: HFD (60 kcal % fat) + pioglitazone (30 mg/kg body weight); HFD + VA: HFD (60 kcal % fat) + vanillic acid (30 mg/kg body weight); (A–C) indicate statistically significant differences $p < 0.05$. Data are presented as mean ± SD (3 rats in each group).

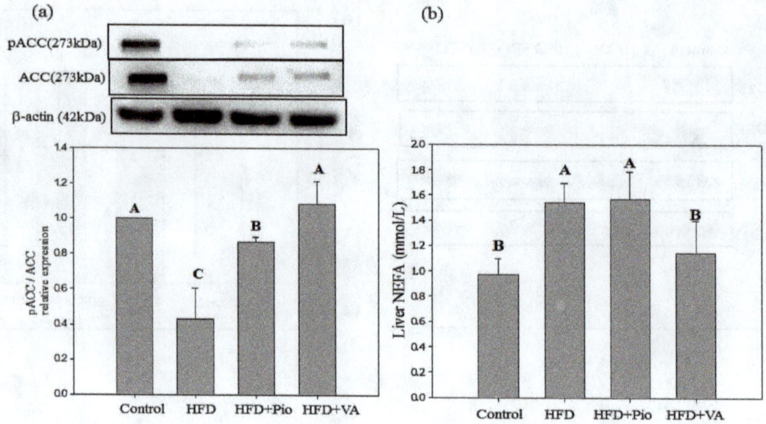

Figure 4. (**a**) Hepatic phosphorylated acetyl-CoA carboxylase/acetyl-CoA carboxylase (pACC/ACC) protein expression; and (**b**) non-esterified free fatty acid (NEFA) in rats fed high-fat diet for 16 weeks and orally administered with vanillic acid during the last 4 weeks. Control: normal diet; HFD: high-fat diet (60 kcal % fat); HFD + Pio: HFD (60 kcal % fat) + pioglitazone (30 mg/kg body weight); HFD + VA: HFD (60 kcal % fat) + vanillic acid (30 mg/kg body weight); NEFA: non-esterified free fatty acid in supernatant of liver homogenate. The liver tissue was homogenized with PBS (1/4; *w/v* and centrifuged at 4 °C for 60 min to obtain the supernatant; (A–C) indicate statistically significant differences $p < 0.05$. Data are presented as mean ± SD (6 rats in each group).

Previous studies indicated that high concentration of NEFA was associated with increased expression of MCP-1 or COX-2 [50,51]. Recent reports also suggest that chronic MCP-1 or COX-2-mediated inflammation in fat is crucial for obesity-linked insulin resistance [52,53]. Phenolic acids were previously reported to exert counteractive effect on inflammation, and prevent the processing of chronic diseases [18]. The results from this study elucidate that VA may reduce hepatic NEFA level, decrease hepatic inflammatory responses and subsequently alleviate insulin resistance in HFD rats.

4. Conclusions

VA is a naturally occurring phenolic acid widely existing in various plant foods. The present study demonstrates that the protective effect of VA against hyperinsulinemia, hyperglycemia and hyperlipidemia is through decreasing hepatic NEFA accumulation, alleviating hepatic inflammation as well as hepatic insulin resistance in HFD-fed rats (Figure 5). Our findings support that VA exerts therapeutic effects and has the potential to be used in clinical medicine or as a dietary supplement for preventing the progression of DM.

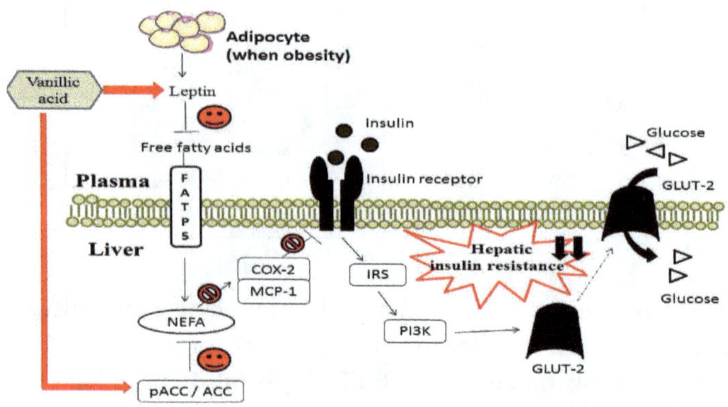

Figure 5. The postulated mechanisms underlying the effect of vanillic acid on hepatic insulin resistance by regulating insulin signaling and inflammation pathways in rats fed an HFD.

Acknowledgments: The authors would like to thank the Ministry of Science and Technology of the Republic of China (ROC), Taiwan, for financially supporting this research under contract No. NSC 100-2313-B-003-001. Our gratitude also goes to the Academic Paper Editing Clinic, National Taiwan Normal University.

Author Contributions: Wen-Chang Chang, James Swi-Bea Wu, Hsu-Min Chien and Szu-Chuan Shen designed the research; Chen-Wen Chen, Po-Ling Kuo and Wen-Chang Chang performed the experimental work; Szu-Chuan Shen, Wen-Chang Chang and Yuh-Tai Wang wrote the manuscript. All authors discussed, edited and approved the final version.

References

1. World Health Organization. Preventing Diabetes is Essential for Keeping Health and Well-Being in Tajikistan. 2011. Available online: http://www.euro.who.int/en/health-topics/noncommunicable-diseases/diabetes/news/news/2011/11/preventing-diabetes-is-essential-for-keeping-health-and-well-being-in-tajikistan (accessed on 21 November 2011).
2. Buettner, R.; Parhofer, K.G.; Woenckhaus, M.; Wrede, C.E.; Kunz-Schughart, L.A.; Scholmerich, J.; Bollheimer, L.C. Defining high-fat-diet rat models: Metabolic and molecular effect of different fat types. *Mol. Endocrinol.* **2006**, *36*, 485–501. [CrossRef] [PubMed]
3. Okabayashi, Y.; Maddux, B.A.; Mcdonald, A.R.; Logsdon, C.D.; Williams, J.A.; Goldfine, I.D. Mechanisms of insulin-induced insulin-receptor downregulation: Decrease of receptor biosynthesis and mRNA levels. *Diabetes* **1989**, *38*, 182–187. [CrossRef] [PubMed]
4. Samuel, V.T. Fructose induced lipogenesis: From sugar to fat to insulin resistance. *Trends Endocrinol. Metab.* **2011**, *22*, 60–65. [CrossRef] [PubMed]
5. Xu, H.; Barnes, G.T.; Yang, Q.; Tan, G.; Yang, D.; Chou, C.J.; Sole, J.; Nichols, A.; Ross, J.S.; Tartaglia, L.A.; *et al.* Chronic inflammation in fat plays a crucial role in the development of obesity-related insulin resistance. *J. Clin. Investig.* **2003**, *112*, 1821–1830. [CrossRef] [PubMed]
6. Arkan, M.C.; Hevener, A.L.; Greten, F.R.; Maeda, S.; Li, Z.W.; Long, J.M.; Wynshaw-Boris, A.; Poli, G.; Olefsky, J.; Karin, M. IKK-β links inflammation to obesity-induced insulin resistance. *Nat. Med.* **2005**, *11*, 191–198. [CrossRef] [PubMed]
7. Cai, D.; Yuan, M.; Frantz, D.F.; Melendez, P.A.; Hansen, L.; Lee, J.; Shoelson, S.E. Local and systemic insulin resistance resulting from hepatic activation of IKKβ and NF-κB. *Nat. Med.* **2005**, *11*, 183–190. [CrossRef] [PubMed]
8. Qatanani, M.; Lazar, M.A. Mechanisms of obesity-associated insulin resistance: Many choices on the menu. *Gene. Dev.* **2007**, *21*, 1443–1455. [CrossRef] [PubMed]
9. Kilmartin, P.A.; Zou, H.; Waterhouse, A.L. A cyclic voltammetry method suitable for characterizing antioxidant properties of wine and wine phenolics. *J. Agric. Food Chem.* **2001**, *49*, 1957–1965. [CrossRef]
10. Adisakwattana, S.; Roengsamarn, S.; Hsu, W.H.; Yibchok-Anun, S. Mechanisms of antihyperglycemic effect of *p*-methoxycinnamic acid in normal and streptozotocin-induced diabetic rats. *Life Sci.* **2005**, *78*, 406–412. [CrossRef] [PubMed]
11. Ohnishi, M.; Matuo, T.; Tsuno, T.; Hosoda, A.; Normura, E.; Taniguchi, H.; Sasaki, H.; Morishita, H. Antioxidation activity and hypoglycemic effect of ferulic acid in STZ-induced diabetic mice and KK-Ay mice. *Biofactors* **2004**, *21*, 315–319. [CrossRef] [PubMed]
12. Jung, U.J.; Lee, M.K.; Park, Y.B.; Jeon, S.M.; Choi, M.S. Antihyperglycemic and antioxidant properties of caffeic acid I *db/db* mice. *J. Pharmacol. Exp. Ther.* **2006**, *318*, 476–483. [CrossRef] [PubMed]
13. Chang, W.C.; Shen, S.C. Effect of water extracts from edible Myrtaceae plants on uptake of 2-(*N*-(7-nitrobenz-2-oxa-1,3-diazol-4-yl)amino)-2-deoxyglucose (2-NBDG) in tumor necrosis factor-α-treated FL83B mouse hepatocytes. *Phytother. Res.* **2013**, *27*, 236–243. [CrossRef] [PubMed]
14. Matthews, D.R.; Hosker, J.P.; Rudenski, A.S.; Naylor, B.A.; Treacher, D.F.; Turner, R.C. Homeostasis model assessment: Insulin resistance and beta-cell function from fasting plasma glucose and insulin concentrations in man. *Diavetologia* **1985**, *28*, 412–419. [CrossRef]
15. Sargent, J.M. The use of the MTT assay to study drug resistance in fresh tumor samples. *Recent Results Cancer Res.* **2003**, *161*, 13–25.
16. Bahorun, T.; Luximon-Ramma, A.; Crozier, A.; Aruoma, O.I. Total phenol, flavonoid, proanthocyanidin and vitamin C levels and antioxidant activities of Mauritian vegetables. *J. Sci. Food Agric.* **2004**, *84*, 1553–1561. [CrossRef]

17. Inoue, M.; Suzuki, R.; Sakaguchi, N.; Li, Z.; Takeda, T.; Ogihara, Y.; Jiang, B.Y.; Chen, Y. Selective induction of cell death in cancer cells by gallic acid. *Biol. Pharm. Bull.* **1995**, *18*, 1526–1530. [CrossRef]
18. Scalbert, A.R.; Johnson, I.T.; Saltmarsh, M. Polyphenols: Antioxidants and beyond. *Am. J. Clin. Nutr.* **2005**, *81*, 215S–217S. [PubMed]
19. Feinstein, R.; Kanety, H.; Papa, M.Z.; Lunenfeld, B.; Karasik, A. Tumor necrosis factor-alpha suppresses insulin-induced tyrosine phosphorylation of insulin receptor and its substrates. *J. Biol. Chem.* **1993**, *268*, 26055–26058.
20. Peraldi, P.; Hotamisligil, G.S.; Buurman, W.A.; White, M.F.; Spiegelman, B.M. Tumor necrosis factor (TNF-α) inhibits insulin signaling through stimulation of the p55 TNF receptor and activation of sphingomyelinase. *J. Biol. Chem.* **1996**, *271*, 13018–13022.
21. Kroder, G.; Bossenmayer, B.; Kellerer, M.; Capp, E.; Stoyanov, B.; Muhlhofer, A.; Berti, L.; Horikoshi, H.; Ullrich, A.; Haring, H. Tumor necrosis factor-alpha and hyperglycemia-induced insulin resistance. *J. Clin. Investig.* **1996**, *97*, 1471–1477. [CrossRef] [PubMed]
22. Yoshioka, K.; Oh, K.B.; Saito, M.; Nemoto, Y.; Matsuoka, H. Evaluation of 2-[*N*-(7-nitrobenz-2-oxa-1,3-diazol-4-yl)amino]-2-deoxy-D-glucose, a new fluorescent derivative of glucose, for viability assessment of yeast *Candida albicans*. *Appl. Microbiol. Biotechnol.* **1996**, *46*, 400–404.
23. Louzao, M.C.; Espiña, B.; Vieytes, M.R.; Vega, F.V.; Rubiolo, J.A.; Baba, O.; Terashima, T.; Botana, L.M. "Fluorescent glycogen" formation with sensibility for *in vivo* and *in vitro* detection. *Glycoconj. J.* **2008**, *25*, 503–510. [CrossRef] [PubMed]
24. Kraegen, E.W.; James, D.E.; Storlien, L.H.; Burleigh, K.M.; Chisholm, D.J. *In vivo* insulin resistance in individual peripheral tissues of the high fat fed rat: Assessment by euglycaemic clamp plus deoxyglucose administration. *Diabetologia* **1986**, *29*, 192–198. [CrossRef]
25. Pedersen, O.; Kahn, C.R.; Flier, J.S.; Kahn, B.B. High fat feeding causes insulin resistance and a marked decrease in the expression of glucose transporters (Glut 4) in fat cells of rats. *Endocrinology* **1991**, *129*, 771–777. [CrossRef] [PubMed]
26. Ahren, B.; Gudbjartsson, T.; Al-Amin, A.N. Islet perturbations in rats fed a high-fat diet. *Pancreas* **1999**, *18*, 75–83. [CrossRef] [PubMed]
27. Kaiyala, K.J.; Prigeon, R.L.; Kahn, S.E.; Woods, S.C.; Porte, D.; Schwartz, M.W. Reduced β-cell function contributes to impaired glucose tolerance in dogs made obese by high-fat feeding. *Am. J. Physiol.* **1999**, *277*, E659–E667. [PubMed]
28. Ginsberg, H.N. Insulin resistance and cardiovascular disease. *J. Clin. Investig.* **2000**, *106*, 453–458. [CrossRef] [PubMed]
29. Jellinger, P.S. Metabolic consequences of hyperglycemia and insulin resistance. *Clin. Cornerstone* **2007**, *8*, S30–S42. [CrossRef]
30. Bahadoran, Z.; Mirmiran, P.; Azizi, F. Potential efficacy of broccoli sprouts as a unique supplement for management of type 2 diabetes and its complications. *J. Med. Food* **2013**, *16*, 375–382. [CrossRef] [PubMed]
31. Hekmatdoost, A.; Mirmiran, P.; Hosseini-Esfahani, F.; Azizi, F. Dietary fatty acid composition and metabolic syndrome in Tehranian adults. *Nutrition* **2011**, *27*, 1002–1007. [CrossRef] [PubMed]
32. Prada, P.O.; Zecchin, H.G.; Gasparetti, A.L.; Torsoni, M.A.; Ueno, M.; Hirata, A.E.; do Amaral, M.E.; Höer, N.F.; Boschero, A.C.; Saad, M.J. Western diet modulates insulin signaling, c-Jun N-terminal kinase activity, and insulin receptor substrate-1ser307 phosphorylation in a tissue-specific fashion. *Endocrinology* **2005**, *146*, 1576–1587. [CrossRef] [PubMed]
33. Huang, B.W.; Chiang, M.T.; Yao, H.T.; Chiang, W. The effect of high-fat and high-fructose diets on glucose tolerance and plasma lipid and leptin levels in rats. *Diabetes Obes. Metab.* **2004**, *6*, 120–126. [CrossRef]
34. Bonora, E.; Targher, G.; Alberiche, M.; Bonadonna, R.C.; Saggiani, F.; Zenere, M.B.; Monauni, T.; Muggeo, M. Homeostasis model assessment closely mirrors the glucose clamp technique in the assessment of insulin sensitivity: Studies in subjects with various degrees of glucose tolerance and insulin sensitivity. *Diabetes Care* **2000**, *23*, 57–63. [CrossRef] [PubMed]
35. Feng, Y.; Carroll, A.R.; Addepalli, R.; Fechner, G.A.; Avery, V.M.; Quinn, R.J. Vanillic acid derivatives from the green algae *Cladophora socialis* as potent protein tyrosine phosphatase 1B inhibitors. *J. Nat. Prod.* **2007**, *70*, 1790–1792. [CrossRef] [PubMed]

36. Fraze, E.; Chiou, M.; Chen, Y.; Reaven, G.M. Age-related changes in postprandial plasma glucose, insulin, and free fatty acid concentrations in nondiabetic individuals. *J. Am. Geriatr. Soc.* **1987**, *35*, 224–228. [CrossRef] [PubMed]
37. Jensen, M.D.; Haymond, M.W.; Rizza, R.A.; Cryer, P.E.; Miles, J.M. Influence of body fat distribution on free fatty acid metabolism in obesity. *J. Clin. Investig.* **1989**, *83*, 1168–1173. [CrossRef] [PubMed]
38. Wang, Y.; Wang, P.Y.; Qin, L.Q.; Davaasambuu, G.; Kaneko, T.; Xu, J.; Murata, S.I.; Katoh, R.; Sato, A. The development of diabetes mellitus in wistar rats kept on a high-fat low-carbohydrate diet for long periods. *Endocrine* **2003**, *22*, 85–92. [CrossRef]
39. Considine, R.V.; Sinha, M.K.; Heiman, M.L.; Kriauciunas, A.; Stephens, T.W.; Nyce, M.R.; Ohannesian, J.P.; Marco, C.C.; Mckee, L.J.; Baur, T.L.; *et al.* Serum immunoreative-leptin concentrations in normal weight and obese human. *N. Engl. J. Med.* **1996**, *334*, 292–295. [CrossRef] [PubMed]
40. Maffei, M.; Halaas, J.; Ravussin, E.; Pratley, R.E.; Lee, G.H.; Zhang, Y.; Fei, H.; Kim, S.; Lallone, R.; Ranganathan, S.; *et al.* Leptin levels in human and rodent: Measurement of plasma leptin and *ob* RNA in obese and weight-reduced subjects. *Nat. Med.* **1995**, *1*, 1155–1161. [CrossRef]
41. Pelleymounter, M.A.; Cullen, M.J.; Baker, M.B.; Hecht, R.; Winters, D.; Boone, T.; Collins, F. Effects of the obese gene product on body weight regulation in ob/ob mice. *Science* **1995**, *269*, 540–543. [CrossRef] [PubMed]
42. Halaas, J.L.; Gajiwala, K.S.; Maffei, M.; Cohen, S.L.; Chait, B.T.; Rabinowitz, D.; Lallone, R.L.; Burley, S.K.; Friedman, J.M. Weight-reducing effects of the plasma protein encoded by the obese gene. *Science* **1995**, *269*, 543–546. [CrossRef]
43. Ghorbani, Z.; Hekmatdoost, A.; Mirmiran, P. Anti-hyperglycemic and insulin sensitizer effects of turmeric and its principle constituent curcumin. *Int. J. Endocrinol. Metab.* **2014**, *12*. [CrossRef] [PubMed]
44. Panzhinskiy, E.; Hua, Y.; Lapchak, P.A.; Topchiy, E.; Lehmann, T.E.; Ren, J.; Nair, S. Novel curcumin derivative CNB-001 mitigates obesity-associated insulin resistance. *J. Pharmacol. Exp. Ther.* **2014**, *349*, 248–257. [CrossRef] [PubMed]
45. Martyn, J.A.; Kaneki, M.; Yasuhara, S. Obesity-induced insulin resistance and hyperglycemia: Etiologic factors and molecular mechanisms. *Anesthesiology* **2008**, *109*, 137–148. [CrossRef] [PubMed]
46. Bose, T.; Alvarenga, J.C.; Tejero, M.E.; Voruganti, V.S.; Proffitt, J.M.; Freeland-Graves, J.H. Association of monocyte chemoattractant protein-1 with adipocyte number, insulin resistance and liver function markers. *J. Med. Primatol.* **2009**, *38*, 418–424. [CrossRef] [PubMed]
47. Weisberg, S.P.; Hunter, D.; Huber, R.; Lemieux, J.; Slaymaker, S.; Vaddi, K.; Charo, I.; Leibel, R.L.; Ferrante, A.W. CCR2 modulates inflammatory and metabolic effects of high-fat feeding. *J. Clin. Investig.* **2006**, *116*, 115–124. [CrossRef] [PubMed]
48. Esposito, E.; Iacono, A.; Bianco, G.; Autore, G.; Cuzzocrea, S.; Vajro, P.; Canani, R.B.; Calignano, A.; Raso, G.M.; Meli, R. Probiotics reduce the inflammatory response induced by a high-fat diet in the liver of young rats. *J. Nutr.* **2009**, *139*, 905–911. [CrossRef] [PubMed]
49. Capurso, C.; Capurso, A. From excess adiposity to insulin resistance: The role of free fatty acids. *Vascul. Pharmacol.* **2012**, *57*, 91–97. [CrossRef] [PubMed]
50. Jiang, C.H.; Yao, N.; Wang, Q.Q.; Zhang, J.H.; Sun, Y.; Xiao, N.; Liu, K.; Huang, F.; Fang, S.Z.; Shang, X.L.; *et al.* Cyclocarya paliurus extract modulates adipokine expression and improves insulin sensitivity by inhibition of inflammation in mice. *J. Ethnopharmacol.* **2014**, *153*, 344–351. [CrossRef] [PubMed]
51. Hsieh, P.S.; Jin, J.S.; Chiang, C.F.; Chan, P.C.; Chen, C.H.; Shih, K.C. COX-2-mediated inflammation in fat is crucial for obesity-linked insulin resistance and fatty liver. *Obesity* **2009**, *17*, 1150–1157. [CrossRef] [PubMed]
52. Lloyd, E.E.; Gaubatz, J.W.; Burns, A.R.; Pownall, H.J. Sustained elevations in NEFA induce cyclooxygenase-2 activity and potentiate THP-1 macrophage foam cell formation. *Atherosclerosis* **2007**, *192*, 49–55. [CrossRef] [PubMed]
53. Mas, S.; Martínez-Pinna, R.; Martín-Ventura, J.L.; Pérez, R.; Gomez-Garre, D.; Ortiz, A.; Fernandez-Cruz, A.; Vivanco, F.; Egido, J. Local non-esterified fatty acids correlate with inflammation in atheroma plaques of patients with type 2 diabetes. *Diabetes* **2010**, *59*, 1292–301. [CrossRef] [PubMed]

14

Diet, Microbiota and Immune System in Type 1 Diabetes Development and Evolution

María E. Mejía-León and Ana M. Calderón de la Barca *

Department Nutrición y Metabolismo, Centro de Investigación en Alimentación y Desarrollo, A.C., Carr. La Victoria, Km. 0.6, Hermosillo, Sonora 83304, Mexico; esther.mejia83@gmail.com

* Correspondence: amc@ciad.mx

Abstract: Type 1 diabetes (T1D) is the second most frequent autoimmune disease in childhood. The long-term micro- and macro-vascular complications of diabetes are associated with the leading causes of disability and even mortality in young adults. Understanding the T1D etiology will allow the design of preventive strategies to avoid or delay the T1D onset and to help to maintain control after developing. T1D development involves genetic and environmental factors, such as birth delivery mode, use of antibiotics, and diet. Gut microbiota could be the link between environmental factors, the development of autoimmunity, and T1D. In this review, we will focus on the dietary factor and its relationship with the gut microbiota in the complex process involved in autoimmunity and T1D. The molecular mechanisms involved will also be addressed, and finally, evidence-based strategies for potential primary and secondary prevention of T1D will be discussed.

Keywords: Type 1 diabetes; autoimmunity; diet; gut microbiota; dysbiosis; *Bacteroides*

---

1. Introduction

Type 1 diabetes (T1D) is one of the two most frequent autoimmune disorders in childhood and adolescence. It is due to the cellular-mediated autoimmune destruction of pancreatic β-cells, which leads to an absolute insulin deficiency, disturbing glucose metabolism [1]. The T1D prevalence of 1:300 is increasing over the world, representing 5%–10% of all diabetes mellitus cases [2].

Long-term micro- and macrovascular complications of diabetes are the leading causes of mortality [3] and disability in young adults. Understanding T1D etiology will allow for the design of preventive strategies to avoid or delay T1D onset and help to keep it under control if developed.

Genetic predisposition is the main determinant involved in T1D development, with the human leucocyte antigen (HLA) DR3-DQ2 and DR4-DQ8 haplotypes as the most common variants involved, which are shared with other autoimmune diseases such as celiac disease [4]. Since pancreatic β-cell autoimmunity appears frequently in the first 6 years of life, and its progression towards T1D can occur in preschoolers or during puberty, the factors investigated as possible triggers are related to early life and the immune system maturation process [5,6]. In addition to genetics, other factors such as birth delivery mode, diet, infections, and the use of antibiotics have been associated with T1D development [7]. However, the causality and possible mechanisms by which these factors relate to T1D remain unclear.

During the last decade, advances in molecular techniques have allowed for the study of gut microbiota in animal models of T1D [8] and, more recently, in children with autoimmunity and T1D [9–15]. The gut microbiota could be the link between environmental factors and the development of autoimmunity and T1D. This has led to the proposal of a possible intestinal origin of T1D [9], and has placed the microbiota as the central factor for its study.

In this review, we are focusing on the dietary element and its relationship with the gut microbiota in the complex process towards autoimmunity and the progression to T1D. The molecular mechanisms involved will also be addressed, and evidence-based strategies for potential primary and secondary prevention of T1D will be discussed.

2. Diet and the Shaping of the Gut Microbiota

The first gut microbiota composition is mostly acquired at birth. The delivery mode determines the type of microorganisms that will colonize the newborn gut. Thus, children born vaginally develop a microbiota composed by *Lactobacillus*, *Prevotella* or *Sneathia* spp. from the maternal vaginal tract. Meanwhile, in those infants born by caesarean section, the bacterial communities from the mothers' or skin or the skin of participants in the surgical procedure, such as *Staphylococcus*, *Corynebacterium*, and *Propionibacterium* spp., will dominate [10].

After delivery, diet is one of the main modulators of infant gut microbiota. Diet acts in a direct way by providing the substrates and sources of bacterial contamination from breast and nipple skin in breastfeeding babies or due to the tools and preparation methods in bottle-fed babies with infant formulas. Diet also contributes indirectly in the regulation of intestinal and pancreatic physiology [11]. During early childhood, microbiota diversity rapidly increases and new strains are acquired. Breastfeeding increases the diversity of lactic acid bacteria, while infant formulas contribute to the acquisition of bacterial communities such as *Staphylococcus aureus*, *Clostridium difficile*, *Bacteroides* spp., and other pathogenic communities. The microbiota structure is very unstable until the age of 2–3 years and it responds to changes in the diet, such as the introduction of solid foods or diseases; in subsequent years, it resembles the adult composition [12,13].

Around the age of 7 years old, the most prevalent phyla are *Firmicutes* and *Bacteroidetes*, representing about 90% of microorganisms, while the remaining 10% consists of *Proteobacteria*, *Tericutes* and *Cyanobacteria*. Three enterotypes have been proposed for the world population, in accordance with with the clustering patterns seen in the variations in the levels of the dominant microbiota genera: *Bacteroides*, *Prevotella*, and *Ruminococcus* [14]. In adults, these enterotypes have been associated with long-term dietary patterns. Thus, the *Bacteroides* enterotype has been correlated with diets dominated by high levels of animal protein and saturated fats, as occurs in the western diet. On the other hand, the *Prevotella* enterotype is more prevalent in people with higher consumption of carbohydrates and simple sugars, as observed in agrarian and vegetarian societies [15]. These enterotypes appear to be stable in adults after 6 months despite changes in saturated fats and fiber in feeding patterns [16].

In the last 5 years, several studies have examined the microbiota of healthy school-age children from different regions around the world. In all cases, the age, dietary patterns, and geography/traditions were the main determinants explaining the differences in gut microbiota composition. For example, microbiota profiles rich in *Prevotella* have been described in children from Burkina Faso [17], Mexico [18], Indonesia [19], Thailand [19,20], Malawi [21], and Amerindians from the Venezuelan Amazon [21]. All of them have common diets with a low content of fat and animal protein, and a high content of starch, fiber, and plant polysaccharides. In contrast, in the same age group of the United States [21], Italy [17], China [19], Japan [19] and Taiwan [19], the present gut microbiota is dominated by *Bacteroides*. In these, the diet is westernized with a high content of animal protein and fat, and a low fiber content.

Recently, the enterotype hypothesis has been questioned and reformulated because, according to Knights *et al.* [22], the stability of microbiotal composition could arise because "people resemble themselves over time in general rather than because there are specific barriers to switching cluster types". They demonstrated a temporal fluidity of enterotypes in a gradient form in which one individual can move across time. Hence, enterotypes can be unstable, continuous, and driven by sampling frame. Therefore, for a better understanding of the way that diet shapes the microbiota and in order to minimize bias, multiple sampling is recommended to avoid isolated "snapshots" of a dynamic process. It would also be useful to know the microbiotal composition throughout the entire gastrointestinal tract; however, this requires invasive techniques that are impractical in healthy people [23].

3. The Immunity-Diet-Microbiome Consortium: Towards T1D in Early Life

The modulation of the immune system by the microbiota begins even before birth. The intrauterine environment of the fetus during pregnancy is not completely sterile. There is evidence that the placenta of a term pregnancy has a non-pathogenic commensal microbiota in low-abundance, similar to the oral microbiome of non-pregnant women [24]. This suggests that from a very early stage, the fetus is exposed to bacterial antigens against which it has to develop tolerance.

The intestinal immune system begins to develop after 11 weeks of gestation. At 16 weeks, there are already functional B and T cells. However, the response to antigens remains blocked to protect the fetus from an overreaction of the immature immune system. This is possible because the amniotic fluid contains endotoxin-neutralizing histones and a lipopolysaccharide-binding protein that prevents the activation of the Toll-like receptor (TLR) pathway [25].

After birth, diet and microbiota are the decisive factors that guide the proper maturation of the immune system. Diet is a source of nutrients, but it is also the main route of entry for antigens to the organism [26]. At the same time, early colonizer microbiota produce stimuli that manage the differentiation of cells and tissues of the immune system [25]. At this stage, the infant immune system learns to distinguish the self from the non-self and to control the balance between regulatory and inflammatory responses in the host, due to the types of bacteria that form the gut microbiota [27].

To accomplish this, the immune system applies two adaptive anti-inflammatory strategies: first, the production of secretory IgA (sIgA) to prevent epithelial penetration and to control colonization over the surface towards the lumen. The second strategy is the development of oral tolerance, which helps to prevent hypersensitivity reactions against innocuous antigens that pass through the intestinal barrier [28].

A mutualistic relationship with the microbiota can occur because the gut epithelial cells express microbe-associated molecular pattern (MAMP) receptors, primarily TLR. The NF-κB pathway is activated by TLRs, producing a pro-inflammatory response. This results in the production of cytokines, chemokines, and antibacterial products, according to the type of TLRs that are activated and the microbiotal patterns that are being recognized. For example, the bacterial lipopolysaccharide (LPS) inhibits the interleukin-1 receptor-associated kinase (IRAK) M, a modulator of IRAK1, which is necessary for NF-κB activation. Similarly, the ubiquitination and degradation of IγB is inhibited by reactive oxygen species (ROS) which is induced by the microbiota and, peroxisome proliferator-activated receptor gamma (PPARγ), a product of the activation of Toll-like recepetor (TLR) 4 by LPS, diverts NF-κB from the cell core [29].

In this process initiated by bacterial recognition, there is also production of sIgA, differentiation of effector T helper (Th) 1, Th2, and Th17 cells, and the development of regulatory T cells (Treg). The differentiation of Tregs can be induced by commensal microbiota in the colon, such as Cluster IV and XIVa *Clostridia*, related to their short-chain fatty acid production, which stimulates the expression of Foxp3 in CD4+ T cells [27]. However, other bacterial communities can induce the production of inflammatory T cells. In this setting, the segmented filamentous bacteria can colonize the gut by getting in direct contact with the epithelium, facilitating their presentation by dendritic cells (DCs). This elicits a specific effector host response, characterized by a cascade of pro-inflammatory signals that culminate with the production of Th17 and Th1 cells, mediated by interleukin (IL)-1, IL-6 and IL-12, which can lead to autoimmunity [29]. Thereby, alterations in this process, such as dysbiosis or an inadequate introduction of foods during the first months of life, may increase susceptibility to and generate the development of autoimmune diseases, allergies and other disorders, locally in the gut or at a systemic level.

Besides this, the microorganisms of the microbiota can regulate the intestinal architecture, altering gut permeability. Epithelial cells are bound within each other by structural proteins such as zonulin, claudin, occluding, and actin [30]. For instance, enteropathogenic *E. coli* acts directly on the distribution of occludin and *Clostridium difficile* through its toxins A and B, can disorganize actin and dissociate the zonulin complex, increasing permeability by a paracellular route. Moreover, *Vibrio cholerae* produces the zonula occludens toxin, which is homologous and competes with zonulin causing loss of the tight junctions [31]. As a result, dietary antigens and microbiotal products can pass through the leaky gut and initiate the development of an autoimmune response in genetically predisposed individuals.

Dietary antigens associated with T1D depend on early feeding regimens, the age of introduction of foods, especially wheat, to the infant's diet, and the current consumption of nutrients [26]. In contrast, breastfeeding has beneficial immunomodulatory effects in the newborn. Studies in mice have confirmed that passive-transferred sIgA prevents the translocation of bacteria in the intestine, promoting gut homeostasis, which protects against infection by pathogens [32]. In contrast, milk formula consumption has been historically associated with T1D.

In Finnish children from the Diabetes Prediction and Prevention (DIPP) study [33] and in Americans from the Diabetes Autoimmunity Study in the Young (DAISY) study [34], it has been found that fat intake from bovine milk products as well as proteins from fresh milk presented an increase in the risk of advanced β-cell autoimmunity and subsequent progression to T1D. The presence of high titers of anti-β-casein at diagnosis of patients with T1D and with latent autoimmune diabetes of adults (LADA) has been shown [35]. The A1, A2, and B variants of the bovine β-casein contain the PGPIP (Pro-Gly-Pro-Ile-Pro) motif repeated several times in their sequence. This motif is also repeated in the glucose transporter GLUT2, present in the pancreas. Therefore, a possible explanation for pancreatic damage is a cross-reaction of the immune system initially directed against a dietary antigen. Meanwhile, in the sequence of human β-casein, proline is replaced with valine, avoiding the immunogenicity against the human protein [26].

In addition, it has been proposed that high-gluten diets could be one of the primary drivers for gut dysbiosis associated with the T1D development [36]. This is related with the timing and amounts of dietary gluten fed to infants. The progressive introduction of gluten-containing foods to the diet, in terms of quantity, between 3 and 7 months after birth, can decrease the risk of T1D-associated autoimmunity [37]. T1D children have an altered T-cell reactivity to wheat antigens in the gut and peripheral tissues [9]. Recently, we found that 96% and 20% of the studied T1D Mexican children presented high titers of IgG isotypes anti-gliadins and IgA anti-gliadins, respectively [38]. This was an expected finding since T1D shares its genetic HLA-associated risk with celiac disease.

The effects of gluten on intestinal homeostasis are multiple. Gluten increases gut permeability, affecting the tight junctions, which is well described in celiac disease patients and recently in T1D. As a result, long gliadin peptides can move between the epithelial cells to the lamina propria. Then, the dendritic cells can detect them and migrate to other sites, such as the pancreatic lymph nodes, to activate autoreactive T cells [37]. In an *in vitro* study by Hamari *et al.* [39], it was found that pre-T1D children with multiple autoantibodies and those newly diagnosed with T1D presented a T-cell response against gliadin in a lower frequency and intensity than healthy controls and patients with long evolution T1D. This finding supports the idea of an aberrant immune response related to the development of T1D.

Considering all the results together, the interplay between diet, microbiota, and immune system could partly explain the origin of T1D in susceptible children. These mechanisms reflects the immune link between the pancreas and intestine, as they both develop from the embryonic endoderm [9].

4. The Diabetogenic Microbiome

Over the past decade, the first microbiotal studies in animal models suggested the novel possibility of T1D prevention in humans through gut microbiota modulation. Among them, the experiment by Brugman *et al.* [40], performed in Bio-Breeding diabetes prone (BB-DP) rats, proved that antibiotic treatment had an effect on the incidence of diabetes, and that the differences in gut bacterial composition were detectable before the rats developed disease. In another work by Wen *et al.* [8], the interaction between intestinal microbiota and the innate immune system was recognized as an epigenetic factor which can modify predisposition to T1D. In their study, specific-pathogen-free (SPF) non-obese diabetic (NOD) mice lacking myeloid differentiation primary response 88 (MyD88) did not develop T1D. The MyD88 protein is an adaptor for TLRs and other innate immune receptors that recognize microbial stimuli. Furthermore, they found that this effect was related to commensal microbiota, as germ-free MyD88-negative NOD mice developed diabetes.

More recently, the antibiotic effects over the development of T1D has been further analyzed. It has been found that both the administration of broad spectrum antibiotics, which almost completely eliminate the commensal microbiota, and the use of selective antibiotics, which affect the microbiotal composition and limit certain bacterial groups, increase the incidence of T1D in NOD mice [41]. Moreover, fecal transplant from NOD to non-obese resistant (NOR) mice produced insulitis in the latter, and antibiotics accelerated the appearance of T1D in this model [42]. These studies suggest that antibiotics could potentiate the diabetogenic effects of the altered microbiome.

Research in this topic has strongly increased in the last five years. Taking advantage of the new high-throughput sequencing techniques and bioinformatics, studies in humans have been conducted, looking for the possibility of a diabetogenic microbiome. In Table 1, a comparison of the published studies to date is shown. It is remarkable that in all of these studies, the presence of dysbiosis has been related to the autoimmune process and its further progression to T1D. In Finnish patients, this imbalance has been associated with a decreased bacterial diversity after seroconversion, before the onset of hyperglycemia [43–45]. The development of β-cell autoimmunity may precede the appearance of hyperglycemia for over 15 years [5]. This represents a window of opportunity for possible microbiota-related therapies that could prevent or delay the development of T1D in autoimmune-presenting children.

The pattern of relative abundance of gut bacteria is different among the conducted studies. However, regardless of ethnicity, age and geography, all studies have detected *Bacteroides* as the main genus leading to T1D-associated dysbiosis. An increased proportion of *Bacteroides* in White Americans [46] and Caucasian children [9–11,13] with beta-cell autoimmunity, as well at the onset of T1D of Mestizo children [18], has been reported. Furthermore, there is a directly proportional relationship between the number of T1D-associated autoantibodies and the abundance of *Bacteroides* [44,45]. Hence, the presence of a higher degree of dysbiosis could contribute to the fast progression towards T1D that occurs in children with multiple autoantibodies [5].

An interesting finding of Davis-Richardson *et al.* [47] was the identification of two specific species causing the increase in gut abundance of *Bacteroides*: *B. dorei and B. vulgatus*, with *B. dorei* significantly increased before seroconversion. Therefore, the authors proposed to use them as predictors of T1D-associated autoimmunity. However, no other studies exist that confirm the increased presence of these species in other populations or their power as a predictor tool for T1D. In addition, we found that T1D Mexican children [18] with more than 2 years of evolution, controlled with insulin, presented a lower *Bacteroides* abundance than children with T1D at onset. These patients also had a relatively increased abundance of *Prevotella*, approaching the microbiotal profile described for healthy children with the same age and population.

Possibly, the full rebalancing of the proportion *Bacteroides* to *Prevotella* was not reached in our study [18] due to the diet of patients with T1D. The American Diabetes Association (ADA) [1] recommends an intensive insulin therapy scheme, using the carbohydrate counting method. This allows the patients to have a close to "normal" diet according to their customs. However, to achieve the goals of glycemic control, it tends to limit the dietary load and glycemic index, reducing carbohydrate intake and increasing fat consumption compared to healthy children. In the study by Virtanen *et al.* [48], 38 Finnish children with T1D were followed to analyze their diet. The proportion of energy from fats increased in these children from 26% at onset of disease to 30% two years later. The American Heart Association recommends limiting the intake of saturated fat to 7% of energy to prevent cardiovascular events [49]. In the same study [48], they found that most of the fat sources consumed by T1D children were of animal origin and the saturated fat consumption was around 11%, high above the recommended level. This suggests that the high fat diet may be maintaining the *Bacteroides* levels, limiting the full recovery of the microbiotal balance.

Table 1. Comparison of microbiota composition in humans with autoimmunity and T1D.

Country/Ethnicity	**Diagnostic (*n*)**	**Age in Years**	**Microbiota Diversity in Autoimmunity/T1D**	**Microbiota Relative Abundance in Autoimmunity/T1D**	**Other Findings**
Finland (DIPP Study)/Caucasians [43,50]	β-cell AI (4) HC (4)	0–2 0–3	Reduced	F/B ratio ↓ Increase in: ***Bacteroides*** genus, mainly *Bacteroides ovatus.* Decrease in: *Prevotella and Faecalibacterium*	Non-butyrate producers avoid optimal mucine synthesis in T1D-associated autoimmunity.
Spain/Caucasians [51]	T1D at onset (16) HC (16)	7.16 ± 0.72 7.48 ± 0.87	Similar to the control group ($p > 0.05$)	F/B ratio ↓ Increase in: *Clostridium*, ***Bacteroides*** *and Veionella.* Decrease in: *Lactobacillus, Bifidobacterium* and *Prevotella.*	Microbiota differences were associated with glycemic level.
Finland (FINDIA and TRIGR studies)/Caucasians [44]	β-cell AI (18) HC (18)	FINDIA/TRIGR: 5.1 ± 1/13.3 ± 1 FINDIA/TRIGR: 5.0 ± 2/12.8 ± 1	Reduced	F/B ratio ↓ Increase in: ***Bacteroides*** genus, *Clostridium perfringens.* Decrease in: *Bifidobacterium adolescentis* and *Bifidobacterium pseudocatenulatum.*	The abundance of lactate- and butyrate-producing bacteria was inversely related to the number of β cell autoantibodies.
Mexico/Mestizos [18]	T1D at onset (8) T1D ≥ 2 years evolution (13) HC (8)	12.3 ± 0.64 11 ± 1.04	Similar to the control group ($p > 0.05$)	Unaltered F/B ratio. Increase in: ***Bacteroides*** genus. Decrease in: *Prevotella, Acidaminococcus* and *Megamonas.*	The glycemic control in the T1D ≥ 2 years treated group partially normalizes the microbiotal profile towards *Prevotella*-dominant profile.
Finland (DIPP Study)/Caucasians [47]	High risk cohort (76): β-cell AI (29) T1D at onset (22) HC (47)	0–2	Reduced	F/B ratio ↓ Increase: in ***Bacteroides*** genus due to *Bacteroides dorei* and *Bacteroides vulgatus.*	*B.dorei* abundance peaked over 8 months prior to the appearance of the first islet auto antibody. It coincided with the introduction of solid foods.
Finland, Estonia (DIABIMMUNE Study)/Caucasians [45]	High risk cohort (33): β-cell AI (7) T1D at onset (4) HC (22)	0–3	Reduced	Increase in: *Blautia, Rikenellaceae, Ruminococcus gnavus* and *Streptococcus infantarius* in T1D cases at the time of alpha-diversity divergence.	Decreased community diversity occurs after seroconversion but before onset of T1D. T1D onset is preceded by increased inflammation-assoc. organisms and pathways.
USA/White Americans (TRIALNET Study) [46]	β-cell AI (21) T1D at onset (35) Seroneg. FDR (32) HC (23)	4–49 2–20 3–45 4–24	Similar to the control group ($p > 0.05$)	Increase in: ***Bacteroides.*** Decrease in: *Prevotella* * In seropositive subjects with multiple *versus* one autoantibody.	The microbiomes of β-cell AI and seroneg. FDRs clustered together but separate from those of T1D at onset and HC.

T1D: Type-1 Diabetes; β-cell AI: β-cell autoimmunity; F/B ratio: Firmicutes/Bacteroidetes ratio; HC: Healthy controls; FDR: First degree relatives. DIPP: Diabetes Prediction and Prevention; FINDIA: Finnish Dietary Intervention Trial for the Prevention of Type 1 Diabetes; TRIGR: Trial to Reduce Type 1 Diabetes in the Genetically at Risk; TRIALNET: Type 1 Diabetes TrialNet; * indicate that these findings (Increase in: *Bacteroides,* Decrease in: *Prevotella)* were only detected in seropositive subjects from the TRIALNET study with multiple versus one autoantibody and there were not considered the seronegative first degree relatives included in the original study design.

5. Microbiota: Molecular Mechanisms in T1D

To explain the pathways and the impact of T1D-associated dysbiosis in the metabolism, it is necessary to study the microbiota structural dynamics as an integral organ [52]. Understanding that the gut microbiota is an organ will make it possible to integrate its relationship with T1D as a key for designing new therapies to prevent and/or improve the T1D control.

Dietary components provide different substrates that may result in several products during the fermentation processes. Changes in the microbiotal structure due to diet modifications are because some of the bacterial communities are "genetically better equipped" to metabolize those substrates. Moreover, the same substrate can be used in different pathways according to the type of bacteria that are colonizing the intestinal niche, or in relation to its abundance and available frequency [13]. An example of the former statement is lactate. This substrate can be transformed into butyrate or, in others, short chain fatty acids (SCFA) such as acetate, succinate, and propionate during its anaerobic bacterial fermentation in the gut, depending on the type of microbiota [50].

The lactate model appears to be the strongest possible explanation for understanding the link between T1D and dysbiosis (Figure 1). According to this model, the presence of lactic acid- and butyrate-producing bacteria such as *Prevotella* and *Akkermansia* helps to maintain a healthy epithelium. This is because butyrate contributes to mucin synthesis and to the assembly of tight junctions [53]. These bacteria were common in the microbiota of healthy children around the world [9–12,15,50]. In contrast, when microorganisms such as *Bacteroides* and *Veillonella* are harbored in abundance, this substrate follows the pathway to succinate, acetate, and propionate. These products compromise mucin synthesis and increase paracellular permeability by altering the tight junctions [50].

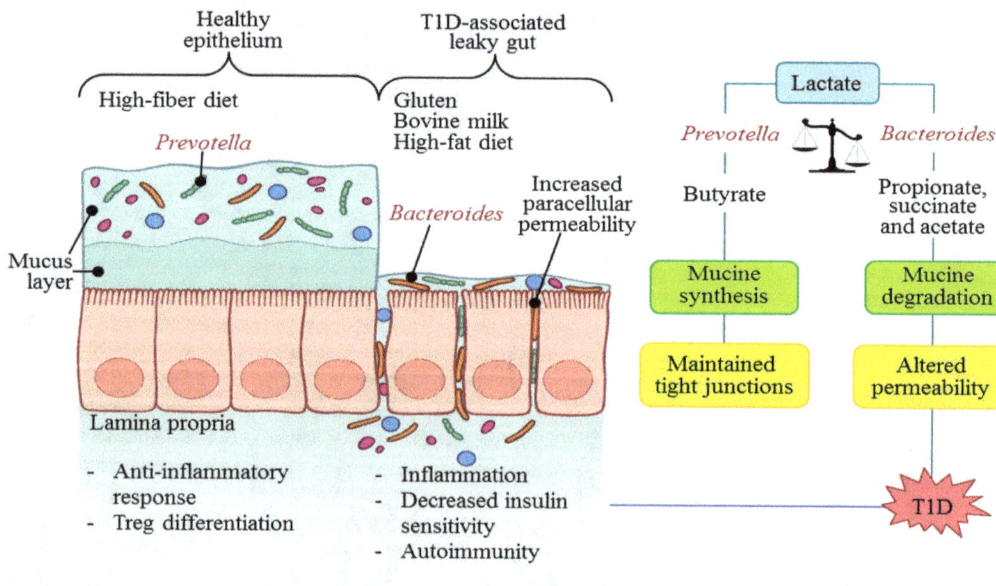

Figure 1. Diet and microbiota associated mechanisms in autoimmunity and type 1 diabetes (T1D) development.

In addition, butyrate may contribute to maintaining the anti-inflammatory response in the healthy gut by inhibiting the activation of NF-κB, signaling through G protein-coupled receptors, and leading to the modulation of antioxidant defense systems, nitric oxide production, and the expression of inflammatory cytokines [28,36]. High-fiber diets have been associated with a decreased risk of inflammatory immune-related diseases. However, it is unknown whether this effect is due to the butyrate itself or to the associated microbial profile [28]. Butyrate also enhances extra-thymic differentiation of Treg cells, while other SCFA, such as acetate, block this process [54]. Treg differentiation seems to be related to histone acetylation in the promoter of the Foxp3 locus, which is also regulated by butyrate [36]. This suggests that microbiota-derived products function as mediators in the communication between bacteria and the host immune system, leading to pro- or anti-inflammatory responses [54], and could be a factor involved in β-cell autoimmunity and T1D.

Systemic effects of intestinal butyrate in the regulatory immune response also occur at the pancreatic level. Butyrate has been associated with the expression of cathelicidin-related antimicrobial peptide (CRAMP) in the β-cells of NOD mice. This peptide has been shown to protect against the development of T1D by inducing a regulatory response and suppressing the inflammatory process in the pancreatic islets of prediabetic mice [55].

Free fatty acid receptor 2 (FFAR2) is one of the G protein-coupled receptors that can be activated by microbiota-derived butyrate. This receptor is involved in the insulin signaling regulation in adipose tissue and in the maintenance of energy homeostasis. Its activation promotes the secretion of GLP-1 in the intestine, the suppression of fat accumulation, and, therefore, increased sensitivity to insulin [56]. This is an interesting mechanism because even though the main problem in T1D is not insulin resistance, the diabetes accelerator theory puts it in context. This theory proposes that in T1D, body constitution, insulin resistance, and autoimmunity are three processes that accelerate the loss of beta-cells by apoptosis [57]. This theory arises when observing that children with autoimmunity that progress more quickly to T1D have greater insulin resistance than those non-progressors [58]. Thus, decreased production of butyrate in children with low levels of *Prevotella* in their gut microbiota could be contributing to T1D development.

Kostic *et al.* [45], in the DIABIMMUNE study, followed children with high genetic risk for T1D from the first days following birth. Their results show associations between the gut bacterial communities and metabolic profile in young children, such as the levels of *Blautia* with long-chain triglycerides and *Ruminococcus* with short-chain triglycerides. Furthermore, these two microorganisms, which were abundant in children who progress to T1D, correlated positively with the presence of branched-chain amino acids such as valine, isoleucine, and leucine. Meanwhile, Oresic *et al.* [59] found that the dysregulation of lipid and amino acid metabolism precedes the appearance of glutamic acid decarboxylase and insulin autoantibodies in children who later developed T1D.

6. T1D Prevention and Control Possibilities

Children born with a genetic risk of T1D represent 30% of all births, but most of them do not develop the disease [60]. The risk increases considerably when β-cell autoimmunity appeared; according to the TEDDY study group [61], this can be attributed to the presence of two or more associated autoantibodies. With the appearance of autoantibodies, the risk for T1D increases up to 75% in the next 10 years and it is almost certain within 20 years [62,63]. Therefore, it is essential to implement effective prevention strategies at three levels of attention: primary prevention, before seroconversion; secondary prevention, when the β-cell autoimmunity is already present, trying to prevent or delay the T1D onset in predisposed children; and tertiary prevention, when the T1D is already present, to avoid complications [62].

6.1. *Primary Prevention of T1D*

Based on the evidence, the primary prevention of T1D should focus on modifiable perinatal factors, which theoretically could help to prevent not only T1D, but other autoimmune and allergic diseases in children. Thus, as the newborn initial microbiota is primarily obtained from the mother during birth and lactation, the possibility of considering maternal microbiome as the starting point has been suggested [52]. Thus, maintaining a healthy maternal microbiota, avoiding unnecessary cesareans, and the promotion of breastfeeding are important activities in which both mothers and health caregivers have to be educated.

Dominguez-Bello *et al.* [64] evaluated the possibility of modulating the gut microbiota from cesarean-born children. The newborns were exposed to a first natural inoculum, obtained from the *Lactobacillus*-dominated vaginas of their healthy mothers, in order to mimic the probable microbiota that they would have acquired if they were born vaginally. Preliminary results show that these babies have bacterial communities with an intermediate pattern between children born vaginally and those born by cesarean not receiving the inoculum. Moreover, regarding lactation, breastfeeding must be encouraged. It is also important that mothers have a varied and balanced diet while nursing. It was recently found that maternal consumption of red meats, meat products, and vegetable oils increases the risk of the baby developing autoimmunity and T1D in the following years [65]. In turn, in those who are exclusively milk formula-fed, supplementation with prebiotics and probiotics have proven to be effective in modifying the intestinal microbiota, resembling the profile of infants who are breastfed, stimulating the proper maturation and function of the immune system [11]. However, the effectiveness of these practices long-term has not yet been proven and it is not known whether they are sufficient to counteract the negative effects associated with the consumption of cow's milk proteins in early life.

Regarding bovine milk proteins contained in milk formulas, an option to prevent the development of autoimmunity in children at high risk might be weaning with a highly casein-hydrolyzed formula. To confirm this, the TRIGR study [66] is evaluating whether or not the use of hydrolyzed formula is safer than conventional milk formulas. The final endpoint of this study is in 2017, when participants turn 10 years old. This is a study with enough power to confirm or reject this theory and to provide the certainty required to direct preventive strategies. The possible benefits of highly hydrolyzed formulas in reducing the risk of autoimmunity with respect to conventional formulas are wide. Among them, they may avoid early exposure to intact bovine insulin, decrease gut permeability and thus the paracellular transit of foreign peptides, induce maturation of Tregs, decrease inflammation, and, with this, potentially contribute to maintaining the diversity of the intestinal microbiota.

6.2. *Secondary and Tertiary Prevention of T1D*

Once the autoimmune process has started, diet is the main known modifiable factor capable of changing the risk of developing T1D. The progression to T1D in children with β-cell autoimmunity is associated with the intake of total sugars, especially from sugar-sweetened beverages in those with a high-risk genotype [67]. The results from the latest clinical and experimental studies suggest that an effective measure in diabetes could be to target the treatment to the modulation of microbiota [68]. Considering the current information, dietary interventions should focus on having a greater impact on the metabolic function of the microbiota rather than on its composition [23]. Still, much remains to be understood about T1D etiology. In other diseases which also have an inflammatory gut background, the use of probiotics and prebiotics has been tested for their management. However, despite these strategies enabling the increase in the abundance of specific bacteria at the genus and species levels, changes in the overall composition of the microbiota are small and are kept only during the intervention period [69].

Other possible practices for prevention and/or treatment include fecal transplantation and the use of mucosa-protective drugs to manage leaky gut syndrome. Although fecal transplant is the only way to completely change microbiome, it is still unknown how unstable the new ecosystem could be, and therefore, the duration and efficacy of its effect in pre-T1D patients. It must also be considered that if fecal transplant would be performed without any dietary intervention, its effect, if significant, would be short-term. In T1D patients, fecal transplant accompanied by diet intervention could help achieve glucose control and recover microbiotal balance. Regarding mucosa-protective drugs, there are new drugs, such as gelatine tannate, that could be used as an intestinal barrier-modulating drug. According to the first trials, this drug may favor a physiological permeability, creating a bioprotective film by forming bonds with mucin, avoiding the aggressive penetration of bacteria, restoring functionality, and thus inducing an indirect anti-inflammatory effect [70].

Finally, in order to treat patients who do not respond adequately to conventional treatment, and investigating the possibility of remission and/or cure of the disease, other therapeutic strategies for T1D are pancreas transplant, pancreatic islet transplant , and, more recently, stem cell therapy [71]. Stem cell therapy seeks to take advantage of the regenerative capacity and immunomodulatory effects of the pluripotent cells. However, none of them have been effective in clinical practice alone in the long term. According to Chhabra and Brayman [72], safe stem cell strategies should be combined with other techniques, such as islet transplant, using the latest gene therapies and novel immunosuppressive and immunomodulatory drugs. In addition, the modulation of intestinal microbiota through fecal transplant and dietary intervention may help maintain the beneficial effects of the discussed techniques long term.

7. Conclusions

The composition of the gut microbiota can be modulated by diet. This modulation can promote the proper maturation of the immune system, or, result in gut dysbiosis and aberrant immune responses that can lead to autoimmunity and T1D in predisposed children. Thus, dietary antigens and microbiota-derived products could be acting as triggers of T1D by promoting a pro-inflammatory and metabolic dysfunctional environment. The genus *Bacteroides* is the largest representative of T1D-associated dysbiosis. Among the possible strategies for prevention and treatment, fecal transplant accompanied by dietary intervention appears to be the most promising option for the prevention of T1D in children with autoimmunity.

Acknowledgments: The work had financial support from the Mexican Council for Science and Technology (CONACYT) grant S0008-2009-01-115212.

Author Contributions: M.E.M. and A.M.C. conceived and wrote the paper. Both authors read and approved the final manuscript.

References

1. American Diabetes Association. Standards of medical care in diabetes—2015: Summary of revisions. *Diabetes Care* **2015**, *38*, S4.
2. Pettitt, D.J.; Talton, J.; Dabelea, D.; Divers, J.; Imperatore, G.; Lawrence, J.M.; Liese, A.D.; Linder, B.; Mayer-Davis, E.J.; Pihoker, C.; *et al.* Prevalence of diabetes in U.S. Youth in 2009: The search for diabetes in youth study. *Diabetes Care* **2014**, *37*, 402–408. [CrossRef] [PubMed]
3. Mathers, C.D.; Loncar, D. Projections of global mortality and burden of disease from 2002 to 2030. *PLoS Med.* **2006**, *3*, e442. [CrossRef] [PubMed]
4. Kantarova, D.; Buc, M. Genetic susceptibility to type 1 diabetes mellitus in humans. *Physiol. Res.* **2007**, *56*, 255–266. [PubMed]
5. Ziegler, A.G.; Rewers, M.; Simell, O.; Simell, T.; Lempainen, J.; Steck, A.; Winkler, C.; Ilonen, J.; Veijola, R.; Knip, M.; *et al.* Seroconversion to multiple islet autoantibodies and risk of progression to diabetes in children. *JAMA* **2013**, *309*, 2473–2479. [CrossRef] [PubMed]
6. Larsson, E.H.; Vehik, K.; Gesualdo, P.; Akolkar, B.; Hagopian, W.; Krischer, J.; Lernmark, Å.; Rewers, M.; Simell, O.; She, J.-X.; *et al.* Children followed in the teddy study are diagnosed with type 1 diabetes at an early stage of disease. *Pediatr. Diabetes* **2014**, *15*, 118–126. [CrossRef] [PubMed]
7. Atkinson, M.A.; Eisenbarth, G.S. Type 1 diabetes: New perspectives on disease pathogenesis and treatment. *Lancet* **2001**, *358*, 221–229. [CrossRef]
8. Wen, L.; Ley, R.E.; Volchkov, P.Y.; Stranges, P.B.; Avanesyan, L.; Stonebraker, A.C.; Hu, C.; Wong, F.S.; Szot, G.L.; Bluestone, J.A.; *et al.* Innate immunity and intestinal microbiota in the development of type 1 diabetes. *Nature* **2008**, *455*, 1109–1113. [CrossRef] [PubMed]
9. Vaarala, O. Is the origin of type 1 diabetes in the gut? *Immunol. Cell Biol.* **2012**, *90*, 271–276. [CrossRef] [PubMed]
10. Dominguez-Bello, M.G.; Costello, E.K.; Contreras, M.; Magris, M.; Hidalgo, G.; Fierer, N.; Knight, R. Delivery mode shapes the acquisition and structure of the initial microbiota across multiple body habitats in newborns. *Proc. Natl. Acad. Sci. USA* **2010**, *107*, 11971–11975. [CrossRef] [PubMed]
11. Guaraldi, F.; Salvatori, G. Effect of breast and formula feeding on gut microbiota shaping in newborns. *Front. Cell. Infect. Microbiol.* **2012**. [CrossRef] [PubMed]
12. Dominguez-Bello, M.G.; Blaser, M.J.; Ley, R.E.; Knight, R. Development of the human gastrointestinal microbiota and insights from high-throughput sequencing. *Gastroenterology* **2011**, *140*, 1713–1719. [CrossRef] [PubMed]

13. Power, S.E.; O'Toole, P.W.; Stanton, C.; Ross, R.P.; Fitzgerald, G.F. Intestinal microbiota, diet and health. *Br. J. Nutr.* **2014**, *111*, 387–402. [CrossRef] [PubMed]
14. Arumugam, M.; Raes, J.; Pelletier, E.; le Paslier, D.; Yamada, T.; Mende, D.R.; Fernandes, G.R.; Tap, J.; Bruls, T.; Batto, J.M.; *et al.* Enterotypes of the human gut microbiome. *Nature* **2011**, *473*, 174–180. [CrossRef] [PubMed]
15. Wu, G.D.; Chen, J.; Hoffmann, C.; Bittinger, K.; Chen, Y.-Y.; Keilbaugh, S.A.; Bewtra, M.; Knights, D.; Walters, W.A.; Knight, R.; *et al.* Linking long-term dietary patterns with gut microbial enterotypes. *Science* **2011**, *334*, 105–108. [CrossRef] [PubMed]
16. Roager, H.M.; Licht, T.R.; Poulsen, S.K.; Larsen, T.M.; Bahl, M.I. Microbial enterotypes, inferred by the prevotella-to-bacteroides ratio, remained stable during a 6-month randomized controlled diet intervention with the new nordic diet. *Appl. Environ. Microbiol.* **2014**, *80*, 1142–1149. [CrossRef] [PubMed]
17. De Filippo, C.; Cavalieri, D.; di Paola, M.; Ramazzotti, M.; Poullet, J.B.; Massart, S.; Collini, S.; Pieraccini, G.; Lionetti, P. Impact of diet in shaping gut microbiota revealed by a comparative study in children from Europe and rural Africa. *Proc. Natl. Acad. Sci. USA* **2010**, *107*, 14691–14696. [CrossRef] [PubMed]
18. Mejia-Leon, M.E.; Petrosino, J.F.; Ajami, N.J.; Dominguez-Bello, M.G.; Calderon de la Barca, A.M. Fecal microbiota imbalance in Mexican children with type 1 diabetes. *Sci. Rep.* **2014**. [CrossRef] [PubMed]
19. Nakayama, J.; Watanabe, K.; Jiang, J.; Matsuda, K.; Chao, S.-H.; Haryono, P.; La-ongkham, O.; Sarwoko, M.-A.; Sujaya, I.N.; Zhao, L.; *et al.* Diversity in gut bacterial community of school-age children in Asia. *Sci. Rep.* **2015**, *5*, 8397. [CrossRef] [PubMed]
20. La-ongkham, O.; Nakphaichit, M.; Leelavatcharamas, V.; Keawsompong, S.; Nitisinprasert, S. Distinct gut microbiota of healthy children from two different geographic regions of Thailand. *Arch. Microbiol.* **2015**, *197*, 561–573. [CrossRef] [PubMed]
21. Yatsunenko, T.; Rey, F.E.; Manary, M.J.; Trehan, I.; Dominguez-Bello, M.G.; Contreras, M.; Magris, M.; Hidalgo, G.; Baldassano, R.N.; Anokhin, A.P.; *et al.* Human gut microbiome viewed across age and geography. *Nature* **2012**, *486*, 222–227. [CrossRef] [PubMed]
22. Knights, D.; Ward, T.L.; McKinlay, C.E.; Miller, H.; Gonzalez, A.; McDonald, D.; Knight, R. Rethinking "enterotypes". *Cell Host Microb.* **2014**, *16*, 433–437. [CrossRef] [PubMed]
23. Graf, D.; di Cagno, R.; Fåk, F.; Flint, H.J.; Nyman, M.; Saarela, M.; Watzl, B. Contribution of diet to the composition of the human gut microbiota. *Microb. Ecol. Health Disease* **2015**, *26*. [CrossRef] [PubMed]
24. Aagaard, K.; Ma, J.; Antony, K.M.; Ganu, R.; Petrosino, J.; Versalovic, J. The placenta harbors a unique microbiome. *Sci. Transl. Med.* **2014**, *6*, 237ra65. [CrossRef] [PubMed]
25. Brugman, S.; Perdijk, O.; van Neerven, R.J.J.; Savelkoul, H.J. Mucosal immune development in early life: Setting the stage. *Arch. Immunol. Ther. Exp.* **2015**, *63*, 251–268. [CrossRef] [PubMed]
26. Calderón de la Barca, A.M.; Mejia-León, M.E. Are dietary caseins related to the onset and evolution of type 1 diabetes and celiac disease? In *Casein: Production, Uses and Health Effects*, 1st ed.; Ventimiglia, A.M., Birkenhäger, J.M., Eds.; Nova Science Publishers, Inc.: New York, NY, USA, 2012; Volume 1, pp. 195–208.
27. Longman, R.S.; Yang, Y.; Diehl, G.E.; Kim, S.V.; Littman, D.R. Microbiota: Host interactions in mucosal homeostasis and systemic autoimmunity. *Cold Spring Harbor Symp. Quant. Biol.* **2013**, *78*, 193–201. [CrossRef] [PubMed]
28. Brandtzaeg, P. The gut as communicator between environment and host: Immunological consequences. *Eur. J. Pharmacol.* **2011**, *668* (Suppl. 1), S16–S32. [CrossRef] [PubMed]
29. Cerf-Bensussan, N.; Gaboriau-Routhiau, V. The immune system and the gut microbiota: Friends or foes? *Nat. Rev. Immunol.* **2010**, *10*, 735–744. [CrossRef] [PubMed]
30. Vaarala, O.; Atkinson, M.A.; Neu, J. The "perfect storm" for type 1 diabetes: The complex interplay between intestinal microbiota, gut permeability, and mucosal immunity. *Diabetes* **2008**, *57*, 2555–2562. [CrossRef] [PubMed]
31. Sharma, R.; Young, C.; Neu, J. Molecular modulation of intestinal epithelial barrier: Contribution of microbiota. *J. Biomed. Biotechnol.* **2010**, *2010*. [CrossRef] [PubMed]
32. Rogier, E.W.; Frantz, A.L.; Bruno, M.E.C.; Wedlund, L.; Cohen, D.A.; Stromberg, A.J.; Kaetzel, C.S. Secretory antibodies in breast milk promote long-term intestinal homeostasis by regulating the gut microbiota and host gene expression. *Proc. Natl. Acad. Sci. USA* **2014**, *111*, 3074–3079. [CrossRef] [PubMed]

34. Lamb, M.M.; Miller, M.; Seifert, J.A.; Frederiksen, B.; Kroehl, M.; Rewers, M.; Norris, J.M. The effect of childhood cow's milk intake and HLA-DR genotype on risk of islet autoimmunity and type 1 diabetes: The diabetes autoimmunity study in the young. *Pediatr. Diabetes* **2015**, *16*, 31–38. [CrossRef] [PubMed]
35. Birgisdottir, B.E.; Hill, J.P.; Thorsson, A.V.; Thorsdottir, I. Lower consumption of cow milk protein A1 β-casein at 2 years of age, rather than consumption among 11- to 14-year-old adolescents, may explain the lower incidence of type 1 diabetes in Iceland than in Scandinavia. *Ann. Nutr. Metab.* **2006**, *50*, 177–183. [CrossRef] [PubMed]
36. Davis-Richardson, A.; Triplett, E. A model for the role of gut bacteria in the development of autoimmunity for type 1 diabetes. *Diabetologia* **2015**, *58*, 1386–1393. [CrossRef] [PubMed]
37. Larsen, J.; Weile, C.; Antvorskov, J.C.; Engkilde, K.; Nielsen, S.M.B.; Josefsen, K.; Buschard, K. Effect of dietary gluten on dendritic cells and innate immune subsets in BALB/c and nod mice. *PLoS ONE* **2015**, *10*, e0118618. [CrossRef] [PubMed]
38. Mejía-León, M.E.; Calderón de la Barca, A.M. Serum IgG subclasses against dietary antigens in children with type 1 diabetes. *Pediatr. Diabetes* **2015**. submitted for publication.
39. Hamari, S.; Kirveskoski, T.; Glumoff, V.; Kulmala, P.; Simell, O.; Knip, M.; Ilonen, J.; Veijola, R. CD4+ T-cell proliferation responses to wheat polypeptide stimulation in children at different stages of type 1 diabetes autoimmunity. *Pediatr. Diabetes* **2015**, *16*, 177–188. [CrossRef] [PubMed]
40. Brugman, S.; Klatter, F.A.; Visser, J.T.J.; Wildeboer-Veloo, A.C.M.; Harmsen, H.J.M.; Rozing, J.; Bos, N.A. Antibiotic treatment partially protects against type 1 diabetes in the bio-breeding diabetes-prone rat. Is the gut flora involved in the development of type 1 diabetes? *Diabetologia* **2006**, *49*, 2105–2108. [CrossRef] [PubMed]
41. Candon, S.; Perez-Arroyo, A.; Marquet, C.; Valette, F.; Foray, A.-P.; Pelletier, B.; Milani, C.; Ventura, M.; Bach, J.-F.; Chatenoud, L. Antibiotics in early life alter the gut microbiome and increase disease incidence in a spontaneous mouse model of autoimmune insulin-dependent diabetes. *PLoS ONE* **2015**, *10*, e0125448. [CrossRef] [PubMed]
42. Brown, K.; Godovannyi, A.; Ma, C.; Zhang, Y.; Ahmadi-Vand, Z.; Dai, C.; Gorzelak, M.A.; Chan, Y.; Chan, J.M.; Lochner, A.; *et al.* Prolonged antibiotic treatment induces a diabetogenic intestinal microbiome that accelerates diabetes in nod mice. *ISME J.* **2015**. [CrossRef] [PubMed]
43. Giongo, A.; Gano, K.A.; Crabb, D.B.; Mukherjee, N.; Novelo, L.L.; Casella, G.; Drew, J.C.; Ilonen, J.; Knip, M.; Hyoty, H.; *et al.* Toward defining the autoimmune microbiome for type 1 diabetes. *ISME J.* **2011**, *5*, 82–91. [CrossRef] [PubMed]
44. De Goffau, M.C.; Luopajärvi, K.; Knip, M.; Ilonen, J.; Ruohtula, T.; Härkönen, T.; Orivuori, L.; Hakala, S.; Welling, G.W.; Harmsen, H.J.; *et al.* Fecal microbiota composition differs between children with β-cell autoimmunity and those without. *Diabetes* **2013**, *62*, 1238–1244. [CrossRef] [PubMed]
45. Kostic, A.D.; Gevers, D.; Siljander, H.; Vatanen, T.; Hyötyläinen, T.; Hämäläinen, A.-M.; Peet, A.; Tillmann, V.; Pöhö, P.; Mattila, I.; *et al.* The dynamics of the human infant gut microbiome in development and in progression toward type 1 diabetes. *Cell Host Microb.* **2015**, *17*, 260–273. [CrossRef] [PubMed]
46. Alkanani, A.K.; Hara, N.; Gottlieb, P.A.; Ir, D.; Robertson, C.E.; Wagner, B.D.; Frank, D.N.; Zipris, D. Alterations in intestinal microbiota correlate with susceptibility to type 1 diabetes. *Diabetes* **2015**, *64*, 3510–3520. [CrossRef] [PubMed]
47. Davis-Richardson, A.G.; Ardissone, A.N.; Dias, R.; Simell, V.; Leonard, M.T.; Kemppainen, K.M.; Drew, J.C.; Schatz, D.; Atkinson, M.A.; Kolaczkowski, B.; *et al.* Bacteroides dorei dominates gut microbiome prior to autoimmunity in Finnish children at high risk for type 1 diabetes. *Front. Microbiol.* **2014**. [CrossRef]
48. Virtanen, S.M.; Ylonen, K.; Rasanen, L.; Ala-Venna, E.; Maenpaa, J.; Akerblom, H.K. Two year prospective dietary survey of newly diagnosed children with diabetes aged less than 6 years. *Arch. Dis. Childh.* **2000**, *82*, 21–26. [CrossRef] [PubMed]
49. Lichtenstein, A.H.; Appel, L.J.; Brands, M.; Carnethon, M.; Daniels, S.; Franch, H.A.; Franklin, B.; Kris-Etherton, P.; Harris, W.S.; Howard, B.; *et al.* Diet and lifestyle recommendations revision 2006: A scientific statement from the american heart association nutrition committee. *Circulation* **2006**, *114*, 82–96. [CrossRef] [PubMed]
50. Dietert, R.R. The microbiome in early life: Self-completion and microbiota protection as health priorities. *Birth Defects Res. Part B Dev. Reprod. Toxicol.* **2014**, *101*, 333–340. [CrossRef] [PubMed]

51. Murri, M.; Leiva, I.; Gomez-Zumaquero, J.M.; Tinahones, F.; Cardona, F.; Soriguer, F.; Queipo-Ortuno, M.I. Gut microbiota in children with type 1 diabetes differs from that in healthy children: A case-control study. *BMC Med.* **2013**, *11*. [CrossRef] [PubMed]
52. Brown, C.T.; Davis-Richardson, A.G.; Giongo, A.; Gano, K.A.; Crabb, D.B.; Mukherjee, N.; Casella, G.; Drew, J.C.; Ilonen, J.; Knip, M.; *et al.* Gut microbiome metagenomics analysis suggests a functional model for the development of autoimmunity for type 1 diabetes. *PLoS ONE* **2011**, *6*, e25792. [CrossRef] [PubMed]
53. Peng, L.; Li, Z.-R.; Green, R.S.; Holzman, I.R.; Lin, J. Butyrate enhances the intestinal barrier by facilitating tight junction assembly via activation of AMP-activated protein kinase in Caco-2 cell monolayers. *J. Nutr.* **2009**, *139*, 1619–1625. [CrossRef] [PubMed]
54. Arpaia, N.; Campbell, C.; Fan, X.; Dikiy, S.; van der Veeken, J.; deRoos, P.; Liu, H.; Cross, J.R.; Pfeffer, K.; Coffer, P.J.; *et al.* Metabolites produced by commensal bacteria promote peripheral regulatory T-cell generation. *Nature* **2013**, *504*, 451–455. [CrossRef] [PubMed]
55. Sun, J.; Furio, L.; Mecheri, R.; van der Does, A.M.; Lundeberg, E.; Saveanu, L.; Chen, Y.; van Endert, P.; Agerberth, B.; Diana, J. Pancreatic β-cells limit autoimmune diabetes via an immunoregulatory antimicrobial peptide expressed under the influence of the gut microbiota. *Immunity* **2015**, *43*, 304–317. [CrossRef] [PubMed]
56. Kasubuchi, M.; Hasegawa, S.; Hiramatsu, T.; Ichimura, A.; Kimura, I. Dietary gut microbial metabolites, short-chain fatty acids, and host metabolic regulation. *Nutrients* **2015**, *7*, 2839–2849. [CrossRef] [PubMed]
57. Fourlanos, S.; Harrison, L.C.; Colman, P.G. The accelerator hypothesis and increasing incidence of type 1 diabetes. *Curr. Opin. Endocrinol. Diabetes Obes.* **2008**, *15*, 321–325. [CrossRef] [PubMed]
58. Fourlanos, S.; Narendran, P.; Byrnes, G.B.; Colman, P.G.; Harrison, L.C. Insulin resistance is a risk factor for progression to type 1 diabetes. *Diabetologia* **2004**, *47*, 1661–1667. [CrossRef] [PubMed]
59. Orešič, M.; Simell, S.; Sysi-Aho, M.; Näntö-Salonen, K.; Seppänen-Laakso, T.; Parikka, V.; Katajamaa, M.; Hekkala, A.; Mattila, I.; Keskinen, P.; *et al.* Dysregulation of lipid and amino acid metabolism precedes islet autoimmunity in children who later progress to type 1 diabetes. *J. Exp. Med.* **2008**, *205*, 2975–2984. [CrossRef] [PubMed]
60. Mejía-León, M.E.; Ruiz-Dyck, K.M.; Calderón de la Barca, A.M. HLA-DQ genetic risk gradient for type 1 diabetes and celiac disease in North-Western Mexico. *Rev. Gastroenterol. de Méx.* **2015**, *80*, 135–143. [CrossRef] [PubMed]
61. Teddy Study Group. The environmental determinants of diabetes in the young (TEDDY) study. *Ann. N. Y. Acad. Sci.* **2008**, *1150*, 1–13.
62. Skyler, J.S. Toward primary prevention of type 1 diabetes. *JAMA* **2015**, *313*, 1520–1521. [CrossRef] [PubMed]
63. Simmons, K.; Michels, A.W. Lessons from type 1 diabetes for understanding natural history and prevention of autoimmune disease. *Rheumatic Dis. Clin. N. Am.* **2014**, *40*, 797–811. [CrossRef] [PubMed]
64. De Jesus-Laboy, K.M.; Cox, L.M.; Rodriguez-Rivera, S.M.; Rivera-Vinas, J.; Mendez, K.; Clemente, J.C.; Knight, R.; Dominguez-Bello, M.G. Restoring the normal microbiota of cesarean-section born infants. In Proceedings of American society for microbiology 114th general meeting, Boston, MA, USA, 18 May 2014; pp. I–741.
65. Niinistö, S.; Takkinen, H.M.; Uusitalo, L.; Rautanen, J.; Vainio, N.; Ahonen, S.; Nevalainen, J.; Kenward, M.G.; Lumia, M.; Simell, O.; *et al.* Maternal intake of fatty acids and their food sources during lactation and the risk of preclinical and clinical type 1 diabetes in the offspring. *Acta Diabetol.* **2015**, *52*, 763–772. [CrossRef] [PubMed]
66. Knip, M.; Virtanen, S.M.; Becker, D.; Dupré, J.; Krischer, J.P.; Åkerblom, H.K. Early feeding and risk of type 1 diabetes: Experiences from the trial to reduce insulin-dependent diabetes mellitus in the genetically at risk (TRIGR). *Am. J. Clin. Nutr.* **2011**, *94*, 1814S–1820S. [CrossRef] [PubMed]
67. Lamb, M.; Frederiksen, B.; Seifert, J.; Kroehl, M.; Rewers, M.; Norris, J. Sugar intake is associated with progression from islet autoimmunity to type 1 diabetes: The diabetes autoimmunity study in the young. *Diabetologia* **2015**, *58*, 2027–2034. [CrossRef] [PubMed]
68. He, C.; Shan, Y.; Song, W. Targeting gut microbiota as a possible therapy for diabetes. *Nutr. Res.* **2015**, *35*, 361–367. [CrossRef] [PubMed]
69. Conlon, M.; Bird, A. The impact of diet and lifestyle on gut microbiota and human health. *Nutrients* **2014**, *7*, 17–44. [CrossRef] [PubMed]

70. Lopetuso, L.R.; Scaldaferri, F.; Bruno, G.; Petito, V.; Franceschi, F.; Gasbarrini, A. The therapeutic management of gut barrier leaking: The emerging role for mucosal barrier protectors. *Eur. Rev. Med. Pharmacol. Sci.* **2015**, *19*, 1068–1076. [PubMed]
71. Vardanyan, M.; Parkin, E.; Gruessner, C.; Rodriguez Rilo, H.L. Pancreas *vs.* Islet transplantation: A call on the future. *Curr. Opin. Organ Transpl.* **2010**, *15*, 124–130. [CrossRef] [PubMed]
72. Chhabra, P.; Brayman, K.L. Stem cell therapy to cure type 1 diabetes: From hype to hope. *Stem Cells Transl. Med.* **2013**, *2*, 328–336. [CrossRef] [PubMed]

The Effect of the Traditional Mediterranean-Style Diet on Metabolic Risk Factors

Marissa Garcia [1], Jessica D. Bihuniak [2], Julia Shook [1], Anne Kenny [3], Jane Kerstetter [1] and Tania B. Huedo-Medina [1,*]

1 Department of Allied Health Sciences, University of Connecticut, Storrs, CT 06269, USA; Marissa.Garcia27@gmail.com (M.G.); Julia.shook@uconn.edu (J.S.); Jane.Kerstetter@uconn.edu (J.K.)
2 NYU Steinhardt, Department of Nutrition and Food Studies, New York University, New York, NY 10003, USA; jdb13@nyu.edu
3 Center on Aging, University of Connecticut Health Center, Farmington, CT06030, USA; kenny@uchc.edu
* Correspondence: Tania.Huedo-Medina@uconn.edu

Abstract: The Mediterranean-style diet (MedSD) has gained attention for its positive effects on health outcomes, including metabolic risk factors. However, it is unknown as to which components of MedSD interventions are most beneficial in reducing risk. The objective of this meta-analysis was to obtain effect sizes for metabolic risk factors and explain the variability across the current literature based on study design, sample, and diet characteristics. Six electronic databases were searched from inception until 9 February 2016. Data from 29 studies ($N = 4133$) were included. There were significant effects in favor of the MedSD for waist circumference, triglycerides, blood glucose, systolic blood pressure, and diastolic blood pressure ($d_+ = -0.54$; $d_+ = -0.46$; $d_+ = -0.50$; $d_+ = -0.72$; $d_+ = -0.94$, respectively). The MedSD was significantly beneficial when the intervention was longer in duration, was conducted in Europe, used a behavioral technique, and was conducted using small groups. The traditional MedSD had significant beneficial effects on five of the six metabolic risk factors. Results from this study provide support for population specific dietary guideline for metabolic risk reduction.

Keywords: Mediterranean diet; metabolic syndrome; meta-analysis

---

1. Introduction

Metabolic syndrome is defined as a group of interrelated risk factors of metabolic origin that appear to directly promote the development of cardiovascular disease (CVD) [1]. The National Cholesterol Education Program's Adult Treatment Panel III report (NCEP ATPIII) [2] identified six components of metabolic syndrome that are related to CVD: (1) abdominal obesity; (2) atherogenic dyslipidemia; (3) elevated blood pressure; (4) insulin resistance; (5) proinflammatory state; and (6) prothrombotic state [2]. According to the ATP III criteria, a diagnosis of metabolic syndrome can be made when three out of five of the following characteristics are present: (1) abdominal obesity characterized by waist circumference (WC) >102 cm for men and >88 cm for women; (2) triglycerides (TG) $\geqslant$150 mg/dL; (3) HDL cholesterol (HDL) <40 mg/dL for men and <50 mg/dL for women; (4) blood pressure $\geqslant$130/$\geqslant$85 mmHg; and (5) fasting glucose (FBG) $\geqslant$110 mg/dL [2]. Metabolic syndrome is a major health concern in the United States. Findings from the Third National Health and Nutrition Examination Survey (NHANES) suggest that according to the NCEP ATP III criteria approximately 34% of adults in the United States have metabolic syndrome [3].

Lifestyle therapies such as diet modification and physical activity are currently recommended as first-line interventions to reduce metabolic risk factors [1]. The Mediterranean-style diet (MedSD) is well-known for its cardio-protective benefits [4] and more recently, has been evaluated for the prevention and treatment of metabolic syndrome [5]. This dietary pattern emphasizes abundance of plant-based foods, a variety of minimally processed and locally grown foods, and olive oil as the principal source of fat [6]. The MedSD also includes daily consumption of low to moderate amounts of cheese and yogurt (low-fat and non-fat versions may be preferable), twice weekly consumption of fish and poultry, consumption of up to seven eggs per week, fresh fruit as dessert, red meat consumption limited to a few times a month, moderate consumption of wine (1 glass/day for women and 1–2 glasses/day for men) and regular physical activity at a level which promotes healthy weight and well-being [6].

To our knowledge, only one meta-analysis has evaluated literature on the effects of a MedSD on metabolic syndrome [7]. This meta-analysis included 35 clinical trials, two prospective studies, and 13 cross-sectional studies with a total of 534,906 participants and found an overall beneficial effect of the Mediterranean diet on reducing metabolic syndrome and its components in adults [7,8]. Further, the Scientific Report of the 2015 [8] found dietary characteristics similar to that of a MedSD, including higher intake of vegetables, fruits, seafood, legumes, and nuts; moderate intake of alcohol (among adults); lower consumption of red and processed meat, and low intake of sugar-sweetened foods and drinks [8], to have a positive effect on metabolic syndrome risk factors (*i.e.*, blood pressure and lipid profiles). Taken together, the findings from the meta-analysis by Kastorini *et al.* [7] noted above and the 2015 Advisory Committee on the Dietary Guidelines for Americans [8] clearly support the positive effects of the MedSD on metabolic risk factors. However, it is currently unclear which specific characteristics of MedSD-based interventions significantly contribute to the previously observed beneficial effects of a traditional MedSD on metabolic risk factors. We therefore conducted a high quality meta-analysis with specific attention to each criteria of metabolic syndrome, each component of the MedSD, and each methodological characteristic which may help to explain the difference in results between published studies.

2. Methods

2.1. Literature Search

The data sources were obtained following the Preferred Reporting Items for Systematic Reviews and Meta-Analyses: The PRISMA Statement [9] guidelines. Original research studies that were published regardless of publication type until 9 February 2016 were included. Language was not restricted. Six computer databases were searched: PubMed, EMBASE (via Scopus), Web of Science, CINAHL, Agricola, and CAB Direct. A comprehensive literature search was conducted with the assistance of the University of Connecticut Health Sciences Librarian (JL) using combinations of Medical Subject Headings and other key words related to the aim of the study. Examples of the key words include: "Mediterranean Diet", "Mediterranean Style Diet", adiposity, "metabolic syndrome", overweight, BMI, "body mass", "waist circumference", obese, obesity, "abdominal fat", and "weight loss". The comprehensive search that was conducted for each database can be found in the supplemental material (S1). In addition to the electronic database search, all studies from Kastorini *et al.* [7] were screened and none of the studies overlap in both meta-analyses due to a difference in inclusion criteria.

2.2. Selection Criteria

Studies had to meet the following criteria to be included: (1) report pre-and post-intervention data on waist circumference (any other metabolic risk factors were additional); and (2) focus on the MedSD as a whole dietary pattern. Studies were excluded if they (1) did not have pre- and post-intervention data on waist circumference; (2) focused on particular components of the Mediterranean diet, such as only olive oil; (3) included exercise in the intervention; (4) included participants <18 years of age; (5) restricted calorie intake; and (6) did not report the information in a way that would allow effect sizes to be calculated using the published information. The relevance of studies was assessed by two independent researchers (M.G. and J.S.) with a hierarchical approach on the basis of title, abstract, and full manuscript. The original search resulted in 1696 abstracts with relevant key words. After screening and hand-searching articles, 29 articles (39 total comparisons) that used the traditional MedSD were included in analysis. Refer to Figure 1 for the PRISMA figure of included and excluded articles. A list of excluded articles is available in the supplemental material (Table S1).

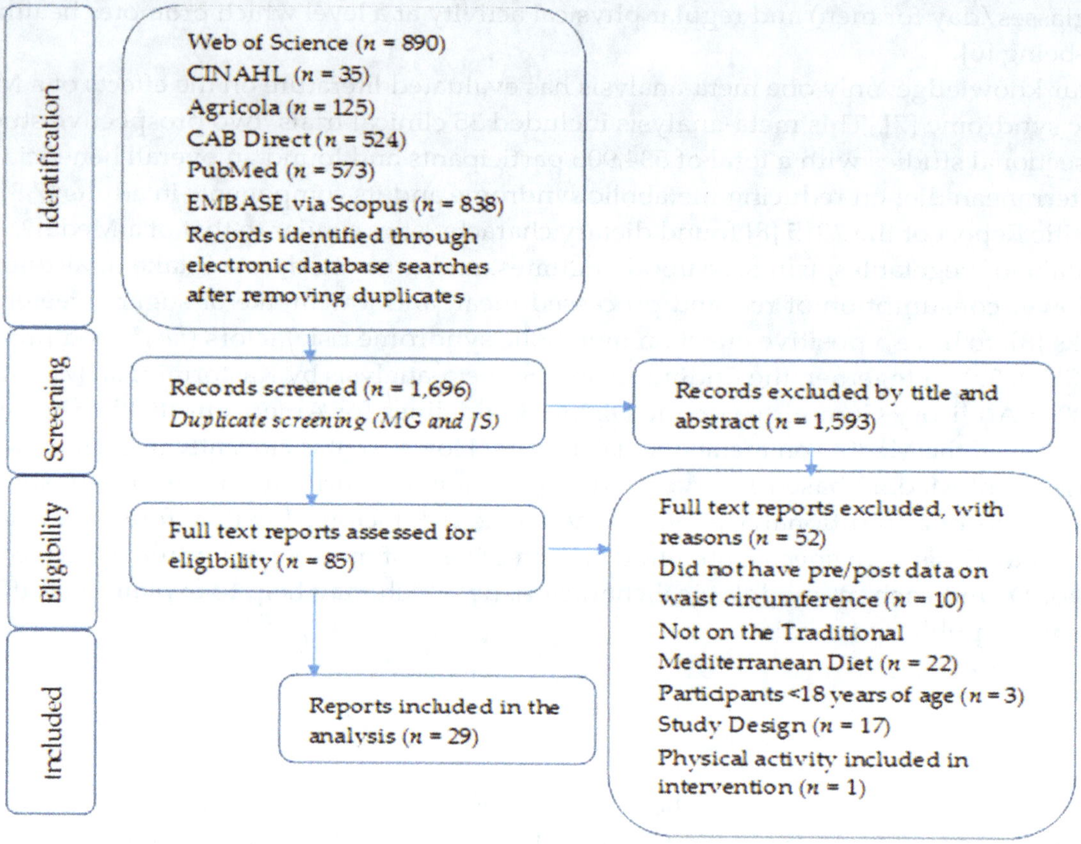

Figure 1. PRISMA Figure outlining the process of study identification, screening, eligibility, and inclusion.

2.3. Data Extraction

A comprehensive and detailed coding form and manual was created by a multidisciplinary team. The coding form includes approximately 330 variables for each study. Various characteristics were extracted from each study: (1) sample characteristics such as ethnicity, number and proportion of females, location of sample, and recruitment details; (2) intervention characteristics such as length of intervention, diet type, distribution of macronutrients, calorie intake, and participation in dietary counseling; and (3) study design characteristics such as number of interventions, type of control group, experimental conditions, and setting. The coding form was pilot-tested by two independent researchers (M.G. and J.S.) and was reviewed by additional experts (J.B., J.K., A.K., T.B.H.-M) before being finalized. The coding form and manual are available upon request to the corresponding author. All 30 studies were independently reviewed and coded by two researchers (M.G. and J.S.) and disagreements were solved by a third-party expert (T.B.H.-M).

2.4. Risk of Bias

The Cochrane Collaboration's tool for assessing risk of bias was used to assess risk of bias within individual studies [10]. In accordance with these guidelines, we report descriptions of internal and external validity summary ratings categorically, converting these to numerical scores as necessary for the purpose of meta-analytic moderator analysis.

Methodological quality (MQ) rankings have been identified as an under-analyzed element of the data reported in meta-analyses [11]. In this meta-analysis, MQ ratings based on the Cochrane risk of bias scale were entered as one or more possible moderators into the mixed-effects meta-regression models.

2.5. Statistical Analysis

Inter-rater reliability was calculated for all continuous and categorical variables. The kappa (κ) coefficient was used to calculate categorical agreement [12] (kappa = 0.94, 96.9% agreement) and Pearson's correlation coefficient was used to calculate continuous agreement [13] ($r = 1$). We tested for asymmetries by using the Begg [14], Egger [15], and trim-and-fill [16] statistical tests as well as the funnel plot [17] graphical technique. Publication bias, descriptive statistics, and reliability tests were calculated using R version 3.1.2 [18] and particularly, "metafor" package [19] for all the meta-analytic analysis.

Effect sizes (ESs) were calculated for each outcome by calculating the standardized mean change [20] for each sample [21], using the standard deviation of the pretest and adjusting by small sample sizes. The data extracted to obtain the individual ESs could be means and standard deviations, F-ANOVA, *t*-test, or mean and standard deviation change. To uphold the assumption of independence, each outcome was analyzed independently when multiple outcomes were reported from the same study. Twenty-two studies report at least three outcomes with the most common outcomes being waist circumference, HDL cholesterol, and triglycerides. Fourteen studies reported all six outcomes of interest. A multivariate approach for multiple subsamples per study was not followed because no more than five comparisons were available per study. Multiple ESs were obtained from the same study when data was reported separately by participant and diet characteristics [22,23]. Only two studies had subsamples based on sex [24,25] and three studies had multiple subsamples for participant characteristics [26–28].

Weighted mean effect size by the inverse of the variance of each study was calculated across all studies under random- and fixed-effects assumptions [29]. To test for heterogeneity, Cochran's Q [30] and I^2 [31] were calculated. To evaluate the sources of heterogeneity of the ESs, moderator analysis using weighted mixed-effects models with maximum likelihood estimation of the random-effects weights was performed testing each variable for study, intervention, and participant characteristics independently. The moving constant technique [32] was used to produce estimates of the ES ($d+$) at meaningful levels of the moderators and their Confidence Intervals (*Cis*) at different levels of interest. This technique was used to demonstrate results at the maximum and minimum values of significant moderators. Two-sided statistical significance was $p < 0.05$. Finally, clinical units of measures were included by transforming arithmetically the standardized ES to its unstandardized version [33].

3. Results

3.1. Description of Included Studies

A description of the included studies can be found in Table 1. Analysis of 29 reports shows that out of 4133 participants, 72% were female with a mean age of 46.93 (SD = 8.30). A majority of the studies were conducted in Europe (55.9%) and published in English (96.9%). Studies varied in design: 33.3% had a non-MedSD comparison group and 58.9% of studies were crossover or pre-/post-test only design. The mean publication year was 2009 (SD = 2.90) with a 12-year range from 2003 to 2015. The mean intervention length was 35.3 (SD = 50.71) weeks with a range from four to 208 weeks. No significant asymmetries were found using any of the statistical tests or the graphical funnel plot.

Table 1. Description of Included Studies.

Study	Country	*N*	% F	Age	Diseases	Recruit-ment	Dietary Assessment	Type of Diet	Duration (Weeks)	Control	Outcome
Aizawa, *et al.* (2009) [26]	Canada	63	51%	53.9	PDM PHTN	Physician referral	Group, unsupervised	MedSD	24	No carotid artery stiffness	Carotid artery stiffness
Bedard, *et al.* (2012) [27]	Canada	67	NR	39	Ob (57%)	NR	Individual, supervised	MedSD	8	Non-Ob	CVDRF
Bekkouche, *et al.* (2014) [34]	Algeria	86	NR	52	MS (67%)	Hospital	Individual, unsupervised	MedSD	12	No MS, healthy	IR, OS, Inflam.
Bos, *et al.* (2010) [35]	Netherlands	60	NR	52.5	Ob (100%)	NR	Individual, unsupervised	MedSD	10	High SFA diet; High MUFA diet	Serum lipids, IS
Connolly, *et al.* (2011) [28]	Great Britain	206	42%	60.4	CVD or CVDRF (100%)	Hospital, physician referral	Individual, unsupervised	MedSD	16	None	CVDRF
Corbalan, *et al.* (2009) [36]	Spain	1406	82%	39	Ob (100%)	Clinic referral	Individual, unsupervised	MedSD	34	None	WT
Esposito, *et al.* (2006) [37]	Italy	65	0%	43.9	MS, ED (100%)	Research database	Individual, unsupervised	MedSD	24	Regular diet	IIEF score
Esposito, *et al.* (2007) [38]	Italy	59	100%	41.9	MS, FSD (100%)	Research Database	Individual, unsupervised	MedSD	24	Regular Diet	FSFI score
Esposito, *et al.* (2004) [39]	Italy	180	45%	43.9	MS (100%)	Clinic	Group, unsupervised	MedSD	104	Regular Diet	Endo func, Vas Infl
Esposito, *et al.* (2009) [40]	Italy	215	51%	52.2	NIDDM (100%)	Clinic	Group, unsupervised	MedSD	208	LF Diet	Glycemic control
Goulet, *et al.* (2003) [41]	Canada	77	100%	47	None, healthy	Newspaper ad.	Individual, unsupervised	MedSD	12	None	Serum lipid, WT
Goulet, *et al.* (2007) [42]	Canada	77	100%	46.7	None, healthy	Newspaper ad.	Individual, unsupervised	MedSD	24	None	WT
Jones, *et al.* (2011) [43]	United States	89	100%	47.5	MS (100%)	NR	Individual, unsupervised	MedSD-MF	12	MD, no MF	MS RF
Kolomvotsou, *et al.* (2013) [44]	Greece	90	48%	50.4	Ob (100%)	Hospital	Individual, unsupervised	MedSD	8	Regular diet	AO intake, plasma AO capacity

Table 1. *Cont.*

Study	Country	*N*	% F	Age	Diseases	Recruit-ment	Dietary Assessment	Type of Diet	Duration (Weeks)	Control	Outcome
Leblanc, *et al.* (2014) [45]	Canada	108	47%	41.4	Ob, MS (100%)	Media advertise-ments	Individual and group, unsupervised and supervised	MedSD	12	None	Dietary intake, Met profile
Leighton, *et al.* (2009) [46]	Chile	145	0%	39	MS (24%)	Maestranza Diesel	Group, supervised	MedSD	52	None	MS RF
Lerman, *et al.* (2010) [47]	United States	24	83%	54.4	MS and high LDL-C (100%)	Previous study by Lerman	NR	MedSD-MF	12	MD, no MF	Plasma lipids
Lindeberg, *et al.* (2007) [48]	Sweden	29	0%	61	IHD, IGT, NIDDM	Hospital	Individual, unsupervised	MedSD	12	Paleolithic Diet	WT, serum glucose
Llaneza, *et al.* (2010) [49]	Spain	116	100%	56.4	IR (100%)	Hospital	Group, unsupervised	MedSD, soy supplement	104	MD, no supp	IR
Papandreou, *et al.* (2012 [50]	Greece	40	NR	41.5	Ob, OSAS (100%)	University Medical School	Group, unsupervised	MedSD	26	Prudent Diet	OSAS
Papandreou, *et al.* (2012) [51]	Greece	21	NR	41.5	Ob, OSAS (100%)	University Medical School	Group, unsupervised	MedSD	26	Prudent Diet	TBARS
Rallidis, *et al.* (2009) [52]	Greece	82	48%	50.4	Ob (100%)	Hospital	Individual, unsupervised	MedSD	8	Regular Diet	Endo func
Richard, *et al.* (2011) [53]	Canada	26	0%	49.4	MS (100%)	NR	Individual, unsupervised	MedSD	35	Western Diet	CVDRF
Rubenfire, *et al.* (2011) [24]	United States	126	68%	51	MS (100%)	Physician referral	Individual, unsupervised	MedSD	12	None	WT, BP, TG, serum glucose
Ryan, *et al.* (2013) [54]	Australia	12	50%	55	NAFLD (100%)	Hospital	Individual, unsupervised	MedSD	6	LF diet	WT, IS
Sanchez-Benito, *et al.* (2012) [55]	Spain	158	87%	48	OverWT (100%)	Pharmacy office	Individual, unsupervised	MedSD	26	None	BMI, BP, cholesterol
Stendall-Hollis, *et al.* (2013) [56]	United States	129	100%	29.7	OverWT (100%)	Magazine, hospital, Craigslist	Individual, unsupervised	MedSD	16	MyPyramid for P & B	WT, Inflam Bio

Table 1. *Cont.*

Study	Country	*N*	% F	Age	Diseases	Recruit-ment	Dietary Assessment	Type of Diet	Duration (Weeks)	Control	Outcome
Timar, *et al.* (2013) [25]	Romania	223	50%	55	NIDDM (100%)	Diabetes Center	Group, unsupervised	MedSD	52	Diabetic Diet	Glycemic control, CVDRF
Van Velden, *et al.* (2007) [57]	South Africa	12	25%	46	MS (100%)	NR	Group, unsupervised	MedSD with red wine	8	MD without red wine	CVDRF

Note. *N*, number of participants at baseline; F, females; NR, not reported; OverWT, Overweight; Ob, Obesity; MedSD, Mediterranean Style Diet; PDM, Pre-diabetes mellitus; PHTN, Pre-hypertension; CVDRF, Cardiovascular Disease risk factors; MS, Metabolic Syndrome; OS, oxidative stress; NIDDM, Non-insulin Dependent Diabetes; IR, insulin resistance; Inflam, Inflammation; SFA, saturated fatty acid; IS, Insulin Sensitivity; ED, Erectile Dysfunction; IIEF, International Index of Erectile Function; FSD, Female Sexual Dysfunction; FSFI, Female Sexual Function Index; Endo Func., endothelial function; Vas Infl, vascular inflammation; MedSD-MF, Low-Glycemic Mediterranean Diet with Medical Food; MS RF, Metabolic Syndrome Risk Factors; AO, antioxidant; WC, waist circumference; IHD, ischaemic heart disease; IGT, impaired glucose tolerance; OSAS, Obstructive Sleep Apnea Syndrome; TBARS, thiobarbituric acid reacting substances; BP, blood pressure; TG, serum triglycerides; Inflam Bio, inflammatory biomarkers; MyPyramid for P&B, USDA MyPyramid Diet for Pregnant and Breastfeeding Women; FVII, activated factor VII; MI, Myocardial Infarction; Met profile, metabolic profile.

Note on Dietary Assessment column:

- *Individual:* A dietitian performed a dietary assessment, providing individualized needs for caloric intake and recommendations, for each participant.
- *Group:* The study provided general dietary recommendations for the participants, such as a range of servings of certain food groups, calories based on sex, as opposed to tailoring diets to individual needs based on weight and height.
- *Supervised:* Participants consumed foods in a supervised setting, where the researchers had control over participant food choices and quantity of food served.
- *Unsupervised:* Participants food consumption was unsupervised by researchers, such as eating at home.

3.2. *Effect Sizes*

The traditional MedSD was found to have a significant beneficial effect on five out of six outcomes of interest (Table 2, Figures S1–S6). Overall ESs under random-effects assumptions indicate that the traditional MedSD had a significant overall effect on WC, TG, FBG, systolic blood pressure (SBP), and diastolic blood pressure (DBP) ($d_+ = -0.54$, 95% CI −0.77 to −0.31; $d_+ = -0.46$, 95% CI −0.72 to −0.21; $d_+ = -0.50$, 95% CI −0.81 to −0.20; $d_+ = -0.72$, 95% CI −1.03 to −0.42; $d_+ = -0.94$, 95% CI −1.45 to −0.44, respectively), but did not have a significant effect on HDL ($d_+ = 0.19$, 95% CI −0.07 to 0.46). There was large heterogeneity between studies with I^2 ranging from 92.98% to 98.42%.

Table 2. Summary of Results, Overall Effect Sizes and Homogeneity.

Outcome	k	d_+ (95% CI)		Homogeneity of d's		
		Fixed-Effects	Random-Effects	Q	I^2 (%)	p-Value
WC	39	−0.44 (−0.48 to −0.41) *	−0.54 (−0.77 to −0.31) *	390.1	96.39	<0.0001
HDL	27	0.15 (0.09 to 0.21) *	0.19 (−0.07 to 0.46)	294.6	93.95	<0.0001
TG	25	−0.34 (−0.40 to −0.28) *	−0.46 (−0.72 to −0.21) *	231.06	93.74	<0.0001
FBG	23	−0.37 (−0.42 to −0.33) *	−0.50 (−0.81 to −0.20) *	281.18	96.69	<0.0001
SBP	25	−0.74 (−0.78 to −0.70) *	−0.72 (−1.03 to −0.42) *	320.11	97.00	<0.0001
DBP	25	−0.99 (−1.06 to −0.93) *	−0.94 (−1.45 to −0.44) *	2263.05	98.42	<0.0001

Note: d_+, overall effect size; WC, waist circumference; HDL, HDL cholesterol; TG, triglycerides, FBG, fasting blood glucose; SBP, systolic blood pressure; DBP, diastolic blood pressure; * indicates a significant effect; k represents the number of interventions for each outcome included in the analysis; Q represents Cochran's Q indicating significance of heterogeneity; I^2 represents the magnitude of heterogeneity; p-value represents the significance of heterogeneity.

3.3. *Moderator Analysis*

All moderation effects are presented in Table 3. In regards to study characteristics, trending associations were found for study region. Studies conducted in Europe showed significant beneficial effects from the traditional MedSD intervention on four of the metabolic risk factors (waist circumference, HDL cholesterol, triglycerides and fasting blood glucose) whereas studies conducted in the United States did not result in significant effect sizes for any of the study characteristics.

Significant associations were found for study design waist circumference, HDL cholesterol, triglycerides, fasting blood glucose and systolic blood pressure. Studies that included a comparison intervention group design (*i.e.*, a different type of diet) had more beneficial significant effect sizes favoring the MedSD compared to those studies using a traditional pre-/post-design or a crossover design.

Studies with a higher *Impact per Publication* (IPP) value showed more significant beneficial effects for waist circumference, HDL cholesterol, triglycerides, and fasting blood glucose with significant positive associations for each.

The length of the intervention (in weeks) significantly explained between 27.89% and 51.13% of the variability between studies for the following outcomes: waist circumference, HDL cholesterol, triglycerides, fasting blood glucose and systolic blood pressure. There was a significant positive association for length of intervention for all six outcomes of interest (Figures S7–S11). The longer the length of the intervention, the more significant the beneficial effect in favor of the traditional MedSD. Additional significant or trending intervention characteristics included the use of a behavioral technique, supervision, and dietary interventions conducted primarily in small groups. The use of a behavioral technique resulted in trending or significant beneficial effects in all of the outcomes of interest compared to the effects when there was no behavioral technique used.

Table 3. Significant Moderator Analysis Results.

Moderator	Outcome	Category	k	d_+ (95% CI)	R^2	p-Value	Clinical Unit of Measure
Study Characteristics							
Region	WC	Europe	19	−0.49 (−1.23 to 0.24)	2.25%	0.19	−1.23 cm
		US	7	−0.33 (−0.96 to 0.29)	2.90%	0.19	−0.83 cm
	HDL	Europe	10	0.80 (0.04 to 1.57)	19.3%	0.04	0.13 mmol/L
		US	6	−0.10 (−0.71 to 0.50)	19.3%	0.04	−0.02 mmol/L
	TG	Europe	9	−0.74 (−1.46 to −0.03)	4.11%	0.12	−0.35 mmol/L
		US	4	−0.13 (−073 to 0.46)	4.11%	0.12	−0.06 mmol/L
	FBG	Europe	9	−0.74 (−1.76 to 0.27)	9.14%	0.15	−0.06 mmol/L
		US	3	−0.18 (−1.05 to 0.69)	9.14%	0.15	−0.01 mmol/L
	SBP	Europe	10	−0.68 (−1.83 to 0.47)	0.36%	0.25	−3.21 mmol/L
		US	4	−0.47 (−1.44 to 0.50)	0.36%	0.25	−2.22 mmol/L
	DBP	Europe	10	−1.13 (−2.02 to 1.14)	2.88%	0.24	−3.47 mmol/L
		US	4	−0.44 (−1.95 to 0.74)	2.88%	0.24	−1.35 mmol/L
Study Design	WC	MedSD *vs.* Other Diet	13	−1.14 (−1.49 to −0.78)	28.71%	<0.0001	−2.87 cm
		Pre/Post or Crossover	23	−0.27 (−0.52 to −0.02)	28.71%	<0.0001	−0.68 cm
	HDL	MedSD *vs.* Other Diet	9	0.79 (0.45 to 1.15)	45.64%	<0.0001	0.13 mmol/L
		Pre/Post or Crossover	16	−0.16 (−0.42 to 0.09)	45.64%	<0.0001	−0.16 mmol/L
	TG	MedSD *vs.* Other Diet	8	−0.98 (−1.39 to −0.59)	28.04%	0.008	−0.46 mmol/L
		Pre/Post or Crossover	15	−0.21 (−0.49 to 0.07)	28.04%	0.008	−0.10 mmol/L
	FBG	MedSD *vs.* Other Diet	7	−1.13 (−1.59 to −0.66)	30.92%	<0.0001	−0.09 mmol/L
		Pre/Post or Crossover	14	−0.27 (−0.59 to 0.06)	30.92%	<0.0001	−0.02 mmol/L
	SBP	MedSD *vs.* Other Diet	7	−1.37 (−1.86 to −0.87)	32.26%	<0.0001	−6.47 mmHg
		Pre/Post or Crossover	16	−0.53 (−0.84 to −0.22)	32.26%	<0.0001	−2.69 mmHg
	DBP	MedSD *vs.* Other Diet	7	−1.32 (−2.31 to −0.32)	0.00%	0.004	−4.06 mmHg
		Pre/Post or Crossover	16	−0.87 (−1.52 to −0.21)	0.00%	0.004	−2.67 mmHg

Table 3. *Cont.*

Moderator	Outcome	Category	k	d_+ (95% CI)	R^2	p-Value	Clinical Unit of Measure
Impact per Publication Metric	WC	0 (minimum)	39	−0.18 (−0.42 to 0.06)	50.13%	<0.0001	−0.45 cm
		16.104 (maximum)	39	−1.89 (−2.43 to −1.37)	50.13%	<0.0001	−4.76 cm
	HDL	0 (minimum)	26	−0.03 (−0.31 to 0.26)	29.44%	0.0006	−0.005 mmol/L
		16.104 (maximum)	26	0.95 (0.38 to 1.52)	29.44%	0.0006	0.15 mmol/L
	TG	0 (minimum)	24	−0.23 (−0.53 to 0.08)	22.65%	<0.0001	−0.11 mmol/L
		16.104 (maximum)	24	−1.09 (−1.68 to −0.52)	22.65%	<0.0001	−0.52 mmol/L
	FBG	0 (minimum)	22	−0.13 (−0.45 to 0.19)	41.52%	0.0004	−0.01 mmol/L
		16.104 (maximum)	22	−1.45 (−2.03 to −0.88)	41.52%	0.0004	−0.11 mmol/L
	SBP	0 (minimum)	24	−0.51 (−0.86 to −0.16)	13.10%	0.13	−2.41 mmHg
		16.104 (maximum)	24	−1.16 (−1.84 to −0.49)	13.10%	0.13	−5.48 mmHg
	DBP	0 (minimum)	23	−0.69 (−1.37 to 0.02)	3.54%	0.18	−2.12 mmHg
		16.104 (maximum)	23	−1.77 (−3.06 to −0.49)	3.54%	0.18	−5.44 mmHg
Intervention Characteristics							
Length of intervention (in weeks)	WC	4 weeks (minimum)	39	−0.24 (−0.45 to −0.03)	46.18%	<0.0001	−0.604 cm
		208 weeks (maximum)	39	−2.50 (−3.29 to −1.71)	46.18%	<0.0001	−6.29 cm
	HDL	4 weeks (minimum)	27	−0.09 (−0.32 to 0.14)	48.04%	<0.0001	−0.01 mmol/L
		208 weeks (maximum)	27	1.79 (1.06 to 2.53)	48.04%	<0.0001	0.29 mmol/L
	TG	4 weeks (minimum)	25	−0.19 (−0.46 to 0.07)	32.1%	0.0009	−0.09 mmol/L
		208 weeks (maximum)	25	−1.73 (−2.51 to −0.95)	32.1%	0.0009	−0.83 mmol/L
	FBG	4 weeks (minimum)	23	−0.19 (−0.45 to 0.07)	51.13%	<0.0001	−0.01 mmol/L
		208 weeks (maximum)	23	−2.22 (−3.02 to −1.41)	51.1%	<0.0001	−0.17 mmol/L
	SBP	4 weeks (minimum)	25	−0.45 (−0.77 to −0.14)	27.89%	0.0004	−2.12 mmHg
		208 weeks (maximum)	25	−2.04 (−2.98 to −1.09)	27.89%	0.004	−9.63 mmHg
	DBP	4 weeks (minimum)	25	−0.67 (−1.26 to −0.08)	6.39%	0.10	−2.06 mmHg
		208 weeks (maximum)	25	−2.37 (−4.15 to −0.59)	6.39%	0.10	−7.28 mmHg

Table 3. *Cont.*

Moderator	Outcome	Category	k	d_+ (95% CI)	R^2	p-Value	Clinical Unit of Measure
Number of Females	WC	0 (minimum)	35	−0.49 (−0.76 to −0.23)	0.00%	0.95	−1.23 cm
		1154 (maximum)	35	−0.54 (−1.91 to 0.83)	0.00%	0.95	−1.36 cm
	HDL	0 (minimum)	25	0.33 (−0.06 to 0.72)	0.00%	0.39	0.06 mmol/L
		1154 (maximum)	25	−3.43 (−11.69 to 4.83)	0.00%	0.39	−0.56 mmol/L
	TG	0 (minimum)	23	−0.45 (−0.87 to −0.03)	0.00%	0.89	−0.22 mmol/L
		1154 (maximum)	23	−1.04 (−10.91 to 8.83)	0.00%	0.91	−0.49 mmol/L
	FBG	0 (minimum)	21	−0.55 (−0.91 to −0.19)	0.00%	0.91	−0.04 mmol/L
		1154 (maximum)	21	−0.46 (−1.94 to 1.01)	0.00%	0.91	−0.04 mmol/L
	SBP	0 (minimum)	23	−0.70 (−1.04 to −0.36)	0.00%	0.79	−3.31 mmHg
		1154 (maximum)	23	−0.91 (−2.36 to 0.53)	0.00%	0.79	−4.29 mmHg
	DBP	0 (minimum)	22	−0.59 (−0.95 to −0.25)	67.92%	<0.0001	−1.81 mmHg
		1154 (maximum)	22	−5.82 (−7.29 to −4.33)	67.92%	<0.0001	−17.89 mmHg
Total sample size	WC	12 (minimum)	39	−0.54 (−0.81 to −0.26)	0.00%	0.97	−1.36 cm
		1406 (maximum)	39	−0.56 (−1.88 to 0.77)	0.00%	0.97	−1.41 cm
	HDL	12 (minimum)	27	−0.18 (−0.63 to 0.27)	13.29%	0.05	−0.03 mmol/L
		1406 (maximum)	27	5.69 (0.10 to 11.29)	13.29%	0.05	0.93 mmol/L
	TG	12 (minimum)	25	−0.20 (−0.66 to 0.26)	4.55%	0.18	−0.09 mmol/L
		1406 (maximum)	25	−4.65 (−10.79 to 1.48)	4.55%	0.18	−2.22 mmol/L
	FBG	12 (minimum)	23	−0.49 (−0.84 to −0.15)	0.00%	0.85	−0.04 mmol/L
		1406 (maximum)	23	−0.64 (−2.05 to −0.78)	0.00%	0.85	−0.05 mmol/L
	SBP	12 (minimum)	25	−0.71 (−1.05 to −0.35)	0.00%	0.79	−3.35 mmHg
		1406 (maximum)	25	−0.93 (−2.38 to 0.53)	0.00%	0.79	−4.39 mmHg
	DBP	12 (minimum)	24	−0.41 (−0.73 to −0.09)	72.14%	<0.0001	−1.26 mmHg
		1406 (maximum)	24	−5.9 (−7.22 to −4.58)	72.14%	<0.0001	−18.14 mmHg

Table 3. *Cont.*

Moderator	Outcome	Category	k	d_+ (95% CI)	R^2	p-Value	Clinical Unit of Measure
Sample size of intervention group	WC	11 (minimum)	39	−0.54 (−0.79 to −0.28)	0.00%	0.99	−1.36 cm
		1154 (maximum)	39	−0.55 (−1.93 to 0.82)	0.00%	0.99	−1.38 cm
	HDL	11 (minimum)	27	0.11 (−0.33 to 0.54)	0.00%	0.60	0.02 mmol/L
		1154 (maximum)	27	2.24 (−5.41 to 9.89)	0.00%	0.60	0.37 mmol/L
	TG	11 (minimum)	25	−0.34 (−0.76 to 0.07)	0.00%	0.47	−0.16 mmol/L
		1154 (maximum)	25	−3.45 (−11.62 to 4.73)	0.00%	0.47	−1.65 mmol/L
	FBG	11 (minimum)	23	−0.50 (−0.84 to −0.17)	0.00%	0.96	−0.04 mmol/L
		1154 (maximum)	23	−0.54 (−1.96 to 0.88)	0.00%	0.96	−0.04 mmol/L
	SBP	11 (minimum)	25	−0.71 (−1.05 to −0.37)	0.00%	0.78	−3.35 mmHg
		1154 (maximum)	25	−0.93 (−2.39 to 0.53)	0.00%	0.78	−4.39 mmHg
	DBP	11 (minimum)	24	−0.51 (−0.82 to −0.20)	71.80%	<0.0001	−1.57 mmHg
		1154 (maximum)	24	−5.91 (−7.25 to −4.58)	71.80%	<0.0001	−18.17 mmHg
Use of a behavioral technique	WC	No	21	−0.43 (−0.74 to −0.11)	0.00%	<0.0001	−1.08 cm
		Yes	18	−0.66 (−1.00 to −0.33)	0.00%	<0.0001	−1.66 cm
	HDL	No	14	−0.08 (−0.42 to 0.26)	13.88%	0.02	−0.01 mmol/L
		Yes	13	0.48 (0.13 to 0.83)	13.88%	0.02	0.08 mmol/L
	TG	No	14	−0.27 (−0.61 to 0.06)	6.26%	0.0003	−0.13 mmol/L
		Yes	11	−0.70 (−1.08 to −0.33)	6.26%	0.0003	−0.33 mmol/L
	FBG	No	12	−0.29 (−0.71 to 0.12)	4.51%	0.001	−0.02 mmol/L
		Yes	11	−0.72 (−1.14 to −0.29)	4.51%	0.001	−0.06 mmol/L
	SBP	No	13	−0.53 (−0.94 to −0.12)	1.71%	<0.0001	−2.50 mmHg
		Yes	12	−0.94 (−1.37 to −0.51)	1.71%	<0.0001	−4.44 mmHg
Level of intervention or supervision during the study	WC	Primarily one-on-one	14	−0.47 (−0.83 to −0.11)	17.28%	<0.0001	−1.18 cm
		Small groups	9	−1.14 (−1.58 to −0.69)	17.28%	<0.0001	−2.87 cm
	HDL	Primarily one-on-one	8	−0.18 (−0.63 to 0.28)	15.73%	0.03	−0.03 mmol/L
		Small groups	9	0.65 (0.23 to 1.07)	15.73%	0.03	0.11 mmol/L

Table 3. *Cont.*

Moderator	Outcome	Category	*k*	d_+ (95% CI)	R^2	*p*-Value	Clinical Unit of Measure
Level of intervention or supervision during the study	TG	Primarily one-on-one	8	−0.14 (−0.55 to 0.27)	16.04%	<0.0001	−0.07 mmol/L
		Small groups	7	−1.03 (−1.45 to −0.59)	16.04%	<0.0001	−0.49 mmol/L
	FBG	Primarily one-on-one	7	−0.19 (−0.69 to 0.32)	19.26%	0.0002	−0.01 mmol/L
		Small groups	7	−1.04 (−1.54 to −0.55)	19.26%	0.0002	−0.08 mmol/L
	SBP	Primarily one-on-one	9	−0.48 (−0.92 to −0.04)	28.65%	<0.0001	−2.26 mmHg
		Small groups	7	−1.43 (−1.93 to −0.94)	28.65%	<0.0001	−6.75 mmHg
	DBP	Primarily one-on-one	9	−0.37 (−1.19 to 0.46)	2.44%	0.002	−1.13 mmHg
		Small groups	7	−1.54 (−2.48 to −0.60)	2.44%	0.002	−4.73 mmHg

Note: WC, waist circumference; HDL, HDL cholesterol; TG, triglycerides, FBG, fasting blood glucose; SBP, systolic blood pressure; DBP, diastolic blood pressure; k is the number of interventions included in the analysis for each outcome; R^2 indicates the percentage of heterogeneity that the moderator accounts for; *p*-value represents the significance of the moderation effect; Clinical Unit of Measure was calculated using a predictive model transforming arithmetically the standardized ES to its unstandardized version.

The level of intervention or supervision during the study (*i.e.*, primarily one-on-one or small groups) resulted in significant or trending associations for waist circumference, HDL cholesterol, triglycerides, fasting blood glucose and systolic blood pressure. Interventions consisting of small groups saw significant beneficial effects for all six outcomes, whereas interventions that were primarily one-on-one resulted in only two significant outcomes.

In regards to specific components of the traditional MedSD interventions, specific macronutrient proportions of the diet, assessment of dietary compliance and participant engagement in dietary counseling did not significantly explain the variability between studies. Participant characteristics, in particular the presence or absence of certain disease states, were also analyzed as moderators. Disease states that were included in this analysis were cardiovascular disease, type II diabetes mellitus, metabolic syndrome, and overweight/obesity. These variables were not considered to be significant moderators.

3.4. Risk of Bias

Risk of bias was unclear for random sequence generation, allocation, blinding, incomplete outcome data, selective reporting, and other potential sources of bias (Figure S12). Moderator analysis was not significant for any of the risk of bias parameters (data not shown). No high or low risk of bias was found for random sequence generation and 3.3% of the articles had low risk of bias for allocation concealment. As for blinding of participants and personnel, 6.7% of the articles had low risk of bias and 13.3% of the articles had high risk of bias. Blinding of outcome assessment had 10% low risk of bias and 10% high risk of bias. Incomplete outcome data in the short-term and long-term both resulted in 6.7% of articles with high risk of bias. No high or low risk of bias was reported for selective reporting. With regard to other bias, 3.3% of articles had low risk of bias whereas 10% had high risk of bias.

4. Discussion

The present meta-analysis of 29 intervention trials found that the traditional MedSD has significant beneficial effects for five out of six of the metabolic risk factors: waist circumference, triglycerides, fasting blood glucose, systolic blood pressure and diastolic blood pressure. The significant heterogeneity between studies was partly attributed to the location of the studies, the length of the intervention, and the IPP value of the journal where the study was published. Significant beneficial associations were found for studies conducted in Europe, those of longer duration, studies using a behavioral technique, studies with a comparison intervention group, and studies conducted primarily in groups for most of the metabolic risk factors. To our knowledge, this is the first meta-analysis to evaluate the effects of the Mediterranean diet on metabolic syndrome that meets 100% of the AMSTAR criteria [58].

Our findings that a traditional MedSD is beneficial in reducing the risk of CVD-associated metabolic parameters complements and extends previous work in this area. Several recent systematic reviews and meta-analyses published on the MedSD and CVD risk have reported similar positive effects on HDL cholesterol [59], triglycerides [59], systolic blood pressure [60,61], diastolic blood pressure [60,61], and fasting blood glucose [60]. These studies also found similar significant positive associations in moderator analysis for studies conducted in Mediterranean countries [7,62], duration of study [7], study design [62], and study quality [4,7].

To our knowledge, only one meta-analysis has been published on the effects of the Mediterranean diet on metabolic syndrome [7]. The meta-analysis by Kastorini *et al.* [7] included 35 clinical trials, two prospective studies, and 13 cross-sectional studies with a total of 534,906 participants. Consistent with our current analysis, Kastorini *et al.* found that the MedSD was associated with reductions in waist circumference, triglycerides and fasting glucose levels. The MedSD was also associated with beneficial effects on HDL cholesterol, whereas there were no association for systolic and diastolic blood pressure [7]. However, in the present meta-analysis we did not find a significant effect for HDL cholesterol and found a significant beneficial association for both systolic and diastolic blood pressure. The literature search employed by Kastorini *et al.* [7] differed from the current meta-analysis in that the search was limited to those manuscripts published in English and to three computer databases. Small literature searches of only a few key terms at a time were conducted rather than one comprehensive literature search. Clinical trials with lack of randomization, lack of a control diet group, and interventions without inclusion of all traditional Mediterranean diet components were excluded from their analysis [7]. For the present meta-analysis, a comprehensive literature search was performed using six electronic databases, language was not restricted and studies without comparison groups or with a lack of randomization were not excluded. Thus, differences in search criteria may have contributed to the reported discrepancies in the associations for the MedSD and HDL cholesterol and the MedSD and blood pressure between the present report and meta-analysis by Kastorini *et al.* [7].

Study Limitation and Strengths

Our meta-analysis had several limitations. There is significant heterogeneity between studies that could not be explained by the moderators included in our analyses. The data reported in our sample of studies did not allow us to control for baseline physical activity or different types and duration of on-going exercise, and thus, physical activity could not be included as a moderator. Weight loss was not the objective in any of the included studies, however, we did not control for weight change among participants. Lastly, ecological fallacy is a possibility as we did not have access to the raw data from the included studies and should be cautious interpreting the group results as individual effects. There are also multiple strengths for this meta-analysis. We used a comprehensive literature search in six electronic databases and an inclusive and comprehensive coding form and manual were used for data extraction. We performed moderation analysis on all variables with sufficient data provided in the published material. We excluded interventions that included exercise, which we believed would have precluded us from solely evaluating diet-associated effects. To our knowledge, this is the first meta-analysis to find significant beneficial associations for MedSD interventions that use behavioral techniques and small group interventions and metabolic risk factors. Lastly, we were able to use the moving constant technique and a predictive model to calculate effect sizes for each significant moderator and transform that effect size into clinical units of measure.

5. Conclusions

The results of the present meta-analysis suggest that the traditional MedSD can have risk reduction effects on a number of metabolic parameters. In addition, the MedSD was significantly beneficial for different metabolic risk factors when, in general the intervention was longer in duration, the study was conducted in Europe, the report was published in a journal with higher Impact per Publication value, the study included a comparison intervention, a behavioral technique was used, and the study was conducted using small groups. More high-quality intervention studies conducted in non-European countries that control for physical activity and changes in weight, and include objective measures of compliance are warranted and would allow for further moderator analyses.

Acknowledgments: The research team would like to acknowledge Jill Livingston, the University of Connecticut Health Science Librarian, for her assistance with the literature search. Hatch Act Formula Fund 2013–2018 obtained by T.B.H.-M., J.K., A.K.

Author Contributions: T.B.H.-M., M.G., J.D.B., A.K., and J.K. conceived and designed the research; T.B.M.-H., M.G. and J.S. conducted the research; T.B.H.-M. and M.G. analyzed the data; T.B.H.-M., M.G., and J.D.B. wrote the paper; T.B.H.-M., M.G., J.D.B., J.S., A.K., and J.K. revised the manuscript for important intellectual content.

Abbreviations

The following abbreviations are used in this manuscript:

MedSD	Mediterranean-style Diet
CVD	Cardiovascular Disease
PRISMA	Preferred Reporting Items for Systematic Reviews and Meta-Analyses
MQ	Methodological Quality
ESs	Effect Sizes
WC	Waist circumference
FBG	Fasting blood glucose
TG	Triglycerides
SBP	Systolic blood pressure
DBP	Diastolic blood pressure
IPP	Impact per publication

References

1. Grundy, S.M.; Cleeman, J.I.; Daniels, S.R.; Donato, K.A.; Eckel, R.H.; Franklin, B.A.; Gordon, D.J.; Krauss, R.M.; Savage, P.J.; Smith, S.C., Jr.; *et al.* Diagnosis and management of the metabolic syndrome: An American Heart Association/National Heart, Lung, and Blood Institute scientific statement. *Curr. Opin. Cardiol.* **2006**, *21*, 1–6. [CrossRef] [PubMed]
2. Grundy, S.M.; Brewer, H.B., Jr.; Cleeman, J.I.; Smith, S.C., Jr.; Lenfant, C.; National Heart, Lung, and Blood Institute; American Heart Association. Definition of metabolic syndrome: Report of the National Heart, Lung, and Blood Institute/American Heart Association conference on scientific issues related to definition. *Arterioscler. Thromb. Vasc. Biol.* **2004**, *24*, e13–e18. [CrossRef] [PubMed]
3. Ervin, R.B. Prevalence of metabolic syndrome among adults 20 years of age and over, by sex, age, race and ethnicity, and body mass index: United States, 2003–2006. In *National Health Statistics Reports*; Center for Disease Control and Prevention: Hyattsville, MD, USA, 2009; pp. 1–7.
4. Sofi, F.; Abbate, R.; Gensini, G.F.; Casini, A. Accruing evidence on benefits of adherence to the Mediterranean diet on health: An updated systematic review and meta-analysis. *Am. J. Clin. Nutr.* **2010**, *92*, 1189–1196. [CrossRef] [PubMed]
5. Babio, N.; Toledo, E.; Estruch, R.; Ros, E.; Martinez-Gonzalez, M.A.; Castaner, O.; Bullo, M.; Corella, D.; Aros, F.; Gomez-Gracia, E.; *et al.* PREDIMED Study Investigators Mediterranean diets and metabolic syndrome status in the PREDIMED randomized trial. *CMAJ* **2014**, *186*, E649–E657. [CrossRef] [PubMed]
6. Mediterranean Diet Pyramid. Oldways: Health through Heritage. Available online: http://oldwayspt.org/resources/heritage-pyramids/mediterranean-pyramid/overview (accessed on 3 August 2014).

7. Kastorini, C.M.; Milionis, H.J.; Esposito, K.; Giugliano, D.; Goudevenos, J.A.; Panagiotakos, D.B. The effect of Mediterranean diet on metabolic syndrome and its components: A meta-analysis of 50 studies and 534,906 individuals. *J. Am. Coll. Cardiol.* **2011**, *57*, 1299–1313. [CrossRef] [PubMed]
8. United States Department of Agriculture (USDA), Center for Nutrition Policy and Promotion. *Report of the Dietary Guidelines Advisory Committee on the Dietary Guidelines for Americans, 2015*; United States Department of Agriculture: Washington, DC, USA, 2015.
9. Moher, D.; Liberati, A.; Tetzlaff, J.; Altman, D.G. Preferred Reporting Items for Systematic Reviews and Meta-Analyses: The PRISMA Statement. *J. Clin. Epidemiol.* **2009**, *62*, 1006–1012. [CrossRef] [PubMed]
10. Higgins, J.P., Green, S., Eds.; *Cochrane Handbook for Systematic Reviews of Interventions*; The Cochrane Collaboration: Chichster, UK, 2011.
11. Johnson, B.T.; Low, R.E.; MacDonald, H.V. Panning for the gold in health research: Incorporating studies' methodological quality in meta-analysis. *Psychol. Health* **2015**, *30*, 135–152. [CrossRef] [PubMed]
12. Cohen, J. Weighted kappa: Nominal scale agreement with provision for scaled disagreement or partial credit. *Psychol. Bull.* **1968**, *70*, 213–220. [CrossRef] [PubMed]
13. Bartko, J.J. The intraclass correlation coefficient as a measure of reliability. *Psychol. Rep.* **1966**, *19*, 3–11. [CrossRef] [PubMed]
14. Begg, C.B.; Mazumdar, M. Operating characteristics of a rank correlation test for publication bias. *Biometrics* **1994**, *50*, 1088–1101. [CrossRef] [PubMed]
15. Egger, M.; Davey Smith, G.; Schneider, M.; Minder, C. Bias in meta-analysis detected by a simple, graphical test. *BMJ* **1997**, *315*, 629–634. [CrossRef] [PubMed]
16. Duval, S.; Tweedie, R. A Nonparametric "Trim and Fill" Method of Accounting for Publication Bias in Meta-Analysis. *J. Am. Stat. Assoc.* **2000**, *95*, 89–98.
17. Sterne, J.A.; Egger, M. Funnel plots for detecting bias in meta-analysis: Guidelines on choice of axis. *J. Clin. Epidemiol.* **2001**, *54*, 1046–1055. [CrossRef]
18. R Development Core Team. *R: A Language and Environment for Statistical Computing*; ISBN: 3-900051-07-0. Available online: http://www.R-project.org/ (accessed on 14 March 2016).
19. Viechtbauer, W. Conducting meta-analyses in R with the meta for package. *J. Stat. Softw.* **2010**, *36*, 59862. [CrossRef]
20. Becker, B.J. Synthesizing standardized mean-change measures. *Br. J. Math. Stat. Psychol.* **1998**, *41*, 257–278. [CrossRef]
21. Huedo-Medina, T.B.; Johnson, B.T. *Estimating the Standardized Mean Difference Effect Size and Its Variance from Different Data Sources: A Spreadsheet*; University of Connecticut: Storrs, CT, USA, 2011.
22. Becker, B.E.A. *Multivariate Meta-Analysis*; Academic Press: San Diego, CA, USA, 2000.
23. Gleser, L.J.; Olkin, I. Stochastically dependent effect sizes. In *The Handbook of Research Synthesis and Meta-Analysis*, 2nd ed.; Russell Sage: New York, NY, USA, 1994; p. 357.
24. Rubenfire, M.; Mollo, L.; Krishnan, S.; Finkel, S.; Weintraub, M.; Gracik, T.; Kohn, D.; Oral, E.A. The metabolic fitness program: Lifestyle modification for the metabolic syndrome using the resources of cardiac rehabilitation. *J. Cardiopulm. Rehabil. Prev.* **2011**, *31*, 282–289. [CrossRef] [PubMed]
25. Timar, R.; Timar, B.; Horhat, F.; Oancea, C. The impact of Mediterranean diet on glycemic control and cardiovascular risk factors in type 2 diabetic patients. *J. Food Agric. Environ.* **2013**, *11*, 561–563.
26. Aizawa, K.; Shoemaker, J.K.; Overend, T.J.; Petrella, R.J. Effects of lifestyle modification on central artery stiffness in metabolic syndrome subjects with pre-hypertension and/or pre-diabetes. *Diabetes Res. Clin. Pract.* **2009**, *83*, 249–256. [CrossRef] [PubMed]
27. Bedard, A.; Dodin, S.; Corneau, L.; Lemieux, S. The impact of abdominal obesity status on cardiovascular response to the Mediterranean diet. *J. Obes.* **2012**, *2012*, 969124. [CrossRef] [PubMed]
28. Connolly, S.; Holden, A.; Turner, E.; Fiumicelli, G.; Stevenson, J.; Hunjan, M.; Mead, A.; Kotseva, K.; Jennings, C.; Jones, J.; *et al.* MyAction: An innovative approach to the prevention of cardiovascular disease in the community. *Br. J. Cardiol.* **2011**, *18*, 171–176.
29. Schmidt, F.L.; Oh, I.S.; Hayes, T.L. Fixed- *versus* random-effects models in meta-analysis: Model properties and an empirical comparison of differences in results. *Br. J. Math. Stat. Psychol.* **2009**, *62*, 97–128. [CrossRef] [PubMed]
30. Higgins, J.P.; Thompson, S.G.; Deeks, J.J.; Altman, D.G. Measuring inconsistency in meta-analyses. *BMJ* **2003**, *327*, 557–560. [CrossRef] [PubMed]

31. Huedo-Medina, T.B.; Sanchez-Meca, J.; Marin-Martinez, F.; Botella, J. Assessing heterogeneity in meta-analysis: Q statistic or I^2 index? *Psychol. Methods* **2006**, *11*, 193–206. [CrossRef] [PubMed]
32. Johnson, B.T.; Huedo-Medina, T.B. Depicting estimates using the intercept in meta-regression models: The moving constant technique. *Res. Synth. Methods* **2011**, *2*, 204–220. [CrossRef] [PubMed]
33. Lipsey, M.W.; Wilson, D.B. *Practical Meta-Analysis*; SAGE: Thousand Oaks, CA, USA, 2001.
34. Bekkouche, L.; Bouchenak, M.; Malaisse, W.J.; Yahia, D.A. The Mediterranean diet adoption improves metabolic, oxidative, and inflammatory abnormalities in Algerian metabolic syndrome patients. *Horm. Metab. Res.* **2014**, *46*, 274–282. [CrossRef] [PubMed]
35. Bos, M.B.; de Vries, J.H.; Feskens, E.J.; van Dijk, S.J.; Hoelen, D.W.; Siebelink, E.; Heijligenberg, R.; de Groot, L.C. Effect of a high monounsaturated fatty acids diet and a Mediterranean diet on serum lipids and insulin sensitivity in adults with mild abdominal obesity. *Nutr. Metab. Cardiovasc. Dis.* **2010**, *20*, 591–598. [CrossRef] [PubMed]
36. Corbalan, M.D.; Morales, E.M.; Canteras, M.; Espallardo, A.; Hernandez, T.; Garaulet, M. Effectiveness of cognitive-behavioral therapy based on the Mediterranean diet for the treatment of obesity. *Nutrition* **2009**, *25*, 861–869. [CrossRef] [PubMed]
37. Esposito, K.; Giugliano, F.; de Sio, M.; Carleo, D.; di Palo, C.; D'Armiento, M.; Giugliano, D. Dietary factors in erectile dysfunction. *Int. J. Impot. Res.* **2006**, *18*, 370–374. [CrossRef] [PubMed]
38. Esposito, K.; Giugliano, D.; Ciotola, M. Mediterranean diet and the metabolic syndrome. *Mol. Nutr. Food Res.* **2007**, *51*, 1268–1274. [CrossRef] [PubMed]
39. Esposito, K.; Marfella, R.; Ciotola, M.; di Palo, C.; Giugliano, F.; Giugliano, G.; D'Armiento, M.; D'Andrea, F.; Giugliano, D. Effect of a Mediterranean-style diet on endothelial dysfunction and markers of vascular inflammation in the metabolic syndrome: A randomized trial. *JAMA* **2004**, *292*, 1440–1446. [CrossRef] [PubMed]
40. Esposito, K.; Maiorino, M.I.; di Palo, C.; Giugliano, D. Adherence to a Mediterranean diet and glycaemic control in Type 2 diabetes mellitus. *Diabet. Med.* **2009**, *26*, 900–907. [CrossRef] [PubMed]
41. Goulet, J.; Lamarche, B.; Nadeau, G.; Lemieux, S. Effect of a nutritional intervention promoting the Mediterranean food pattern on plasma lipids, lipoproteins and body weight in healthy French-Canadian women. *Atherosclerosis* **2003**, *170*, 115–124. [CrossRef]
42. Goulet, J.; Lapointe, A.; Lamarche, B.; Lemieux, S. Effect of a nutritional intervention promoting the Mediterranean food pattern on anthropometric profile in healthy women from the Quebec city metropolitan area. *Eur. J. Clin. Nutr.* **2007**, *61*, 1293–1300. [CrossRef] [PubMed]
43. Jones, J.L.; Ackermann, D.; Barona, J.; Calle, M.; Andersen, C.; Kim, J.E.; Volek, J.S.; McIntosh, M.; Najm, W.; Lerman, R.H.; *et al.* A Mediterranean low-glycemic-load diet alone or in combination with a medical food improves insulin sensitivity and reduces inflammation in women with metabolic syndrome. *Br. J. Med. Med. Res.* **2011**, *1*, 356–370. [CrossRef]
44. Kolomvotsou, A.I.; Rallidis, L.S.; Mountzouris, K.C.; Lekakis, J.; Koutelidakis, A.; Efstathiou, S.; Nana-Anastasiou, M.; Zampelas, A. Adherence to Mediterranean diet and close dietetic supervision increase total dietary antioxidant intake and plasma antioxidant capacity in subjects with abdominal obesity. *Eur. J. Nutr.* **2013**, *52*, 37–48. [CrossRef] [PubMed]
45. Leblanc, V.; Bégin, C.; Hudon, A.M.; Royer, M.M.; Corneau, L.; Dodin, S.; Lemieux, S. Gender differences in the long-term effects of a nutritional intervention program promoting the Mediterranean diet: Changes in dietary intakes, eating behaviors, anthropometric and metabolic variables. *Nutr. J.* **2014**, *13*, 107. [CrossRef] [PubMed]
46. Leighton, F.; Polic, G.; Strobel, P.; Pérez, D.; Martínez, C.; Vásquez, L.; Castillo, O.; Villarroel, L.; Echeverría, G.; Urquiaga, I.; *et al.* Health impact of Mediterranean diets in food at work. *Public Health Nutr.* **2009**, *12*, 1635–1643. [CrossRef] [PubMed]
47. Lerman, R.H.; Minich, D.M.; Darland, G.; Lamb, J.J.; Chang, J.; Hsi, A.; Bland, J.S.; Tripp, M.L. Subjects with elevated LDL cholesterol and metabolic syndrome benefit from supplementation with soy protein, phytosterols, hops rho iso-alpha acids, and Acacia nilotica proanthocyanidins. *J. Clin. Lipidol.* **2010**, *4*, 59–68. [CrossRef] [PubMed]
48. Lindeberg, S.; Jonsson, T.; Granfeldt, Y.; Borgstrand, E.; Soffman, J.; Sjostrom, K.; Ahren, B. A Palaeolithic diet improves glucose tolerance more than a Mediterranean-like diet in individuals with ischaemic heart disease. *Diabetologia* **2007**, *50*, 1795–1807. [CrossRef] [PubMed]

49. Llaneza, P.; Gonzalez, C.; Fernandez-Inarrea, J.; Alonso, A.; Diaz-Fernandez, M.J.; Arnott, I.; Ferrer-Barriendos, J. Soy isoflavones, Mediterranean diet, and physical exercise in postmenopausal women with insulin resistance. *Menopause* **2010**, *17*, 372–378. [CrossRef] [PubMed]
50. Papandreou, C.; Schiza, S.E.; Bouloukaki, I.; Hatzis, C.M.; Kafatos, A.G.; Siafakas, N.M.; Tzanakis, N.E. Effect of Mediterranean diet *versus* prudent diet combined with physical activity on OSAS: A randomised trial. *Eur. Respir. J.* **2012**, *39*, 1398–1404. [CrossRef] [PubMed]
51. Papandreou, C.; Schiza, S.E.; Tzatzarakis, M.N.; Kavalakis, M.; Hatzis, C.M.; Tsatsakis, A.M.; Kafatos, A.G.; Siafakas, N.M.; Tzanakis, N.E. Effect of Mediterranean diet on lipid peroxidation marker TBARS in obese patients with OSAHS under CPAP treatment: A randomised trial. *Sleep Breath* **2012**, *16*, 873–879. [CrossRef] [PubMed]
52. Rallidis, L.S.; Lekakis, J.; Kolomvotsou, A.; Zampelas, A.; Vamvakou, G.; Efstathiou, S.; Dimitriadis, G.; Raptis, S.A.; Kremastinos, D.T. Close adherence to a Mediterranean diet improves endothelial function in subjects with abdominal obesity. *Am. J. Clin. Nutr.* **2009**, *90*, 263–268. [CrossRef] [PubMed]
53. Richard, C.; Couillard, C.; Royer, M.-M.; Desroches, S.; Couture, P.; Lamarche, B. Impact of the Mediterranean diet with and without weight loss on plasma cell adhesion molecule concentrations in men with the metabolic syndrome. *Mediterr. J. Nutr. Metab.* **2011**, *4*, 33–39. [CrossRef]
54. Ryan, M.C.; Itsiopoulos, C.; Thodis, T.; Ward, G.; Trost, N.; Hofferberth, S.; O'Dea, K.; Desmond, P.V.; Johnson, N.A.; Wilson, A.M. The Mediterranean diet improves hepatic steatosis and insulin sensitivity in individuals with non-alcoholic fatty liver disease. *J. Hepatol.* **2013**, *59*, 138–143. [CrossRef] [PubMed]
55. Sánchez-Benito, J.L.; Pontes Torrado, Y.; González Rodríguez, A. Weight loss intervention has achieved a significant decrease of blood pressure and cholesterol. *Clin. Investig. Arterioscler.* **2012**, *24*, 241–249. [CrossRef]
56. Stendell-Hollis, N.R.; Thompson, P.A.; West, J.L.; Wertheim, B.C.; Thomson, C.A. A comparison of Mediterranean-style and MyPyramid diets on weight loss and inflammatory biomarkers in postpartum breastfeeding women. *J. Women's Health (Larchmt.)* **2013**, *22*, 48–57. [CrossRef] [PubMed]
57. Van Velden, D.P.; van der Merwe, S.; Fourie, E.; Kidd, M.; Blackhurst, D.M.; Kotze, M.J.; Mansvelt, E.P.G. The short-term influence of a Mediterranean-type diet and mild exercise with and without red wine on patients with the metabolic syndrome. *S. Afr. J. Enol. Vitic.* **2007**, *28*, 44–49.
58. Shea, B.J.; Grimshaw, J.M.; Wells, G.A.; Boers, M.; Andersson, N.; Hamel, C.; Porter, A.C.; Tugwell, P.; Moher, D.; Bouter, L.M. Development of AMSTAR: A measurement tool to assess the methodological quality of systematic reviews. *BMC Med. Res. Methodol.* **2007**, *7*. [CrossRef] [PubMed]
59. Ajala, O.; English, P.; Pinkney, J. Systematic review and meta-analysis of different dietary approaches to the management of type 2 diabetes. *Am. J. Clin. Nutr.* **2013**, *97*, 505–516. [CrossRef] [PubMed]
60. Nordmann, A.J.; Suter-Zimmermann, K.; Bucher, H.C.; Shai, I.; Tuttle, K.R.; Estruch, R.; Briel, M. Meta-Analysis Comparing Mediterranean to Low-Fat Diets for Modification of Cardiovascular Risk Factors. *Am. J. Med.* **2011**, *124*, 841–851. [CrossRef] [PubMed]
61. Nordmann, A. Mediterranean or low-fat diets to reduce cardiovascular risk? *Praxis (Bern 1994)* **2011**, *100*, 1283–1288. [CrossRef] [PubMed]
62. Psaltopoulou, T.; Sergentanis, T.N.; Panagiotakos, D.B.; Sergentanis, I.N.; Kosti, R.; Scarmeas, N. Mediterranean diet and stroke, cognitive impairment, depression: A meta-analysis. *Ann. Neurol.* **2013**, *74*, 580–591. [CrossRef] [PubMed]

16

NO-Rich Diet for Lifestyle-Related Diseases

Jun Kobayashi *, Kazuo Ohtake and Hiroyuki Uchida

Division of Pathophysiology, Department of Clinical Dietetics and Human Nutrition, Faculty of Pharmaceutical Science, Josai University, Saitama 350-0295, Japan; kazuo@josai.ac.jp (K.O.); mrhiro@josai.ac.jp (H.U.)

* Correspondence: junkoba@josai.ac.jp

Abstract: Decreased nitric oxide (NO) availability due to obesity and endothelial dysfunction might be causally related to the development of lifestyle-related diseases such as insulin resistance, ischemic heart disease, and hypertension. In such situations, instead of impaired NO synthase (NOS)-dependent NO generation, the entero-salivary nitrate-nitrite-NO pathway might serve as a backup system for NO generation by transmitting NO activities in the various molecular forms including NO and protein *S*-nitrosothiols. Recently accumulated evidence has demonstrated that dietary intake of fruits and vegetables rich in nitrate/nitrite is an inexpensive and easily-practicable way to prevent insulin resistance and vascular endothelial dysfunction by increasing the NO availability; a NO-rich diet may also prevent other lifestyle-related diseases, including osteoporosis, chronic obstructive pulmonary disease (COPD), and cancer. This review provides an overview of our current knowledge of NO generation through the entero-salivary pathway and discusses its safety and preventive effects on lifestyle-related diseases.

Keywords: lifestyle-related disease; nitric oxide (NO); nitrate; nitrite; insulin resistance; ischemia/reperfusion injury; chronic obstructive pulmonary disease (COPD); osteoporosis; cancer

---

1. Introduction

Health problems, such as insulin resistance, cardiovascular disease, osteoporosis, and cancer share some common risk factors, including unhealthy and excessive nutrition, a lack of physical activity, smoking and heavy drinking [1]. So-called lifestyle-related diseases are now the leading causes of mortality and morbidity in developed countries [2]. Healthy diets and exercise training are low-cost and easily-practicable lifestyle changes to be recommended for patients with these conditions before starting pharmacological therapy. Recent prospective and epidemiologic studies have shown that among the various foods, green leafy vegetables are undoubtedly protective against coronary heart disease, hypertension [3–6], and ischemic stroke [7]. This may be because vegetables and fruits rich in nitrate can provide a physiological substrate for reduction to form nitrite and nitric oxide (NO). The beneficial effects of these foods on the diseases resulting from circulatory disturbances are attributed to the cyclic guanosine monophosphate (cGMP)-dependent actions of NO, including vasodilation and vascular endothelial protection from platelet aggregation and leukocyte adhesion [8]. However, in addition to these classical functions of NO, recent studies have indicated novel functions for NO through cGMP-independent and protein *S*-nitrosylation-dependent intracellular signaling pathways [9]. *S*-nitrosylation is associated with the activation of transcription factors, the regulation of a number of signal transduction molecules [10] and redox protein modification [11], mitochondrial functions [12,13], and cell apoptosis [14], which could explain how the dietary nitrate exerts preventive effects against the development of lifestyle-related metabolic, inflammatory, and proliferative disorders. This review provides an overview of our current knowledge of NO production through the dietary nitrate-nitrite-NO pathway and its physiological aspect, then discusses the safety and efficacy of dietary nitrate, as well as its preventive effects on lifestyle-related diseases.

2. The Dietary Nitrate-nitrite-NO Pathway and Its Physiological Aspect

In addition to endogenous NO generation through the L-arginine-NO synthase (NOS) pathway, NO is also generated through the NOS-independent nitrate-nitrite-NO pathway [15] (Figure 1). Green leafy vegetables such as lettuce, spinach and beetroot all contain high concentrations of nitrate [16] (Table 1). Vegetables account for 60%–80% of the daily nitrate intake in a Western diet [17], and substantial elevations in the plasma nitrite levels can occur through increasing the dietary nitrate intake [18]. One serving of such a vegetable contains more nitrate than what is endogenously generated by NOS isoforms during a full day in humans [19]. As shown in Figure 2, the ingested dietary nitrate is absorbed in the upper gastrointestinal tract and reaches the peak plasma level around 30–60 min after ingestion [20] (Table 2). Approximately 25% of the absorbed nitrate is delivered to the salivary gland and secreted into saliva in the oral cavity [21], which is then reduced to nitrite by commensal anaerobic bacteria on the tongue [22]. In the acidic environment of the stomach, part of the swallowed nitrite is immediately protonated to nitrous acid ($NO_2^- + H^+ \rightarrow HNO_2$), then decomposed to form a variety of nitrogen oxides such as NO, nitrogen dioxides (NO_2), and dinitrogen trioxide (N_2O_3) ($2\ HNO_2 \rightarrow N_2O_3 + H_2O$, $N_2O_3 \rightarrow NO + NO_2$) [23]. These nitrogen oxides form additional bioactive adducts, such as *S*-nitrosothiols and *N*-nitrosoamines, following reactions with protein thiols and amines, respectively, in the dietary products. In particular, the NO production in the stomach is greatly enhanced in the presence of dietary polyphenols [24] and ascorbic acid [15], whereas because of its lower stability and shorter half-life relative to *S*-nitrosothiols, the released NO in the stomach is thought to locally contribute to increasing the gastric mucosal blood flow and mucous thickness to ensure the normal gastric physiology, and serves as the first-line host defense against swallowed pathogens [25,26]. However, some of the nitrite escapes the protonation in the acidic milieu of the stomach and enters the systemic circulation, and then reaches the peripheral organs, including skeletal muscles, where it acts in an endocrine manner to exert NO-like activity [18] (Figure 2). Because the plasma levels of nitrite are highly dependent on the amount of salivary nitrate and its reduction to nitrite, the use of an antibacterial mouthwash [27] and frequent spitting of saliva consequently decrease the plasma levels of nitrite [20].

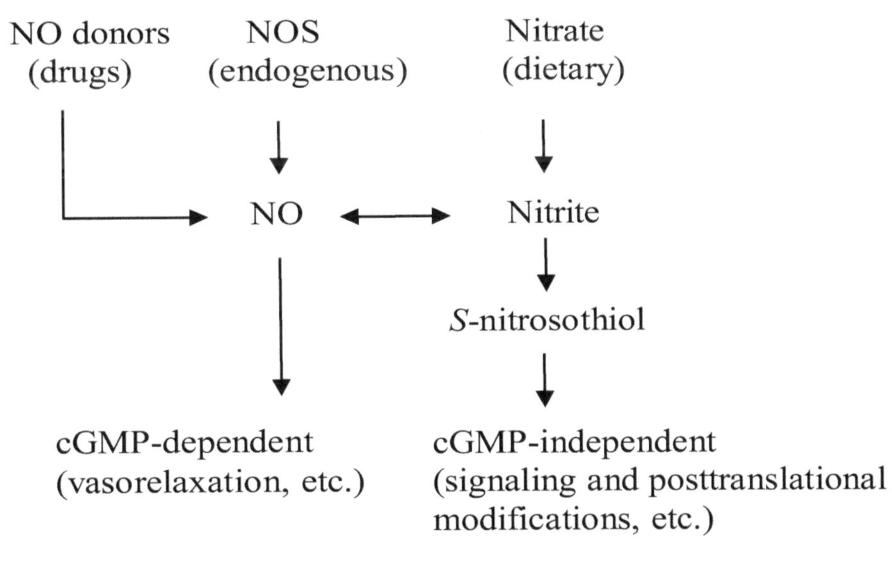

Figure 1. The NO pathways. NO is originated from the diet, drugs, and the endogenous NOS enzyme. The activities of NO are exerted through cGMP-dependent and independent ways. NO donor drugs, such as nitroglycerin and sodium nitroprusside, directly release NO. NOS endogenously generates NO, which is linked to the cGMP-dependent functions of NO. Dietary nitrate/nitrite produce NO and *S*-nitrosothiol, mainly for cGMP-independent functions. NO: nitric oxide, NOS: NO synthase, cGMP: cyclic guanosine monophosphate.

Table 1. Nitrate and nitrite contents of food products.

Food product	Nitrate concentration (mg/100 g) Mean	Range	Nitrite concentration (mg/100 g) Mean	Range	Reference
Beets	275.6	168–359	1.00	0.21–2.98	
Spinach	233.3	53.5–366	0.70	0.0–1.29	
Radishes	168.0	76.4–250	0.01	0.0–0.1	
Celery	154.4	31.6–332	0.16	0.0–0.52	
Lettuce	85.0	7.9–217.1	0.06	0.001–0.97	
Iceberg lettuce	78.6	34.7–108	0.02	0.0–0.17	
Mushroom	59.0	1.9–8.5	0.80	0.0–3.8	[16]
Cabbage	57.3	19.3–97.6	0.24	0.0–1.26	
Broccoli	39.4	2.9–114	0.06	0.001–0.95	
Green beans	38.6	16.5–61.1	0.05	0.0–0.25	
Strawberries	17.3	10.5–29.3	0.20	0.0–0.71	
Banana	13.7	8.8–21.4	0.21	0.0–0.95	
Green pepper	3.3	0.8–5.5	0.04	0.0–0.3	
Spinach	741.0	-	0.02	-	
Mustard greens	116.0	-	0.003	-	
Salad mix	82.1	-	0.13	-	
Cole slaw	55.9	-	0.07	-	
Broccoli	39.5	-	0.07	-	
Tomato	39.2	-	0.03	-	
Vegetable soup	20.9	-	0.001	-	
Hot dog	9.0	-	0.05	-	
Bacon	5.5	-	0.38	-	
Banana	4.5	-	0.009	-	
Pork tenderloin	3.3	-	0.0	-	
Bacon nitrite-free	3.0	-	0.68	-	
French fries	2.0	-	0.17	-	
Ham	0.9	-	0.89	-	[28]
Fruit mix	0.9	-	0.08	-	
Orange	0.8	-	0.02	-	
Apple sauce	0.3	-	0.008	-	
Ketchup	0.1	-	0.13	-	
Carrots	0.1	-	0.006	-	
	Nitrate concentration (mg/L)		**Nitrite concentration (mg/L)**		
Carrot juice	27.55	-	0.036	-	
Vegetable juice *	26.17	-	0.092	-	
Pomegranate juice	12.93	-	0.069	-	
Cranberry juice	9.12	-	0.145	-	
Acai juice	0.56	-	0.013	-	
Green tea	0.23	-	0.007	-	

* V8; Campbell Soup Co (Camden, NJ, USA); Table is reproduced from the reference [16] and [28].

Table 2. Saliva and plasma levels of nitrite, nitrate, and *S*-nitrosothiol before and 30 min after oral administration of sodium nitrate (10 mg/kg) in healthy volunteers.

		0 Min	**30 Min**
Saliva	Nitrite (μM)	104 ± 21	713 ± 150
	Nitrate (mM)	0.19 ± 0.03	8.2 ± 1
	S-NO (nM)	25 ± 9.8	297
Plasma	Nitrite (μM)	123 ± 19	229 ± 46
	Nitrate (mM)	30 ± 4	432 ± 44
	S-NO (nM)	6.3 ± 1.4	No significant change

Data from reference 20, *S*-NO: *S*-nitrosothiol.

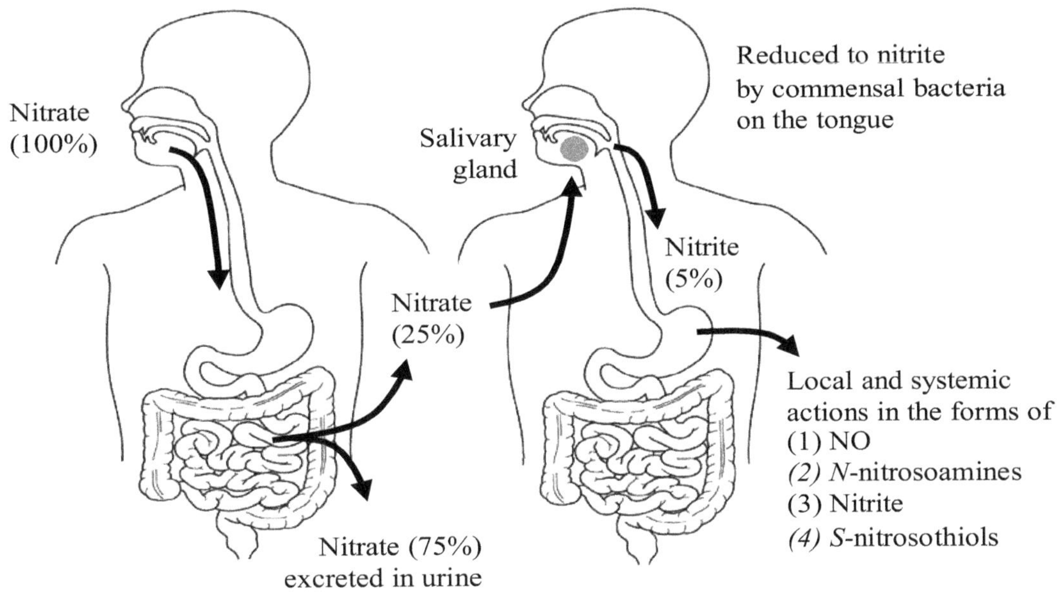

Figure 2. The entero-salivary nitrate-nitrite-NO pathway. Twenty-five percent of the ingested dietary nitrate is recycled to the saliva, and 20% of the nitrate in saliva is converted to nitrite by oral commensal bacteria. Approximately 5% of the originally ingested nitrate is swallowed into the stomach, and provides for NO activities in various forms. (1) NO for local vasodilation, mucus formation, and antimicrobial activity; (2) *N*-nitrosoamines for local carcinogenesis; (3) Nitrite for nitrite pool and transnitrosylation in the peripheral tissues; (4) *S*-nitrosothiols for transnitrosylation in the peripheral tissues.

The plasma nitrite which reaches peripheral tissues is stored in various organs. Although there have been few reports dealing with the tissue levels of nitrate/nitrite following dietary nitrate supplementation in humans, animal studies show that dietary nitrate certainly increases the tissue levels of nitrate/nitrite following increase in the plasma levels of nitrate/nitrite (Table 3), which accordingly exerts therapeutic efficacy for animal models of various disease conditions. Interestingly, while acute dietary nitrate intake increases the plasma levels of nitrite in rodents and humans [10,20], chronic dietary nitrate intake does not always increase the plasma and tissue levels of nitrite, but increases the tissue levels of nitrate and *S*-nitrosylated products (Table 3). Although the mechanism underlying this finding is yet to be clarified, there might be some redox equilibrium of nitrate-nitrite-NO after chronic dietary nitrate intake, resulting in oxidation or reduction of the tissue nitrite to form nitrate or *S*-nitrosylated species, respectively. On the other hand, animal models chronically fed a diet deficient in nitrate/nitrite exhibit significantly diminished plasma and tissue levels of nitrate/nitrite, resulting in increased ischemia-reperfusion injuries in heart and liver compared with the animal models fed a normal diet [29,30]. These results suggest that dietary nitrate intake is important in the maintenance of steady-state tissue levels of nitrate/nitrite for NO-mediated cytoprotection.

Various enzyme/protein-dependent reductions to NO have been proposed under physiological and pathological conditions, which include deoxyhemoglobin [31], deoxymyoglobin in the skeletal, vascular [32], and cardiac muscles [33], xanthine oxidase in endothelial cells, aldehyde oxidase, aldehyde dehydrogenase 2 [34], cytochrome P-450, and mitochondrial nitrite reductases (such as mitochondrial electron transport complexes) in all cells. In contrast to NOS-dependent NO production, which requires molecular oxygen, this nitrite reduction to NO is enhanced under hypoxic and acidic conditions. Because the nitrite-reducing factors are rich in skeletal muscles, tissue hypoxia during submaximal exercise kinetically favors nitrite reduction to NO, thus providing an alternative NO source for vascular dilation and efficient O_2 consumption in the working muscles [35,36].

Table 3. The effects of chronic dietary nitrate supplementation on tissue levels of nitrate/nitrite and therapeutic efficacy for experimental animal models.

Animal Model	Dietary Nitrate	Tissues	Effects of Dietary Nitrate	References
Uninephrectomized hypertension rat with high-salt diet.	Diets with 0.1 mM and 1 mM nitrate/kg/day for 8–11 weeks.	Kidney Heart Liver	Increase in plasma and tissue levels of nitrate and tissue levels of nitrosylation products. Reduction of oxidative stress and attenuation of renal injury, hypertension, cardiac hypertrophy and fibrosis.	[37]
C57BLK6 male mice with hypoxia-induced pulmonary hypertension.	0.6 mM, 15 mM, and 45 mM nitrate/L in drinking water for 3 weeks.	Lung	Increase in plasma and lung levels of nitrite and cGMP. Reduction of right ventricular pressure and hypertrophy, and pulmonary vascular remodeling.	[38]
Male Wistar rat with hypoxic heart damage.	0.7 mM/L nitrate in drinking water for 2 weeks.	Heart	Increase in plasma levels of nitrate and tissue levels of nitrite. Alleviation of metabolic abnormalities in the hypoxic heart. Improvement of myocardial energetics.	[39]

Although elevated plasma levels of nitrite certainly affect the cGMP production in systemic organs, providing an important signaling role in mammalian biology [10], dietary nitrate/nitrite also transmit biological signals via cGMP-independent mechanisms, such as transnitrosylation, a posttranslational modification analogous to phosphorylation, in order to regulate the protein function [40] (Figures 1 and 1). Here, the questions are raised. What is the carrier of NO activity to the peripheral organs, *S*-nitrosothiol, NO itself, or nitrite, and also, how does this carrier transnitrosylate in the peripheral organs? Lundberg *et al.*, showed that oral intake of sodium nitrate (10 mg/kg) in healthy volunteers significantly increased plasma levels of nitrite, but did not increase *S*-nitrosothiol in plasma [20] (Table 2). In addition, Bryan *et al.*, showed that protein *S*-nitrosylation in organs following intraperitoneal nitrite injection to rat, could not be inhibited by NO scavenging with carboxy-2-phenyl-4,4,5,5-tetramethylimidazolin-1-oxyl-3-oxide (cPTIO), suggesting that the nitrite-mediated transnitrosylation in the organs might occur mainly directly through nitrite rather than through either circulating *S*-nitrosothiol or NO itself [10].

Bryan *et al.*, also showed that the increase in plasma nitrite within the physiological concentration rage of 0.2–2 μM after nitrite administration (plasma concentration of nitrite far lower than those required for vasodilation) enhanced *S*-nitrosothiol in the organs (heart, kidney, liver, lung, and aorta) with the subsequent modulation of signaling and gene expressions of cGMP, cytochrome P-450, heat shock protein 70, and heme oxygenase-1 in these organs. Interestingly, they also showed that a switch of the standard chow to the low nitrate/nitrite diet for two days in rats decreased nitrite levels substantially in all tissues and represented changes of the signaling and gene expressions in a direction opposite to those found with nitrite administration [10].

These observations indicate that the nitrite-induced transnitrosylation in organs might be an alternative *in vivo* nitrite signaling for the mammalian biology including protection of protein thiols from irreversible oxidation, transcriptional modulation, and posttranslational regulation of most classes of proteins present in all cells [9] (Figure 3), and also that changes in plasma nitrite levels even within the physiological ranges (e.g., postprandial and fasting) can affect tissue levels of *S*-nitrosothiol and subsequent cellular biology.

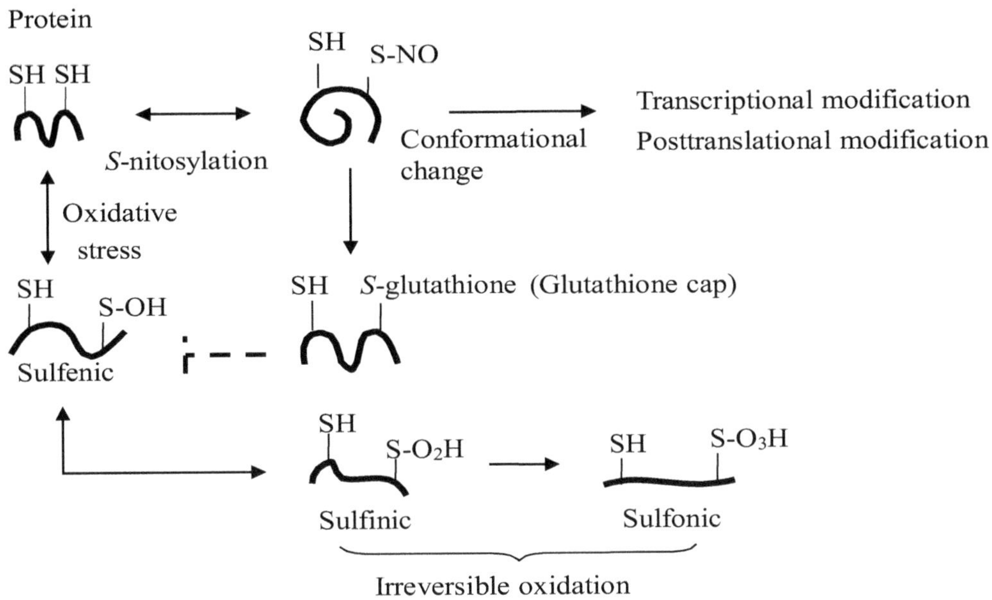

Figure 3. Protein *S*-nitrosylation. *S*-nitrosylation of protein elicits its regulatory effect by adding the NO moiety on the active thiol (SH of cysteine residue) of the protein (e.g., transcriptional factors and enzymes), and cell protection by the subsequent posttranslational addition of glutathione to the protein thiols (so-called glutathione cap), which shields the cysteine residues from further irreversible protein oxidation [11].

3. Safety and Efficacy of Dietary Nitrate

Very high concentrations of nitrate in drinking water may cause methemoglobinemia in infants (blue baby syndrome) [41]. In the 1940s, Comly first reported cases of cyanotic infants who received formula prepared with well water containing a high nitrate content [42]. Based on the subsequent analyses of the infantile cases of methemoglobinemia, the US Environmental Protection Agency (EPA) set a Maximum Contaminant Level (MCL) for nitrate of 44 mg/L (equal to 10 mg/L nitrogen in nitrate). However, it is now thought that methemoglobinemia *per se* was not caused by nitrate itself, but by fecal bacteria that infected infants and produced NO in their gut. A recent report by Avery has argued that it is unlikely that nitrate causes methemoglobinemia without bacterial contamination, and also that the 40–50 mg/L limit on nitrate in drinking water is not necessary [43]. However, there are now legal limits to the concentrations of nitrate and nitrite in both food and drinking water. The WHO showed that the Acceptable Daily Intake for humans (ADI) for nitrate and nitrite were 3.7 and 0.07 mg/kg body weight/day, respectively, which were based on the calculations from the doses of <500 mg of sodium nitrate/kg body weight that were harmless to rats and dogs. The international estimates of nitrate intake from food are 31–185 mg/day in Europe and 40–100 mg/day in the United States [44,45]. However, the Ministry of Health, Labour and Welfare of Japan reported that the average intake of nitrate in the Japanese populations is around 200–300 mg/day, which is one and a half times to two times the ADI. Furthermore, according to a report by Hord [28], in which the daily nitrate and nitrite intakes were calculated based on the variations using the vegetable and fruit components of the DASH (Dietary Approaches to Stop Hypertension) dietary pattern [46], the level easily exceeds 1,200 mg/day nitrate. This is more than five-fold higher than the WHO's ADI of 3.7 mg nitrate/kg body weight/day, and more than two-fold the US Environmental Protection Agency's level of 7.0 mg nitrate/kg body weight/day for a 60 kg individual [28]. Furthermore, as indicated in Figure 2, approximately 25% of the ingested nitrate is secreted in saliva, and 20% of the secreted nitrate in saliva is converted to nitrite by commensal bacteria on the tongue [22], indicating that about 5% of the originally ingested nitrate is swallowed into the stomach (Figure 1). Therefore, for a DASH diet containing 1200 mg nitrate, an individual would be expected to swallow approximately 45 mg of nitrite a day, which easily exceeds the ADI of nitrite. Therefore, a comprehensive reevaluation of the health effects of dietary sources of nitrate/nitrite might be required in the near future [28]. Another major health concern regarding dietary nitrate/nitrite is whether dietary nitrate can cause cancer. In fact, nitrate and nitrite themselves are not carcinogenic, but nitrite which is formed from dietary nitrate might react with dietary amines to form carcinogenic nitrosoamines. This phenomenon will be discussed in detail below.

4. Protective Effects of Dietary Nitrate/Nitrite on Lifestyle-Related Diseases

Lifestyle-related disease is a chronic disease characterized by oxidative and proinflammatory state with reduced NO bioavailability [47]. The cellular redox balance in these patients shifts toward a more oxidizing state which affects a number of protein functions at the transcriptional and posttranslational levels, consequently disrupting the cellular homeostasis [11,40]. However, increased NO bioavailability can improve the intracellular redox environment by *S*-nitrosylation-mediated modulation of most classes of proteins present in all cells [9,40]. Recently, accumulating evidence has suggested that dietary nitrate/nitrite improves the features of lifestyle-related diseases by enhancing NO availability, and thus provides potential options for prevention and therapy for these patients [28]. Based on the recent evidence, the beneficial effects of a diet rich in these components are discussed below, focusing on insulin resistance, hypertension, cardiac ischemia/reperfusion injury, chronic obstructive pulmonary disease (COPD), cancer, and osteoporosis.

4.1. Insulin Resistance

The insulin receptor shares a signaling pathway with the activation of endothelial NOS (eNOS) [19,48–52] to regulate the postprandial blood flow and efficient nutrient disposition to peripheral tissues (Figure 4). Therefore, insulin resistance is always associated with impaired NO availability, suggesting that a reciprocal relationship exists between insulin activation and endothelial function [50,53]. Insulin resistance is improved by NO at various levels including insulin secretion [54,55], mitochondrial function [56], modulation of inflammation [57], insulin signaling [58] and glucose uptake [59]. For example, insulin-stimulated NO production has physiological consequences resulting in capillary recruitment and increased blood flow in skeletal muscle, leading to efficient glucose disposal [52].

However, the most important mechanism to improve insulin resistance might be at the post-receptor level of insulin signaling [60] (Figure 4). In diabetic states, increased adiposity releases free fatty acids and produces excessive reactive oxygen species (ROS) through a toll-like receptor 4 (TLR4)-mediated mechanism, which activates a number of kinases and phosphatases [61], and then disrupts the balance of protein phosphorylation/dephosphorylation associated with insulin signaling [62]. The mechanisms underlying the NO-mediated beneficial effects on insulin resistance are as follows (Figure 4): First, NO suppresses the TLR4-mediated inflammation and ROS production by inactivating IkB kinase-β/nuclear factor-κB (IκκB/NF-κβ) [9,63], the main trigger for the induction of a number of proinflammatory cytokines. Second, Wang *et al.*, indicated that NO mediates the *S*-nitrosylation of protein-tyrosine phosphatase 1B (PTPB1) and enhances the effects of insulin [52]. Because PTPB1 dephosphorylates the insulin receptor and its substrates, attenuating the insulin effect, its phosphatase activity tends to be suppressed by eNOS-mediated *S*-nitrosylation. In contrast, when the vascular eNOS activity is impaired, PTPB1 suppresses the downstream signaling to PI3K/Akt, leading to insulin resistance. Therefore, NO might act as a key regulatory mediator for the downstream signaling linking glucose transporter 4 (GLUT4) translocation and glucose uptake [58,64]. Third, Jiang recently reported that NO-dependent nitrosylation of GLUT4 facilitates GLUT4 translocation to the membrane for glucose uptake, and improves insulin resistance [65]. Fourth, excess nutrients also overproduce superoxide in the mitochondrial respiratory chain, leading to the subsequent formation of ROS. NO can inhibit mitochondrial ROS production through the *S*-nitrosylation of mitochondrial respiratory chain complex 1 enzyme and by improving the efficiency of oxidative phosphorylation in the mitochondria [12].

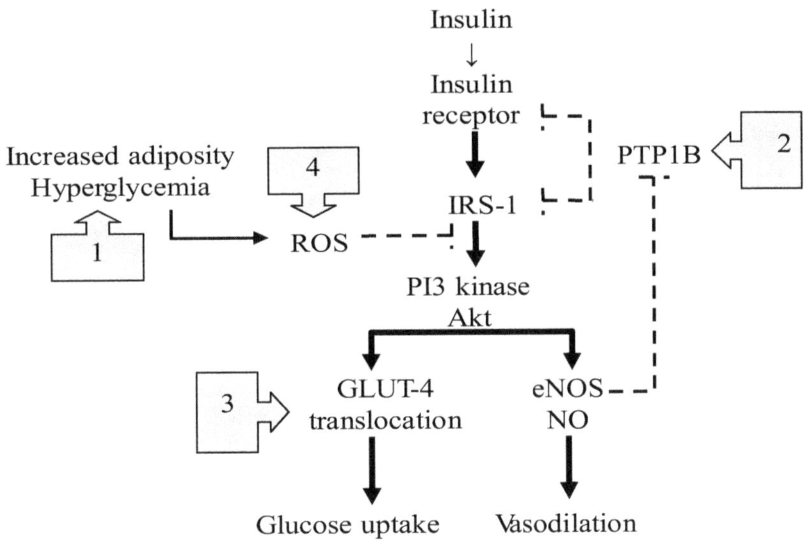

Figure 4. The NO-mediated actions on insulin signaling pathway. The boxes with arrows indicate the sites of NO-mediated actions against insulin resistance. Dotted lines represent inhibition, and solid lines represent stimulation. (**1**) NO suppresses TLR4-mediated inflammation and ROS production; (**2**) NO enhances the effects of insulin through the *S*-nitrosylation-mediated inhibition of phosphatase activity of PTPB1; (**3**) NO-dependent nitrosylation of GLUT4 facilitates glucose uptake; (**4**) NO inhibits mitochondrial ROS production through *S*-nitrosylation of the mitochondrial respiratory chain complex. IRS-1: insulin receptor substrate-1, ROS: reactive oxygen species, NO: nitric oxide, eNOS: endothelial NO synthase, GLUT4: glucose transporter 4, PI3 kinase: phosphatidylinositol 3-kinase, PTPB1: protein-tyrosine phosphatase B1, TLR4: toll like receptor 4.

Indeed, the therapeutic potential of dietary nitrate/nitrite has been supported by recent studies demonstrating the improvements of insulin resistance in humans and animals as a result of its enhancing the NO availability in plasma and tissues [65–68]. As mentioned above, insulin resistance always accompanies metabolic and endothelial dysfunction, which lead to hypertension and atherosclerosis [50,51,53,69,70]. Enhancement of the availability of NO might therefore be a promising strategy for the prevention and treatment of patients with not only insulin resistance, but also endothelial dysfunction [71].

4.2. Hypertension

Increased consumption of fruits and vegetables is associated with a reduction of the risk of cardiovascular disease [72–74]. The DASH studies recommended the consumption of diets rich in vegetables and low-fat dairy products to lower blood pressure, and these effects are thought to be attributable to the high calcium, potassium, polyphenols and fiber and low sodium content in these food items [75,76]. However, vegetable diets containing high nitrate levels increase the plasma levels of nitrate and nitrite [77], which are the physiological substrates for NO production. Accumulating evidence has recently indicated that the nitrate/nitrite content of the fruits and vegetables could contribute to their cardiovascular health benefits in animals [29,33,78–83] and humans [31,84–86].

A number of publications have demonstrated that dietary nitrate reduces blood pressure in humans [87–89]. Larsen *et al.*, reported that the diastolic blood pressure in healthy volunteers was reduced by dietary sodium nitrate (at a dose of 0.1 mmol/kg body weight per day) corresponding to the amount normally found in 150 to 250 g of a nitrate-rich vegetable, such as spinach, beetroot, or lettuce [84]. Webb *et al.*, studied the blood pressure and flow-mediated dilation of healthy volunteers, and showed that the vasoprotective effects of dietary nitrate (a single dose of 500 mL of beetroot juice containing 45.0 ± 2.6 mmol/L nitrate), were attributable to the activity of nitrite converted from the ingested nitrate [86]. Kapil *et al.*, also showed a similar finding that consuming 250 mL of beetroot juice

(5.5 mmol nitrate) enhanced the plasma levels of nitrite and cGMP with a consequent decrease in blood pressure in healthy volunteers, indicating that there was soluble guanylate cyclase-cGMP-mediated vasodilation following a conversion of the nitrite to bioactive NO [85]. They later presented the effects of dietary nitrate on hypertension, and showed the first evidence that daily dietary nitrate supplementation (250 mL of beetroot juice daily) for four weeks reduced the blood pressure, with improvements in the endothelial function and arterial stiffness in patients with hypertension [90]. Because arterial vascular remodeling is the major histological finding associated with aging, these vascular structural changes represent vascular wall fibrosis with increased collagen deposits and reduced elastin fibers, which result in arterial stiffening and subsequent hypertension in elderly patients. Sindler *et al.*, recently demonstrated that dietary nitrite (50 mg/L in drinking water) was effective in the treatment of vascular aging in mice, which was evidenced by a reduction of aortic pulse wave velocity and normalization of NO-mediated endothelium-dependent dilation. They showed that these improvements were mediated by reduction of oxidative stress and inflammation, which were linked to mitochondrial biogenesis and health as a result of increased dietary nitrite. These beneficial effects were also evident with dietary nitrate in their study [91], suggesting that dietary nitrate/nitrite may be useful for the prevention and treatment of chronic age-associated hypertension.

In addition, hypertension is also a major cause of ischemic heart and cardiac muscle remodeling, which lead to congestive heart failure. Bhushan *et al.*, reported that dietary nitrite supplementation in drinking water (50 mg/L sodium nitrite, for nine weeks) increased the cardiac nitrite, nitrosothiol, and cGMP levels, which improved the left ventricular function during heart failure in mice with hypertension produced by transverse aortic constriction. They also showed that dietary nitrite improved the cardiac fibrosis associated with pressure-overloaded left ventricular hypertrophy through NO-mediated cytoprotective signaling [92]. Although a number of studies on the acute effects of dietary nitrate have been conducted using animal models and healthy humans, more evidence in patients with hypertension, as well as additional studies on the long-term effects of dietary nitrate, will be needed in the future.

4.3. Cardiac Ischemia/Reperfusion Injury

During heart ischemia, ATP is progressively depleted in cardiac muscle cells, which impairs ion pumps, leads to the accumulation of calcium ion, and consequently damages the cell membrane stability. On reperfusion, the cardiac muscle cells are further injured, because in the mitochondria, ROS are produced in large quantities due to massive electron leaks and the formation of superoxide with the resupplied oxygen, which denatures cytosolic enzymes and destroys cell membranes by lipid peroxidation. ROS-mediated dysfunction of the sarcoplasmic reticulum also induces massive intracellular calcium overload, leading to the opening of the mitochondrial permeability transition pore and causing cell apoptosis or necrosis, depending on the intracellular ATP levels [93,94]. The availability of vascular NO would thus be expected to be impaired due to the reduced NOS activity in ischemia and subsequent consumption by superoxide during reperfusion [95], resulting in severe ischemia/reperfusion injury [30].

Nitrite, nitrate, and NO-related compounds (e.g., *S*-nitrosothiols) are constitutively present in blood and tissues. The nitrite level in cardiac tissue is a couple of times higher than that in plasma due to an unknown form of active transport from blood to tissues or due to the oxidation of endogenously generated-NO to nitrite by ceruloplasmin [96], and serves as a significant extravascular pool for NO during tissue hypoxia [97]. Carlström *et al.*, showed that dietary nitrate increased the tissue levels of nitrite and *S*-nitrosothiols in the heart, and attenuated oxidative stress and prevented cardiac injury in Sprague-Dawley rats subjected to unilateral nephrectomy and a high-salt diet [37]. Shiva *et al.*, recently showed that the nitrite stored in the heart and liver via systemic and oral routes augmented the tolerance to ischemia/reperfusion injury in the mouse heart and liver [33].

Although the genetic overexpression of eNOS in mice attenuates myocardial infarction [98], in general, the protective effects of NO on cardiac ischemia/reperfusion injury depend on the local stock of nitrite and its subsequent reduction to NO at the critical moment when NOS activity is lacking under hypoxic conditions. Indeed, the tissue levels of *S*-nitrosothiols (NO-mediated signaling molecules) are enhanced through the nitrite reduction due to NOS inhibition, hypoxia, and acidosis [97], suggesting that the tissue nitrite stores can be regarded as a backup and on-demand NO donor. There are a number of factors that have been demonstrated to reduce nitrite in the tissues, including deoxyhemoglobin, deoxymyoglobin, xanthine oxidoreductase, heme-based enzymes in the mitochondria and acidosis during ischemia [99,100]. In patients with coronary heart disease, the different consequences of myocardial infarction may depend on the patient's daily intake of nitrate/nitrite. Indeed, Bryan *et al.*, showed that dietary nitrite (50 mg/L) or nitrate (1 g/L) supplementation in drinking water for seven days maintained higher steady-state levels of nitrite and nitroso compounds, as well as nitrosyl-heme, in mouse cardiac muscle, and these mice exhibited a smaller cardiac infarct size after ischemia/reperfusion injury compared with control mice fed a diet deficient in nitrate/nitrite for seven days. These findings suggest that this protective nitrate/nitrite may be derived at least in part from dietary sources [29].

Shiva *et al.*, demonstrated that the cytoprotective effects of nitrite on ischemia/reperfusion injury are mediated by post-translational *S*-nitrosylation of complex 1 in the mitochondrial respiratory chain, which consequently inhibits the overall mitochondrial ROS formation and apoptotic events [101]. Another possible cytoprotective effects of nitrite may be mediated by the effects of *S*-nitrosylation on the intracellular Ca^{2+} handling, which decreases Ca^{2+} entry by inhibiting L-type Ca^{2+} channels and increasing the sarcoendoplasmic reticulum (SR) Ca^{2+} uptake by activating SR Ca^{2+} transport ATPase (SERCA2a) [102]. These effects will lead to an attenuation of the increase in cytosolic Ca^{2+} during ischemia and Ca^{2+} overload during reperfusion.

Intriguingly, recent large-scale epidemiological studies reported the preventive effects of antioxidant supplementations including vitamins E, C, and beta carotene rich in fruits and vegetables on cardiovascular disease, whereas no beneficial effects were shown in other studies, and in some cases a decrease in cardiovascular protection with these supplementations was observed [103–105]. On the other hand, a number of epidemiological studies have shown the preventive effects of fruits and vegetables on coronary heart disease [3–6,106]. It should be noted that the consumption of an appropriate amount of fruits and vegetables, which might contain balanced doses of nitrate/nitrite and vitamins, might be more effective with regard to health maintenance and improvement than antioxidant supplementation alone.

4.4. *Chronic Obstructive Pulmonary Disease (COPD)*

COPD is considered to be a lifestyle-related disease, because long-term tobacco smoking and subsequent chronic bronchitis are causally associated with this disease [107]. Varraso *et al.*, recently reported the importance of a healthy diet in multi-interventional programs to prevent COPD [108]. They showed that high intake of whole grains, polyunsaturated fatty acids, nuts, and long chain omega-3 fats, and low intake of red/processed meats, refined grains and sugar-sweetened drinks, were associated with a lower risk of COPD in both women and men.

Because cured meats such as bacon, sausage and ham contain high doses of nitrite for preservation, antimicrobial and color fixation, epidemiological studies have demonstrated that the consumption of cured meats is positively linked to the risk of newly diagnosed COPD [109–111]. Nitrite generates reactive nitrogen species, which may cause nitrosative damage to the lungs, eventually leading to structural changes like emphysema [111]. This is supported by an animal study in which rats chronically exposed to 2000 and 3000 mg/L of sodium nitrite in their drinking water for two years showed distinct lung emphysema [112]. However, the dose of nitrite used in that study was 250–350 mg/kg/day, which was too high to compare with those achieved in standard human diets [113].

In fact, cured meats have been reported to generally comprise only 4.8% of the daily nitrite intake, and surprisingly, 93% of the total ingestion of nitrite is derived from saliva [114], suggesting that cured meats provide minimal contributions to the human intake of nitrite, even if they are frequently consumed. In addition, the recent nitrite levels in processed meats have been approximately 80% lower than those in the mid-1970s in the US [115]. Therefore, discussions encompassing all ingested sources of nitrite should consider whether or not the nitrite derived only from the consumption of cured meats might be responsible for the development of COPD.

On the other hand, a number of epidemiological studies have shown the beneficial effects of *n*-3 fatty acids, vitamins, fruits and vegetables on lung functions and the risk of COPD [108,116–122]. Although it may be difficult to isolate the specific effects of these dietary nutrients, as discussed above, the nitrate and nitrite derived from vegetables and fruits are reduced to NO, which is followed by the formation of *S*-nitrosothiols [123], rather than the formation of nitrosamines especially in the presence of reducing agents such as vitamin C and E in the stomach [28,124]. It has been shown that high dietary nitrate intake does not cause the expected elevation of the gastric nitrite concentrations or appreciable changes in the serum nitrite concentrations [125].

As mentioned above, different from the effects of the direct elevation of nitrite concentration in the plasma, the entero-salivary route of dietary nitrate/nitrite might enhance the availability of NO through the formation of *S*-nitrosothiols and its transnitrosylation to the other thiol residues of proteins, suggesting that, depending on the tissues and organs, separate metabolic pathways might exist for NO availability in this entero-salivary route. Consistent with this idea, Larsen *et al.*, recently demonstrated that acute intravenous infusion of nitrite enhanced the plasma levels of nitrite, whereas it did not affect the oxygen consumption (VO_2) or the resting metabolic rate (RMR) in humans. Instead, dietary nitrate significantly reduced the VO_2 and RMR by improving the mitochondrial respiratory chain function and enhancing efficient O_2 consumption, suggesting that rather than direct nitrite infusion to enhance the plasma nitrite levels, biologically active nitrogen oxide (including the *S*-nitrosothiols produced in the stomach) might be an important molecule for the transfer of biological NO activity for cardiopulmonary function [126]. Because COPD is a state of protein-energy malnutrition due to an increased resting metabolic rate and VO_2, the effects of dietary nitrate on the reduction of the RMR and VO_2 might be advantageous for patients with COPD.

Whether the role of NO in COPD is protective or pathogenic depends on the origin and concentration range of NO. NO activity derived from dietary nitrate and constitutive NOS might be protective against COPD largely through the *S*-nitrosothiol-mediated mechanism including inhibition of the noncholinergic nonadrenergic nerve activity, bronchial smooth muscle relaxation, reduction of airway hyperresponsiveness, downregulation of the proinflammatory activity of T lymphocytes, and antimicrobial defense [127]. However, the deleterious effects of NO on the development of COPD might be derived from iNOS-mediated pro-inflammatory signaling [128], which is consequently (not causally) reflected by the huge amount of NO in the exhaled air of patients with COPD [129].

Recent human studies have demonstrated that dietary nitrate (beetroot juice containing approximately 200–400 mg of nitrate) improved the exercise performance and reduced blood pressure in COPD patients [130,131]. However, large-scale epidemiological evidence of the impact of nitrate is still lacking.

4.5. Cancer

In the stomach, swallowed nitrite is decomposed to form a variety of nitrogen compounds, including *N*-nitrosoamines [132]. In the 1950s, Magree *et al.*, first reported that *N*-nitrosodimethylamine caused malignant primary hepatic tumors in rats [133]. After this report, a number of studies followed in relation to the carcinogenic effects of *N*-nitroso compounds in animal models [134,135]. In particular, the dietary intake of red and cured meats was found to be associated with an increased risk of certain types of cancer due to the relatively large amounts of nitrite added. However, the methodological aspects have been challenged concerning the high dose of nitrosatable amines, and the physiological difference between animals and humans [136].

In the stomach, the nitrosonium ion (NO^+) derived from nitrite can bind to thiol compounds (R-SH) and amines (especially secondary amines: R_1-NH-R_2), forming *S*-nitrosothiol and

N-nitrosamine, respectively. However, while *N*-nitrosamine formation occurs even at neutral or basic pH, *S*-nitrosothiol formation tends to occur only under acidic conditions. In addition, this reaction kinetically occurs much more easily than *N*-nitrosamine formation, particularly in the presence of vitamins C and E and polyphenols, which are highly present in fruits and vegetables, which also eliminate potent nitrosating agents such as the N_2O_3 formed from nitrite by decomposing them to NO. This might partly explain why patients with achlorhydria and non-vegetarians eating large amounts of cured meats are at risk of developing gastric cancer [137–142].

However, this idea appears to be inconsistent with the belief that dietary nitrite is a major cause of cancer. This is because, according to the average nitrate/nitrite intake of adults in the US, most of the daily nitrate intake (around 90%) comes from vegetables, and the nitrite intake is primarily derived from recycled nitrate in the saliva (5.2–8.6 mg/day nitrite), with very little coming from cured meats (0.05–0.6 mg/day nitrite in 50g/day cured meats) and other dietary sources (0–0.7 mg/day nitrite) [136], suggesting that the entero-salivary route may be the more important source of nitrosamine exposure than exogenous intake including cured meats, that is, spitting out saliva all day long might prevent cancer development more effectively than cutting cured meats. However, recent experimental and epidemiological studies could not demonstrate a positive relationship between nitrate consumption and the risk of cancer [121,134], and the Joint Food and Agriculture Organization/World Health Organization Expert Committee on Food Additives concluded in 2008 that there was no evidence that nitrate was carcinogenic in humans. Consistent with this, recent studies have found no link between dietary nitrate and cancer [143,144].

Bradbury *et al.*, reported a large-scale study (>500,000 participants) of the associations between fruit, vegetable, or fiber consumption and the risk of cancer at 14 different sites. They showed that there was an inverse association between fruit intake and the risk of upper gastrointestinal tract and lung cancer, as well as an inverse association between fiber intake and liver cancer. The dietary intake of vegetables, as well as fruits and fiber, was inversely associated with the risk of colorectal cancer, suggesting that there is little evidence that vegetable intake is associated with the risk of any of the individual cancer sites reviewed [145].

However, chronic inflammation, including inflammatory bowel disease and *Helicobacter pylori*-induced gastritis induce inducible NOS (iNOS) and generate large quantities of NO [22,146,147], forming nitrosating and oxidant species such as N_2O_3 and peroxynitrite, which might cause mutagenesis through deamination, nitration of DNA, or inhibition of the DNA repair system [148,149]. Depending on the sites and amounts of NO generation, NO might represent a double-edged sword in the sense that it confers both protective and deleterious effects on cancer development [150,151].

Meta-analyses of primary and secondary cancer prevention trials of dietary antioxidant supplements, such as beta carotene, vitamins A, C, and E, showed a lack of efficacy, and on the contrary, an increased risk of mortality [104]. Although the general role of NO in carcinogenesis is complicated, and many unknown mechanisms remain to be resolved, the dietary nitrate/nitrite (at least that obtained from plant-based foods such as fruits and vegetables) have obvious inhibitory effects on cancer risk by playing some synergistic role with other nutrients in these foods.

4.6. Osteoporosis

Lifestyle habits, such as smoking, alcohol intake, little or no exercise, and an inadequate amount of calcium intake all influence the calcium-vitamin D metabolism [152–155] and bone mineral density, in some cases leading to osteoporosis, particularly in postmenopausal women [156]. The implications of NOS-mediated NO in the regulation of bone cell function have been well described in a number of publications [157]. For example, iNOS-induced NO production following stimulation with proinflammatory cytokines, such as interleukin 1 (IL-1) and tumor necrosis factor-α (TNF-α), inhibits bone resorption and formation, resulting in osteoporosis in patients with inflammatory diseases such as rheumatoid arthritis [158]. On the other hand, eNOS, a constitutive NO synthase, plays an important role in regulating osteoblast activity and bone formation, because eNOS knockout mice exhibit osteoporosis due to defective bone formation, and eNOS gene polymorphisms were reported to be causally linked to osteoporosis in postmenopausal women [159].

In addition, Wimalawansa *et al.*, showed that some of the beneficial effects of estrogen on bone metabolism are mediated through a NO-cGMP-mediated pathway [160], suggesting that NO donor therapy might provide a promising alternative to estrogen therapy. In this context, it has been shown that organic nitrate NO donors, such as glycerol trinitrate, isosorbide dinitrate and mononitrate all have beneficial effects on experimental and clinical osteoporosis [161–163], and a number of epidemiological studies also indicated that a high fruit and vegetable intake appears to have a protective effect against osteoporosis in men and pre- and postmenopausal women [164–166]. However, few studies have been conducted to evaluate the detailed mechanism by which inorganic nitrate/nitrite prevents osteoporosis at the molecular level, and thus further basic research will be needed for this purpose.

5. Conclusions

Dietary nitrate, which is provided by fruits and vegetables, can transmit NO activities in various molecular forms, including NO, nitrite, and *S*-nitrosothiols, through the entero-salivary pathway. Although the role of diet-derived NO activity in lifestyle-related diseases is complex and remains to be fully elucidated, the intake of nitrate as a nutrient in vegetables might be beneficial to human health as a result of synergistic effects with other nutrients present in vegetables, and would be recommended as a nutritional approach to the prevention and treatment of the lifestyle related diseases.

Acknowledgments: The authors thank for the financial supports from Josai University. The authors would like to thank the editors and anonymous reviewers for their valuable comments and suggestions to improve the quality of the paper.

Author Contributions: Jun Kobayashi wrote the manuscript. Kazuo Ohtake and Hiroyuki Uchida reviewed the manuscript.

References

1. O'Donoghue, G.; Cunninggham, C.; Murphy, F.; Woods, C.; Aagaard-Hansen, J. Assessment and management of risk factors for the prevention of lifestyle-related disease: A cross-sectional survey of current activities, barriers and perceived training needs of primary care physiotherapists in the Republic of Ireland. *Physiotharapy* **2014**, *100*, 116–122. [CrossRef] [PubMed]
2. Ford, E.S.; Bergmann, M.M.; Boeing, H.; Capewell, S. Healthy lifestyle behaviors and all-cause mortality among adults in the United States. *Prev. Med.* **2012**, *55*, 23–27. [CrossRef] [PubMed]
3. Liu, S.; Manson, J.E.; Lee, I.M.; Cole, S.R.; Hennekens, C.H.; Willett, W.C.; Buring, J. Fruit and vegetable intake and risk of cardiovascular disease: The women's health study. *Am. J. Cin. Nutr.* **2000**, *72*, 922–928.
4. Joshipura, K.J.; Hu, F.B.; Manson, J.E.; Stampfer, M.J.; Rimm, E.B.; Speizer, F.E.; Colditz, G.; Ascherio, A.; Rosner, B.; Spiegelman, D.; *et al.* The effect of fruit and vegetable intake on risk for coronary heart disease. *Ann. Intern. Med.* **2001**, *134*, 1106–1114. [CrossRef] [PubMed]
5. Bazzano, L.A.; He, J.; Ogden, L.G.; Loria, C.M.; Vupputuri, S.; Myers, L.; Whelton, P.K. Fruit and vegerable intake and risk of cardiovascular disease in US adults: The first National Health and Nutrition Examination Survey Epidemiologic Follow-up Study. *Am. J. Clin. Nutr.* **2002**, *76*, 93–99. [PubMed]
6. Daucher, L.; Amouyel, P.; Hercberg, S.; Dallongeville, J. Fruit and vegetable consumption and risk of coronary heart disease: A meta-analysis of cohort studies. *J. Nutr.* **2006**, *136*, 2588–2593.
7. Joshipura, K.J.; Ascherio, A.; Manson, J.E.; Stampfer, M.J.; Rimm, E.B.; Speizer, F.E.; Hennekens, C.H.; Spiegelman, D.; Willett, W.C. Fruit and vegetable intake in relation to risk of ischemic stroke. *JAMA* **1999**, *282*, 1233–1239. [CrossRef] [PubMed]
8. Davignon, J.; Ganz, P. Role of endothelial dysfunction in atherosclerosis. *Circulation* **2004**, *109*, III-27–III-32. [CrossRef] [PubMed]
9. Hess, D.T.; Matsumoto, A.; Kim, S.O.; Marshall, H.E.; Stamler, J.S. Protein *S*-nitrosylation: Purview and parameters. *Nat. Rev. Mol. Cell Biol.* **2005**, *6*, 150–165. [CrossRef] [PubMed]

10. Bryan, N.S.; Fernandez, B.O.; Bauer, S.M.; Garcia-Saura, M.F.; Milsom, A.B.; Rassaf, T.; Maloney, R.E.; Bharti, A.; Rodriguez, J.; Feelisch, M. Nitrite is a signaling molecule and regulator of gene expression in mammalian tissues. *Nat. Chem. Biol.* **2005**, *1*, 290–297. [CrossRef] [PubMed]
11. West, M.B.; Hill, B.G.; Xuan, Y.T.; Bhatnagar, A. Protein glutathiolation by nitric oxide: An intracellular mechanism regulating redox protein modification. *FASEB J.* **2006**, *20*, E1049–E1060. [CrossRef] [PubMed]
12. Larsen, F.J.; Schiffer, T.A.; Borniquel, S.; Sahlin, K.; Ekblom, B.; Lundberg, J.O.; Weitzberg, E. Dietary inorganic nitrate improves mitochondrial efficiency in humans. *Cell Metab.* **2011**, *13*, 149–159. [CrossRef] [PubMed]
13. Nair, K.S.; Irving, B.A.; Lanza, I.R. Can dietary nitrates enhance the efficiency of mitochondria? *Cell Metab.* **2011**, *13*, 117–118. [CrossRef] [PubMed]
14. Melino, G.; Bernassola, F.; Knight, R.A.; Corasaniti, M.T.; Nistico, G.; Finazzi-Agro, A. *S*-nitrosylation regulates apoptosis. *Nature* **1997**, *388*, 432–433. [CrossRef] [PubMed]
15. Weitzberg, E.; Lundberg, J.O. Nonenzymatic nitric oxide production in humans. *Nitric Oxide* **1998**, *2*, 1–7. [CrossRef] [PubMed]
16. Sindelar, J.J.; Milkowski, A.L. Human safety controversies surrounding nitrate and nitrite in the diet. *Nitric Oxide* **2012**, *26*, 259–266. [CrossRef] [PubMed]
17. Ysart, G.; Miller, P.; Barrett, G.; Farrington, D.; Lawrance, P.; Harrison, M. Dietary expoures to nitrate in the UK. *Food Addit. Contamin.* **1999**, *16*, 521–532. [CrossRef] [PubMed]
18. Lundberg, J.O.; Weitzberg, E.; Gladwin, M.T. The nitrate-nitrite-nitric oxide pathway in physiology and therapeutics. *Nat. Rev. Drug Discov.* **2008**, *7*, 156–167. [CrossRef] [PubMed]
19. Lundberg, J.O.; Gladwin, M.T.; Ahluwalia, A.; Benjamin, N.; Bryan, N.S.; Butler, A.; Cabrales, P.; Fago, A.; Feelisch, M.; Ford, P.C.; *et al.* Nitrate and nitrite in biology, nutrition and therapeutics. *Nat. Chem. Biol.* **2009**, *5*, 865–869. [CrossRef] [PubMed]
20. Lundberg, J.O.; Govoni, M. Inorganic nitrate is a possible source for systemic generation of nitric oxide. *Free Radic. Biol. Med.* **2004**, *37*, 395–400. [CrossRef] [PubMed]
21. Spiegelhalder, B.; Eisenbrand, G.; Preussmann, R. Influence of dietary nitrate on nitrite content of human saliva: Possible relevance to *in vivo* formation of *N*-nitroso compounds. *Food Cosmet. Toxicol.* **1976**, *14*, 545–548. [CrossRef]
22. Lundberg, J.O.; Hellstrom, P.M.; Lundberg, J.M.; Alving, K. Greatly increased luminal nitric oxide in ulcerative colitis. *Lancet* **1994**, *344*, 1673–1674. [CrossRef]
23. McKnight, G.M.; Smith, L.M.; Drummond, R.S.; Duncan, C.W.; Golden, M.; Benjamin, N. Chemical synthesis of nitric oxide in the stomach from dietary nitrate in humans. *Gut* **1997**, *40*, 211–214. [CrossRef] [PubMed]
24. Takahama, U.; Oniki, T.; Hirota, S. Oxidation of quercetin by salivary components. Quercetin-dependent reduction of salivary nitrite under acidic conditions producing nitric oxide. *J. Agric. Food Chem.* **2002**, *50*, 4317–4322. [CrossRef] [PubMed]
25. Björne, H.; Peterson, J.; Phillipson, M.; Weitzberg, E.; Holm, L.; Lundberg, J.O. Nitrite in saliva increases gastric mucosal blood flow and mucus thickness. *J. Clin. Investig.* **2004**, *113*, 106–114. [CrossRef] [PubMed]
26. Petersson, J.; Phillipson, M.; Jansson, E.A.; Patzak, A.; Lundberg, J.O.; Holm, L. Dietary nitrate increases gastric mucosal blood flow and mucosal defence. *Am. J. Physiol. Gastrointest. Liver Physiol.* **2007**, *292*, G718–G724. [CrossRef] [PubMed]
27. Govoni, M.; Jansson, E.A.; Weitzberg, E.; Lundberg, J.O. The increase in plasma nitrite after a dietary nitrate load is markedly attenuated by an antibacterial mouthwash. *Nitric Oxide* **2008**, *19*, 333–337. [CrossRef] [PubMed]
28. Hord, N.G.; Tang, Y.; Bryan, N.S. Food sources of nitrates and nitrites: The physiologic context for potential health benefits. *Am. J. Clin. Nutr.* **2009**, *90*, 1–10. [CrossRef] [PubMed]
29. Bryan, N.S.; Calvert, J.W.; Elrod, J.W.; Gundewar, S.; Ji, S.Y.; Lefer, D.J. Dietary nitrite supplementation protects against ischemia-reperfusion injury. *Proc. Natl. Acad. Sci. USA* **2007**, *104*, 19144–19149. [CrossRef] [PubMed]
30. Raat, N.J.H.; Noguchi, A.C.; Liu, V.B.; Raghavachari, N.; Liu, D.; Xu, X.; Shiva, S.; Munson, P.J.; Gladwin, M.T. Dietary nitrate and nitrite modulate blood and organ nitrite and the cellular ischemic stress response. *Free Radic. Biol. Med.* **2009**, *47*, 510–517. [CrossRef] [PubMed]
31. Cosby, K.; Partovi, K.S.; Crawford, J.H.; Patel, R.P.; Reiter, C.D.; Martyr, S.; Yang, B.K.; Waclawiw, M.A.; Zalos, G.; Xu, X.; *et al.* Nitrite reduction to nitric oxide by deoxyhemoglobin vasodilates the human circulation. *Nat. Med.* **2003**, *9*, 1498–1505. [CrossRef] [PubMed]

32. Ormerod, J.O.M.; Ashrafian, H.; Maher, A.R.; Arif, S.; Steeples, V.; Born, G.V.R.; Egginton, S.; Feelisch, M.; Watkins, H.; Frenneaux, M.P. The role of vascular myoglobin in nitrite-mediated blood vessel relaxation. *Cardiovasc. Res.* **2011**, *89*, 560–565. [CrossRef] [PubMed]
33. Shiva, S.; Sack, M.N.; Greer, J.J.; Duranski, M.; Ringwood, L.A.; Burwell, L.; Wang, X.; MacArthur, P.H.; Shoja, A.; Raghavachari, N.; *et al.* Nitrite augments tolerance to ischemia/reperfusion injury via the modulation of mitochondrial electron transfer. *J. Exp. Med.* **2007**, *204*, 2089–2102. [CrossRef] [PubMed]
34. Sonoda, K.; Ohtake, K.; Kubo, Y.; Uchida, H.; Uchida, M.; Natsume, H.; Kobayashi, M.; Kobayashi, J. Aldehyde dehydrogenase 2 partly mediates hypotensive effect of nitrite on L-NAME-induced hypertension in normoxic rat. *Clin. Exp. Hypertens.* **2014**, *36*, 410–418. [CrossRef] [PubMed]
35. Richardson, R.S.; Noyszewski, E.A.; Kendrick, K.F.; Leigh, J.S.; Wagner, P.D. Myoglobin O_2 desaturation during exercise. Evidence of limited O_2 transport. *J. Clin. Investig.* **1996**, *96*, 1916–1926. [CrossRef] [PubMed]
36. Larsen, F.J.; Weitzberg, E.; Lundberg, J.O.; Ekblom, B. Dietary nitrate reduces maximal oxygen consumption while maintaining work performance in maximal exercise. *Free Radic. Biol. Med.* **2010**, *48*, 342–347. [CrossRef] [PubMed]
37. Carlström, M.; Persson, A.E.G.; Larsson, E.; Hezel, M.; Scheffer, P.G.; Teerlink, T.; Weitzberg, E.; Lundberg, J.O. Dietary nitrate attenuates oxidative stress, prevents cardiac and renal injuries, and reduces blood pressure in salt-induced hypertension. *Cardiovasc. Res.* **2011**, *89*, 574–585. [CrossRef] [PubMed]
38. Baliga, R.S.; Milsom, A.B.; Ghosh, S.M.; Trinder, S.L.; MacAllister, R.J.; Ahluwalia, A.; Hobbs, A.J. Dietary nitrate ameliorates pulmonary hypertension cytoprotective role for endothelial nitric oxide synthase and xanthine oxidoreductase. *Circulation* **2012**, *125*, 2922–2932. [CrossRef] [PubMed]
39. Ashmore, T.; Fernandez, B.O.; Branco-Price, C.; West, J.A.; Cowburn, A.S.; Heather, L.C.; Griffin, J.L.; Johnson, R.S.; Feelisch, M.; Murray, A.J. Dietary nitrate increases arginine availability and protects mitochondrial complex I and energetics in the hypoxic rat heart. *J. Physiol.* **2014**, *592*, 4715–4731. [CrossRef] [PubMed]
40. Stamler, J.S.; Lamas, S.; Fang, F.C. Nitrosylation: The prototypic redox-based signaling mechanism. *Cell* **2001**, *106*, 675–683. [CrossRef]
41. Knobeloch, L.; Salna, B.; Hogan, A.; Postle, J.; Anderson, H. Blue babies and nitrate-contaminated well water. *Environ. Health Perspect.* **2000**, *108*, 675–678. [CrossRef] [PubMed]
42. Comly, H.H. Cyanosis in infants caused by nitrates in well water. *JAMA* **1945**, *129*, 112–116. [CrossRef]
43. Avery, A.A. Infantile methemoglobinemia: Reexamining the role of drinking water nitrates. *Environ. Health Perspect.* **1999**, *107*, 583–586. [CrossRef] [PubMed]
44. Mensinga, T.T.; Speijers, G.J.; Meulenbelt, J. Health implications of exposure to environmental nitrogenous compounds. *Toxicol. Rev.* **2003**, *22*, 41–51. [CrossRef] [PubMed]
45. Gangolli, S.D.; van den Brandt, P.A.; Feron, V.J.; Janzowskyd, C.; Koemane, J.H.; Speijersf, G.J.A.; Spiegelhalderg, B.; Walkerh, R.; Wishnoki, J.S. Nitrate, nitrite and *N*-nitroso compounds. *Eur. J. Pharmacol.* **1994**, *292*, 1–38. [CrossRef] [PubMed]
46. Lin, P.H.; Aickin, M.; Champagne, C.; Craddick, S.; Sacks, F.M.; McCarron, P.; Most-Windhauser, M.M.; Rukenbrod, F.; Haworth, L.; Dash-Sodium Collaborative Research Group. Food group sources of nutrients in the dietary pattern s of the DASH-Sodium trial. *J. Am. Diet. Assoc.* **2003**, *103*, 488–496. [PubMed]
47. Kobayashi, J. Nitric oxide and insulin resistance. *Immunoendocrinology* **2015**, *2*, 1.
48. Das, U.N. Insulin: An endogenous cardioprotector. *Curr. Opin. Crit. Care* **2003**, *9*, 375–383. [CrossRef] [PubMed]
49. Abel, E.D. Insulin signaling in heart muscle: Lessons from genetically engineered mouse models. *Curr. Hypertens. Rep.* **2004**, *6*, 416–423. [CrossRef] [PubMed]
50. Kim, J.; Montagnani, M.; Koh, K.K.; Quon, M.J. Reciprocal relationships between insulin resistance and endothelial dysfunction: Molecular and pathphysiological mechanismns. *Circulation* **2006**, *113*, 1888–1904. [CrossRef] [PubMed]
51. Yu, Q.; Gao, F.; Ma, X.L. Insulin says NO to cardiovascular disease. *Cardiovasc. Res.* **2011**, *89*, 516–524. [CrossRef] [PubMed]
52. Wang, H.; Wang, A.X.; Aylor, K.; Barrett, E.J. Nitric oxide directly promotes vascular endothelial insulin transport. *Diabetes* **2013**, *62*, 4030–4042. [CrossRef] [PubMed]

53. Kim, F.; Pham, M.; Rizzo, N.O.; Morton, G.J.; Wisse, B.E.; Kirk, E.A.; Chait, A.; Schwartz, M.W. Vascular inflammation, insulin resistance and reduced nitric oxide production precede the onset of peripheral insulin resistance. *Arterioscler. Thromb. Vasc. Biol.* **2008**, *28*, 1982–1988. [CrossRef] [PubMed]
54. Laffranchi, R.; Gogvadze, V.; Richter, C.; Spinas, G.A. Nitric oxide (nitrogen monoxide, NO) stimulates insulin secretion by inducing calcium release from mitochondria. *Biochem. Biophys. Res. Commun.* **1995**, *217*, 584–591. [CrossRef] [PubMed]
55. Nystrom, T.; Ortsater, H.; Huang, Z.; Zhang, F.; Larsen, F.J.; Weitzberg, E.; Lundbergb, J.O.; Sjöholma, A. Inorganic nitrite stimulates pancreatic islet blood flow and insulin secretion. *Free Radic. Biol. Med.* **2012**, *53*, 1017–1023. [CrossRef] [PubMed]
56. Lee, W.J.; Kim, H.S.; Park, H.S.; Kim, M.O.; Kim, M.; Yun, J.Y.; Kim, E.H.; Lee, S.A.; Lee, S.H.; Koh, E.H.; *et al.* Nitric oxide increases Insulin sensitivity in skeletal muscle by improving mitochondrial function and insulin signaling. *Korean Diabetes J.* **2009**, *33*, 198–205. [CrossRef]
57. Rizzo, N.O.; Maloney, E.; Pham, M.; Luttrell, I.; Wessells, H.; Tateya, S.; Daum, G.; Handa, P.; Schwartz, M.W.; Kim, F. Reduced NO-cGMP signaling contributes to vascular inflammation and insulin resistance induced by high-fat feeding. *Arterioscler. Thromb. Vasc. Biol.* **2010**, *30*, 758–765. [CrossRef] [PubMed]
58. Richey, J.M. The vascular endothelium, a benign restrictive barrier? No! Role of nitric oxide in regulating insulin action. *Diabetes* **2013**, *62*, 4006–4008. [CrossRef] [PubMed]
59. Khoo, N.K.H.; Mo, L.; Zharikov, S.; Kamga, C.; Quesnelle, K.; Golin-Bisello, F.; Li, L.; Wang, Y.; Shiva, S. Nitrite augments glucose uptake in adipocytes through the protein kinase A-dependent stimulation of mitochondrial fusion. *Free Radic. Biol. Med.* **2014**, *70*, 45–53. [CrossRef] [PubMed]
60. Draznin, B. Molecular mechanisms of insulin resistance: Serine phosphorylation of insulin receptor substrate-1 and increased expression of p85α. The two sides of a coin. *Diabetes* **2006**, *55*, 2392–2397. [CrossRef] [PubMed]
61. Carvalho-Filho, M.A.; Ueno, M.; Hirabara, S.M.; Seabra, A.B.; Carvalheria, J.B.C.; Oliveira, M.G.; Velloso, L.A.; Curi, R.; Saad, M.J.A. *S*-nitrosation of the insulin receptor, insulin receptor substrate 1, and protein kinase B/Akt: A novel mechanism of insulin resistance. *Diabetes* **2005**, *54*, 959–967. [CrossRef] [PubMed]
62. Fisher-Wellman, K.H.; Neufer, P.D. Linking mitochondrial bioenergetics to insulin resistance via redox biology. *Trends Endocrinol. Metab.* **2012**, *23*, 142–152. [CrossRef] [PubMed]
63. De Luca, C.; Olefsky, J.M. Inflammation and insulin resistance. *FEBS Lett.* **2008**, *582*, 97–105. [CrossRef] [PubMed]
64. Hsu, M.F.; Meng, T.C. Enhancement of insulin responsiveness by nitric oxide-mediated inactivation of protein-tyrosine phosphatases. *J. Biol. Chem.* **2010**, *285*, 7919–7928. [CrossRef] [PubMed]
65. Jiang, H.; Torregrossa, A.C.; Potts, A.; Pierini, D.; Aranke, M.; Garg, H.K.; Bryan, N.S. Dietary nitrite improves insulin signaling through GLUT4 translocation. *Free Rad. Biol. Med.* **2014**, *67*, 51–57. [CrossRef] [PubMed]
66. Carlström, M.; Larsen, F.J.; Nystrom, T.; Hazel, M.; Borniquel, S.; Weitzberg, E.; Lundberg, J.O. Dietary inorganic nitrate reverses features of metabolic syndrome in endothelial nitric oxide synthase-deficient mice. *Proc. Natl. Acad. Sci. USA* **2010**, *107*, 17716–17720. [CrossRef] [PubMed]
67. Ohtake, K.; Nakano, G.; Ehara, N.; Sonoda, K.; Ito, J.; Uchida, H.; Kobayashi, J. Dietary nitrite supplementation improves insulin resistance in type 2 diabetic KKA(y) mice. *Nitric Oxide* **2015**, *44*, 31–38. [CrossRef] [PubMed]
68. Khalifi, S.; Rahimipour, A.; Jeddi, S.; Ghanbari, M.; Kazerouni, F.; Ghasemi, A. Dietary nitrate improves glucose tolerance and lipid profile in an animal model of hyperglycemia. *Nitric oxide* **2015**, *44*, 24–30. [CrossRef] [PubMed]
69. Biasucci, L.M.; Graziani, F.; Rizzello, V.; Liuzzo, G.; Guidone, C.; Caterina, A.R.D.; Brugaletta, S.; Mingrone, G.; Crea, F. Paradoxical preservation of vascular function in severe obesity. *Am. J. Med.* **2010**, *123*, 727–734. [CrossRef] [PubMed]
70. Assar, M.E.I.; Adana, J.C.R.D.; Angulo, J.; Martinez, M.L.P.; Matias, A.H.; Rodriguez-Manas, L. Preserved endothelial function in human obesity in the absence of insulin resistance. *J. Transl. Med.* **2013**, *11*, 1–11. [CrossRef] [PubMed]
71. Sansbury, B.E.; Cummins, T.D.; Tang, Y.; Hellmann, J.; Holden, C.R.; Harbeson, H.M.A.; Chen, Y.; Patel, R.P.; Spite, M.; Bhatnagar, A.; *et al.* Overexpression of endothelial nitric oxide synthase prevents diet-induced obesity and regulates adipocyte phenotype. *Circ. Res.* **2012**, *111*, 1176–1189. [CrossRef] [PubMed]

72. Ness, A.R.; Powles, J.W. Fruit and vegetables, and cardiovascular disease: A review. *Int. J. Epidemiol.* **1997**, *26*, 1–13. [CrossRef] [PubMed]
73. Van't Veer, P.; Jansen, M.C.; Klerk, M.; Kok, F.J. Fruits and vegetables in the prevention of cancer and cardiovascular disease. *Public Health Nutr.* **2000**, *3*, 103–107. [CrossRef] [PubMed]
74. Bazzano, L.A.; Serdula, M.K.; Liu, S. Dietary intake of fruits and vegetables and risk of cardiovascular disease. *Curr. Atheroscler. Rep.* **2003**, *5*, 492–499. [CrossRef] [PubMed]
75. Sacks, F.M.; Svetkey, L.P.; Vollmer, W.M.; Appel, L.J.; Bray, G.A.; Harsha, D.; Obarzanek, E.; Conlin, P.R.; Miller, E.R., 3rd; Simons-Morton, D.G.; *et al.* Effects on blood pressure of reduced dietary sodium and the Dietary Approaches to Stop Hypertension (DASH) diet. *N. Engl. J. Med.* **2001**, *344*, 3–10. [CrossRef] [PubMed]
76. Appel, L.J.; Moore, T.J.; Obarzanek, E.; Vollmer, W.M.; Svetkey, L.P.; Sacks, F.M.; Bray, G.A.; Vogt, T.M.; Cutler, J.A.; Windhauser, M.M.; *et al.* A clinical trial of the effects of dietary patterns on blood pressure. *N. Engl. J. Med.* **1997**, *336*, 1117–1124. [CrossRef] [PubMed]
77. Ashworth, A.; Mitchell, K.; Blackwell, J.; Vanhatalo, A.; Jones, A.M. High-nitrate vegetable diet increases nitrate and nitrite concentrations and reduces blood pressure in healthy women. *Public Health Nutr.* **2015**. [CrossRef] [PubMed]
78. Gonzalez, F.M.; Shiva, S. Nitrite anion provides potent cytoprotective and antiapoptotic effects as adjunctive therapy to reperfusion for acute myocardial infarction. *Circulation* **2008**, *117*, 2986–2994. [CrossRef] [PubMed]
79. Duranski, M.R.; Greer, J.J.; Dejam, A. Cytoprotective effects of nitrite during *in vivo* ischemia-reperfusion of the heart and liver. *J. Clin. Investig.* **2005**, *115*, 1232–1240. [CrossRef] [PubMed]
80. Webb, A.; Bond, R.; McLean, P.; Uppal, R.; Benjamin, N.; Ahluwalia, A. Reduction of nitrite to nitric oxide during ischemia protects against myocardial ischemia-reperfusion damage. *Proc. Natl. Acad. Sci. USA* **2004**, *101*, 13683–13688. [CrossRef] [PubMed]
81. Baker, J.E.; Su, J.; Fu, X.; Hsu, A.; Gross, G.J.; Tweddell, J.S.; Hogg, N. Nitrite confers protection against myocardial infarction: Role of xanthine oxidoreductase, NADPH oxidase and K(ATP) channels. *J. Mol. Cell Cardiol.* **2007**, *43*, 437–444. [CrossRef] [PubMed]
82. Bryan, N.S.; Calvert, J.W.; Gundewar, S.; Lefer, D.J. Dietary nitrite restores NO homeostasis and is cardioprotective in endothelial nitric oxide synthase-deficient mice. *Free Radic. Biol. Med.* **2008**, *45*, 468–474. [CrossRef] [PubMed]
83. Johnson, G., III; Tsao, P.S.; Mulloy, D.; Lefer, A.M. Cardioprotective effects of acidified sodium nitrite in myocardial ischemia with reperfusion. *J. Pharmacol. Exp. Ther.* **1990**, *252*, 35–41. [PubMed]
84. Larsen, F.J.; Ekblom, B.; Sahlin, K.; Lundberg, J.O.; Weitzberg, E. Effects of dietary nitrate on blood pressure in healthy volunteers. *N. Engl. J. Med.* **2006**, *355*, 2792–2793. [CrossRef] [PubMed]
85. Kapil, V.; Milsom, A.B.; Okorie, M.; Maleki-Toyserkani, S.; Akram, F.; Rehman, F.; Arghandawi, S.; Pearl, V.; Benjamin, N.; Loukogeorgakis, S.; *et al.* Inorganic nitrate supplementation lowers blood pressure in humans: Role for nitrite-derived NO. *Hypertension* **2010**, *56*, 274–281. [CrossRef] [PubMed]
86. Webb, A.J.; Patel, N.; Loukogeorgakis, S.; Okorie, M.; Aboud, Z.; Misra, S.; Rashid, R.; Miall, P.; Deanfield, J.; Benjamin, N.; *et al.* Acute blood pressure lowering, vasoprotective, and antiplatelet properties of dietary nitrate via bioconversion to nitrite. *Hypertension* **2008**, *51*, 784–790. [CrossRef] [PubMed]
87. Vanhatalo, A.; Bailey, S.J.; Blackwell, J.R.; DiMenna, F.J.; Pavey, T.G.; Wilkerson, D.P.; Benjamin, N.; Winyard, P.G.; Jones, A.M. Acute and chronic effects of dietary nitrate supplementation on blood pressure and the physiological responses to moderate-intensity and incremental exercise. *Am. J. Physiol. Regul. Integr. Comp. Physiol.* **2010**, *68*, R1121–R1131. [CrossRef] [PubMed]
88. Hobbs, D.A.; George, T.W.; Lovegrove, J.A. The effects of dietary nitrate on blood pressure and endothelial function: A review of human intervention studies. *Nutr. Res. Rev.* **2013**, *26*, 210–222. [CrossRef] [PubMed]
89. Siervo, M.; Lala, J.; Ogbonmwan, I.; Mathers, J.C. Inorganic nitrate and beetroot juice supplementation reduces blood pressure in adults: A systematic review and meta-analysis. *J. Nutr.* **2013**, *143*, 818–826. [CrossRef] [PubMed]
90. Kapil, V.; Khambata, R.S.; Robertson, A.; Caulfield, M.J.; Ahluwalia, A. Dietary nitrate provides sustained blood pressure lowering in hypertensive patients. *Hypertension* **2015**, *65*, 320–327. [CrossRef] [PubMed]
91. Sindler, A.L.; DeVan, A.E.; Fleenor, B.S.; Seals, D.R. Inorganic nitrite supplementation for healthy arterial aging. *J. Appl. Physiol.* **2014**, *116*, 463–477. [CrossRef] [PubMed]

92. Bhushan, S.; Kondo, K.; Polhemus, D.J.; Otsuka, H.; Nicholson, C.K.; Tao, Y.X.; Huang, H.; Georgiopoulou, V.V.; Murohara, T.; Calvert, J.W.; *et al.* Nitrite therapy improves left ventricular function during heart failure via restoration of nitric oxide-mediated cytoprotective signaling. *Circ. Res.* **2014**, *114*, 1281–1291. [CrossRef] [PubMed]
93. Leist, M.; Single, B.; Castoldi, A.F.; Kuhnle, S.; Nicotera, P. Intracellular adenosine triphosphate (ATP) concentration: A switch in the decision between apoptosis and necrosis. *J. Exp. Med.* **1997**, *185*, 1481–1486. [CrossRef] [PubMed]
94. Eguchi, Y.; Shimizu, S.; Tsujimoto, Y. Intracellular ATP levels determine cell death fate by apoptosis or necrosis. *Cancer Res.* **1997**, *57*, 1835–1840. [PubMed]
95. Murata, I.; Nozaki, R.; Ooi, K.; Ohtake, K.; Kimura, S.; Ueda, H.; Nakano, G.; Sonoda, K.; Inoue, Y.; Uchida, H.; *et al.* Nitrite reduces ischemia/reperfusion-induced muscle damage and improves survival rates in rat crush injury model. *J. Trauma Acute Care Surg.* **2012**, *72*, 1548–1554. [CrossRef] [PubMed]
96. Shiva, S.; Wang, X.; Ringwood, L.A.; Xu, X.; Yuditskaya, S.; Annavajjhala, V.; Miyajima, H.; Hogg, N.; Harris, Z.L.; Gladwin, M.T. Ceruloplasmin is a NO oxidase and nitrite synthase that determines endocrine NO homeostasis. *Nat. Chem. Biol.* **2006**, *9*, 486–493. [CrossRef] [PubMed]
97. Bryan, N.S.; Rassaf, T.; Maloney, R.E.; Rodriguez, C.M.; Saijo, F.; Rodriguez, J.R.; Feelisch, M. Cellular targets and mechanisms of nitros(yl)ation: An insight into their nature and kinetics *in vivo*. *Proc. Natl. Acad. Sci. USA* **2004**, *101*, 4308–4313. [CrossRef] [PubMed]
98. Jones, S.P.; Greer, J.J.M.; Kakkar, A.K.; Ware, P.D.; Turnage, R.H.; Hicks, M.; van Haeren, R.; de Crom, R.; Kawashima, S.; Yokoyama, M.; *et al.* Endothelial nitric oxide synthase overexpression attenuates myocardial reperfusion injury. *Am. J. Physiol. Heart Circ. Physiol.* **2004**, *286*, H276–H282. [CrossRef] [PubMed]
99. Rassaf, T.; Flögel, U.; Drexhage, C.; Hendgen-Cotta, U.; Kelm, M.; Schrader, J. Nitrite reductase function of deoxymyoglobin: Oxygen sensor and regulator of cardiac energetics and function. *Circ. Res.* **2007**, *100*, 1749–1754. [CrossRef] [PubMed]
100. Hendgen-Cotta, U.B.; Merx, M.W.; Shiva, S.; Schmitz, J.; Becher, S.; Klare, J.P.; Steinhoff, H.J.; Goedecke, A.; Schrader, J.; *et al.* Nitrite reductase activity of myoglobin regulates respiration and cellular viability in myocardial ischemia-reperfusion injury. *Proc. Natl. Acad. Sci. USA* **2008**, *105*, 10256–10261. [CrossRef] [PubMed]
101. Shiva, S.; Gladwin, M.T. Nitrite mediates cytoprotection after ischemia-reperfusion by modulating mitochondrial function. *Basic Res. Cardiol.* **2009**, *104*, 113–119. [CrossRef] [PubMed]
102. Calvert, J.W.; Lefer, D.J. Myocardial protection by nitrite. *Cardiovasc. Res.* **2009**, *83*, 195–203. [CrossRef] [PubMed]
103. Vivekananthan, D.; Penn, M.S.; Sapp, S.K.; Hsu, A.; Topol, E.J. Use of antioxidant vitamins for the prevention of cardiovascular disease: Meta-analysis of randomized trials. *Lancet* **2003**, *361*, 2017–2023. [CrossRef]
104. Bjelakovic, G.; Nikolova, D.; Gluud, L.L.; Simonetti, R.G.; Gluud, C. Mortality in randomized trials of antioxidant supplements for primary and secondary prevention: Systemic review and meta-analysis. *JAMA* **2007**, *297*, 842–857. [CrossRef] [PubMed]
105. Sesso, H.D.; Buring, J.E.; Christen, W.G.; Kurth, T.; Belanger, C.; MacFadyen, J.; Bubes, V.; Manson, J.E.; Glynn, R.J.; Gaziano, J.M. Vitamins E and C in the prevention of cardiovascular disease in men. *JAMA* **2008**, *300*, 2123–2133. [CrossRef] [PubMed]
106. Hung, H.C.; Joshipura, K.J.; Jiang, R.; Hu, F.B.; Hunter, D.; Smith-Warner, S.A.; Colditz, G.A.; Rosner, B.; Spiegelman, D.; Willett, W.C. Fruit and vegetable intake and risk of major chronic disease. *J. Natl. Cancer Inst.* **2004**, *96*, 1577–1584. [CrossRef] [PubMed]
107. Wedzicha, J.A.; Seemungal, T.A.R. COPD exacerbations: Defining their cause and prevention. *Lancet* **2007**, *370*, 786–796. [CrossRef]
108. Varraso, R.; Chiuve, S.E.; Fung, T.T.; Barr, R.G.; Hu, F.B.; Willett, W.C.; Camargo, C.A. Alternate healthy eating index 2010 and risk of chronic obstructive pulmonary disease among US women and men: Prospective study. *Brit. Med. J.* **2015**, *350*, h286. [CrossRef] [PubMed]
109. Jiang, R.; Paik, D.C.; Hankinson, J.L.; Barr, R.G. Cured meat consumption, lung function, and chronic obstructive pulmonary disease among United States adult. *Am. J. Respir. Crit. Care Med.* **2007**, *175*, 798–804. [CrossRef] [PubMed]

110. De Batlle, J.; Mendez, M.; Romieu, I.; Balcells, E.; Benet, M.; Donaire-Gonzalez, D.; Ferrer, J.J.; Orozco-Levi, M.; Anto, J.M.; Garcia-Aymerich, J. Cured meat consumption increases risk of readmission in COPD patients. *Eur. Respir. J.* **2012**, *40*, 555–560. [CrossRef] [PubMed]
111. Varraso, R.; Jiang, R.; Barr, R.G.; Willett, W.C.; Carlos, A. Prospective study of cured meats consumption and risk of chronic obstructive pulmonary disease in men. *Am. J. Epidemiol.* **2007**, *166*, 1438–1445. [CrossRef] [PubMed]
112. Shuval, H.I.; Gruener, N. Epidemiological and toxicological aspects of nitrates and nitrites in the environment. *Am. J. Public Health* **1972**, *62*, 1045–1052. [CrossRef] [PubMed]
113. Hsu, J.; Arcot, J.; Lee, N.A. Nitrate and nitrite quantification from cured meat and vegetables and their estimated dietary intake in Australians. *Food Chem.* **2009**, *115*, 334–339. [CrossRef]
114. Archer, D.L. Evidence that ingested nitrate and nitrite are beneficial to health. *J. Food Prot.* **2002**, *65*, 872–875. [PubMed]
115. Cassens, R.G. Residual nitrite in cured meat. *Food Technol.* **1997**, *51*, 53–55.
116. Romieu, I.; Trenga, C. Diet and obstructive lung diseases. *Epidemiol. Rev.* **2001**, *23*, 268–287. [CrossRef] [PubMed]
117. Romieu, I. Nutrition and lung health. *Int. J. Tuberc. Lung Dis.* **2005**, *9*, 362–374. [PubMed]
118. Denny, S.I.; Thompson, R.L.; Margetts, B.M. Dietary factors in the pathogenesis of asthma and chronic obstructive pulmonary disease. *Curr. Allergy Asthma Rep.* **2003**, *3*, 130–136. [CrossRef] [PubMed]
119. McKeever, T.M.; Scrivener, S.; Broadfield, E.; Jones, Z.; Britton, J.; Lewis, S.A. Prospective study of diet and decline in lung function in a general population. *Am. J. Respir. Crit. Care Med.* **2002**, *165*, 1299–1303. [CrossRef] [PubMed]
120. Butland, B.K.; Fehily, A.M.; Elwood, P.C. Diet, lung function, and lung function decline in a cohort of 2512 middle aged men. *Thorax* **2000**, *55*, 102–108. [CrossRef] [PubMed]
121. Smit, H.A.; Grievink, L.; Tabak, C. Dietary influences on chronic obstructive lung disease and asthma: A review of the epidemiological evidence. *Proc. Nutr. Soc.* **1999**, *58*, 309–319. [CrossRef] [PubMed]
122. Carey, I.M.; Strachan, D.P.; Cook, D.G. Effects of changes in fresh fruit consumption on ventilator function in healthy British adults. *Am. J. Respir. Crit. Care Med.* **1998**, *158*, 728–733. [CrossRef] [PubMed]
123. Weitzberg, E.; Lundberg, J.O. Novel aspects of dietary nitrate and human health. *Annu. Rev. Nutr.* **2013**, *33*, 129–159. [CrossRef] [PubMed]
124. Bartsch, H.; Ohshima, H.; Pignatelli, B. Inhibitors of endogenous nitrosation. Mechanisms and implications in human cancer prevention. *Mutat. Res.* **1988**, *202*, 307–324. [CrossRef]
125. Pannala, A.S.; Mani, A.R.; Spencer, J.P.E.; Skinner, V.; Bruckdorfer, K.R.; Moore, K.P.; Rice-Evans, C.A. The effect of dietary nitrate on salivery, plasma, and urinary nitrate metabolism in humans. *Free Radic. Biol. Med.* **2003**, *34*, 576–584. [CrossRef]
126. Larsen, F.J.; Schiffer, T.A.; Ekblom, B.; Mattsson, M.P.; Checa, A.; Wheelock, C.E.; Nystrom, T.; Lundberg, J.O.; Weitzberg, E. Dietary nitrate reduces resting metabolic rate: A randomized, crossover study in humans. *Am. J. Clin. Nutr.* **2014**, *99*, 843–850. [CrossRef] [PubMed]
127. Ricciardolo, F.L.M.; Sterk, P.J.; Gaston, B.; Folkerts, G. Nitric oxide in health and disease of the respiratory system. *Physiol. Rev.* **2004**, *84*, 731–765. [CrossRef] [PubMed]
128. Hansel, T.T.; Kharitonov, S.A.; Donnelly, L.E.; Erin, E.M.; Currie, M.G.; Moore, W.M.; Manning, P.T.; Recker, D.P.; Barnes, P.J. A selective inhibitor of inducible nitric oxide synthase inhibits exhaled breath nitric oxide in healthy volunteers and asthmatics. *FASEB J.* **2003**, *17*, 1298–1300. [CrossRef] [PubMed]
129. Brindicci, C.; Ito, K.; Resta, O.; Pride, N.B.; Barnes, P.J.; Kharitonov, S.A. Exhaled nitric oxide from lung periphery is increased in COPD. *Eur. Respir. J.* **2005**, *26*, 52–59. [CrossRef] [PubMed]
130. Berry, M.J.; Justus, N.W.; Hauser, J.I.; Case, A.H.; Helms, C.C.; Basu, S.; Rogers, Z.; Lewis, M.T.; Miller, G.D. Dietary nitrate supplementation improves exercise performance and decreases blood pressure in COPD patients. *Nitric Oxide* **2014**. [CrossRef] [PubMed]
131. Kerley, C.P.; Cahill, K.; Bolger, K.; McGowan, A.; Burke, C.; Faul, J.; Cormican, L. Dietary nitrate supplementation in COPD: An acute, double-blind, randomized, placebo-controlled, crossover trial. *Nitric Oxide* **2015**, *44*, 105–111. [CrossRef] [PubMed]
132. Iijima, K.; Grant, J.; McElroy, K.; Fyfe, V.; Preston, T.; McColl, K.E. Novel mechanism of nitrosative stress from dietary nitrate with relevance to gastro-oesophageal junction cancers. *Cartinogenesis* **2003**, *24*, 1951–1960. [CrossRef] [PubMed]

133. Magee, P.N.; Barnes, J.M. The production of malignant primary hepatic tumours in the rat by feeding dimethylnitrosamine. *Br. J. Cancer* **1956**, *10*, 114–122. [CrossRef] [PubMed]
134. Mirvish, S.S. *N*-nitroso compounds: Their chemical and *in vivo* formation and possible importance as environmental carcinogenesis. *J. Toxicol. Environ. Health* **1977**, *2*, 1267–1277. [CrossRef] [PubMed]
135. Mirvish, S.S. Role of *N*-nitroso compounds (NOC) and *N*-nitrosation in etiology of gastric, esophageal, nasopharyngeal and bladder cancer and contribution to cancer of known exposures to NOC. *Cancer Lett.* **1995**, *93*, 17–48. [CrossRef]
136. Bryan, N.S.; Alexander, D.D.; Coughlin, J.R.; Milkowski, A.L.; Boffetta, P. Ingested nitrate and nitrite and stomach cancer risk: An updated review. *Food Chem. Toxicol.* **2012**, *50*, 3646–3665. [CrossRef] [PubMed]
137. Buiatti, E.; Palli, D.; Decarli, A.; Amadori, D.; Avellini, C.; Bianchi, S.; Biserni, R.; Cipriani, F.; Cocco, P.; Giacosa, A.; *et al.* A case-control study of gastric cancer and diet in Italy. *Int. J. Cancer* **1989**, *44*, 611–616. [CrossRef] [PubMed]
138. Ward, M.H.; López-Carrillo, L. Dietary factors and the risk of gastric cancer in Mexico city. *Am. J. Epidemiol.* **1999**, *149*, 925–932. [CrossRef] [PubMed]
139. Van den Brandt, P.A.; Botterweck, A.A.M.; Goldbohm, A. Salt intake, cured meat consumption, refrigerator use and stomach cancer incidence: A prospective cohort study (Netherlands). *Cancer Cause Control* **2003**, *14*, 427–438. [CrossRef]
140. Kuhnle, G.G.C.; Story, G.W.; Reda, T.; Mani, A.R.; Moore, K.P.; Lunn, J.C.; Bingham, S.A. Diet-induced endogenous formation of nitroso compounds in the GI tract. *Free Radic. Biol. Med.* **2007**, *43*, 1040–1047. [CrossRef] [PubMed]
141. Hogg, N. Red meat and colon cancer: Heme proteins and nitrite in the gut. A commentary on "Diet-induced endogenous formation of nitroso compounds in the GI tract". *Free Radic. Biol. Med.* **2007**, *43*, 1037–1039. [CrossRef] [PubMed]
142. McEvoy, C.T.; Temple, N.; Woodside, J.V. Vegetarian diets, low-meat diets and health: A review. *Public Health Nutr.* **2012**, *15*, 2287–2294. [CrossRef] [PubMed]
143. Gilchrist, M.; Winyard, P.G.; Benjamin, N. Dietary nitrate-good or bad? *Nitric Oxide* **2010**, *22*, 104–109. [CrossRef] [PubMed]
144. Milkowski, A.; Garg, H.K.; Coughlin, J.R.; Bryan, N.S. Nutritional epidemiology in the context of nitric oxide biology: A risk-benefit evaluation for dietary nitrite and nitrate. *Nitric Oxide* **2010**, *15*, 110–119. [CrossRef] [PubMed]
145. Bradbury, K.E.; Appleby, P.N.; Key, T.J. Fruit, vegetable, and fiber intake in relation to cancer risk: Findings from the European Prospective Investigation into Cancer and Nutrition (EPIC). *Am. J. Clin. Nutr.* **2014**, *100*, 394S–398S. [CrossRef] [PubMed]
146. Lim, J.W.; Kim, H.; Kim, KH. NF-κB, inducible nitric oxide synthase and apoptosis by *Helicobacter pylori* infection. *Free Radic. Biol. Med.* **2001**, *31*, 355–366. [CrossRef]
147. Wilson, K.T.; Ramanujam, K.S.; Mobley, H.L.; Musselman, R.F.; James, S.P.; Meltzer, S.J. *Helicobacter pylori* stimulates inducible nitric oxide synthase expression and activity in a murine macrophage cell line. *Gastroenterology* **1996**, *111*, 1524–1533. [CrossRef]
148. Jaiswal, M.; LaRusso, N.F.; Gores, G.J. Nitric oxide in gastrointestinal epithelial cell cartinogenesis: Linking inflammation to oncogenesis. *Am. J. Physiol. Gastrointest. Liver physiol.* **2001**, *281*, G626–G634. [PubMed]
149. Zhao, K.; Whiteman, M.; Spencer, J.P.; Halliwell, B. DNA damage by nitrite and peroxynitrite: Protection by dietary phenols. *Methods Enzymol.* **2001**, *335*, 296–307. [PubMed]
150. Wink, D.A.; Vodovotz, Y.; Laval, J.; Laval, F.; Dewhirst, M.W.; Mitchell, J.B. The multifaceted roles of nitric oxide in cancer. *Carcinogenesis* **1998**, *19*, 711–721. [CrossRef] [PubMed]
151. Lancaster, J.R.; Xie, K. Tumors face NO problems? *Cancer Res.* **2006**, *66*, 6459–6462. [CrossRef] [PubMed]
152. Brot, C.; Jorgensen, N.R.; Sorensen, O.H. The influence of smoking on vitamin D status and calcium metabolism. *Eur. J. Clin. Nutr.* **1999**, *53*, 920–926. [CrossRef] [PubMed]
153. Maurel, D.B.; Boisseau, N.; Benhamou, C.L.; Jaffre, C. Alcohol and bone: Review of dose effects and mechanisms. *Osteoporos. Int.* **2012**, *23*, 1–16. [CrossRef] [PubMed]
154. Holbrook, T.L.; Barrett-Connor, E.; Wingard, D.L. Dietary calcium and risk of hip fracture: 14-year prospective population study. *Lancet* **1988**, *332*, 1046–1049. [CrossRef]
155. Feskanich, D.; Willett, W.C.; Colditz, G.A. Calcium, vitamin D, milk consumption, and hip fractures: A prospective study among postmenopausal women. *Am. J. Clin. Nutr.* **2003**, *77*, 504–511. [PubMed]

156. Muraki, S.; Yamamoto, S.; Ishibashi, H.; Oka, H.; Yoshimura, N.; Kawaguchi, H.; Nakamura, K. Diet and lifestyle associated with increased bone mineral density: Cross-sectional study of Japanese elderly women at an osteoporosis outpatient clinic. *J. Orthop. Sci.* **2007**, *12*, 317–320. [CrossRef] [PubMed]
157. Van't Hof, R.J.; Ralston, S.H. Nitric oxide and bone. *Immunology* **2001**, *103*, 255–261. [CrossRef] [PubMed]
158. Armour, K.E.; van't Hof, R.J.; Grabowski, P.S.; Reid, D.M.; Ralston, S.H. Evidence for pathogenic role of nitric oxide in inflammation-induced osteoporosis. *J. Bone Miner. Res.* **1999**, *14*, 2137–2142. [CrossRef] [PubMed]
159. Liu, S.; Yan, H.; Hou, W.; Wu, P.; Tian, J.; Tian, L.; Zhu, B.; Ma, J.; Lu, S. Relationships between endothelial nitric oxide synthase gene polymorphisms and osteoporosis in postmenopausal women. *J. Zhejiang. Univ. Sci. B* **2009**, *10*, 609–618. [CrossRef] [PubMed]
160. Wimalawansa, S.J. Nitric oxide: Novel therapy for osteoporosis. *Expert Opin. Pharmacother.* **2008**, *9*, 1–20. [CrossRef] [PubMed]
161. Wimalawansa, S.J.; de Marco, G.; Gangula, P.; Yallampalli, C. Nitric oxide donor alleviates ovariectomy-induced bone loss. *Bone* **1996**, *18*, 301–304. [CrossRef]
162. Hao, Y.J.; Tang, Y.; Chen, F.B.; Pei, F.X. Different doses of nitric oxide donor prevent osteoporosis in ovariectomized rats. *Clin. Orthop. Relat. Res.* **2005**, *435*, 226–231. [CrossRef] [PubMed]
163. Jamal, S.A.; Reid, L.S.; Hamilton, C.J. The effects of organic nitrates on osteoporosis: A systematic review. *Osteoporos. Int.* **2013**, *24*, 763–770. [CrossRef] [PubMed]
164. Prynne, C.J.; Mishra, G.D.; O'Connell, M.A.; Muniz, G.; Laskey, M.A.; Yan, L.; Prentice, A.; Ginty, F. Fruit and vegetable intakes and bone mineral status: A cross sectional study in 5 age and sex cohorts. *Am. J. Clin. Nutr.* **2006**, *83*, 1420–1428. [PubMed]
165. Tucker, K.L.; Hannan, M.T.; Chen, H.; Cupples, L.A.; Wilson, P.W.; Kiel, D.P. Potassium, magnesium, and fruit and vegetable intakes are associated with greater bone mineral density in elderly men and women. *Am. J. Clin. Nutr.* **1999**, *69*, 727–736. [PubMed]
166. Macdonald, H.M.; New, S.A.; Golden, M.H.; Campbell, M.K.; Reid, D.M. Nutritional associations with bone loss during the menopausal transition: Evidence of a beneficial effect of calcium, alcohol, and fruit and vegetable nutrients and of a detrimental effect of fatty acids. *Am. J. Clin.* **2004**, *79*, 155–165.

Permissions

All chapters in this book were first published by MDPI; hereby published with permission under the Creative Commons Attribution License or equivalent. Every chapter published in this book has been scrutinized by our experts. Their significance has been extensively debated. The topics covered herein carry significant findings which will fuel the growth of the discipline. They may even be implemented as practical applications or may be referred to as a beginning point for another development.

The contributors of this book come from diverse backgrounds, making this book a truly international effort. This book will bring forth new frontiers with its revolutionizing research information and detailed analysis of the nascent developments around the world.

We would like to thank all the contributing authors for lending their expertise to make the book truly unique. They have played a crucial role in the development of this book. Without their invaluable contributions this book wouldn't have been possible. They have made vital efforts to compile up to date information on the varied aspects of this subject to make this book a valuable addition to the collection of many professionals and students.

This book was conceptualized with the vision of imparting up-to-date information and advanced data in this field. To ensure the same, a matchless editorial board was set up. Every individual on the board went through rigorous rounds of assessment to prove their worth. After which they invested a large part of their time researching and compiling the most relevant data for our readers.

The editorial board has been involved in producing this book since its inception. They have spent rigorous hours researching and exploring the diverse topics which have resulted in the successful publishing of this book. They have passed on their knowledge of decades through this book. To expedite this challenging task, the publisher supported the team at every step. A small team of assistant editors was also appointed to further simplify the editing procedure and attain best results for the readers.

Apart from the editorial board, the designing team has also invested a significant amount of their time in understanding the subject and creating the most relevant covers. They scrutinized every image to scout for the most suitable representation of the subject and create an appropriate cover for the book.

The publishing team has been an ardent support to the editorial, designing and production team. Their endless efforts to recruit the best for this project, has resulted in the accomplishment of this book. They are a veteran in the field of academics and their pool of knowledge is as vast as their experience in printing. Their expertise and guidance has proved useful at every step. Their uncompromising quality standards have made this book an exceptional effort. Their encouragement from time to time has been an inspiration for everyone.

The publisher and the editorial board hope that this book will prove to be a valuable piece of knowledge for researchers, students, practitioners and scholars across the globe.

List of Contributors

Sidra Sarfaraz, Aileen Hawke and D. Dan Ramdath
Guelph Research and Development Centre, Agriculture and Agri-Food Canada, Guelph, ON N1G 5C9, Canada

Shamjeet Singh
School of Pharmacy, Faculty of Medical Sciences, The University of the West Indies, St. Augustine, Trinidad and Tobago

Sandra T. Clarke
Applied Bioscience Graduate Program and Faculty of Science, University of Ontario Institute of Technology, Oshawa, ON L1G 0C5, Canada

Kyung Won Lee, Dayeon Shin and Won O. Song
Department of Food Science and Human Nutrition, Michigan State University, 469 Wilson Road, Trout FSHN Building, East Lansing, MI 48824, USA

Tung Po Wong, Leo Ka Yu Chan and Po Sing Leung
School of Biomedical Sciences, Faculty of Medicine, The Chinese University of Hong Kong, Shatin, Hong Kong, China

Concha F. García-Prieto
The Rolf Luft Research Center for Diabetes and Endocrinology, Karolinska Institutet, Stockholm 17176, Sweden

María S. Fernández-Alfonso
Instituto Pluridisciplinar and Facultad de Farmacia, Universidad Complutense, Madrid 28040, Spain

Yan-Chuan Li, Jia-Yue Qi, Dan Shi, Shan-Shan Du, Li-Yan Liu, Ren-Nan Feng and Chang-Hao Sun
Department of Nutrition and Food Hygiene, School of Public Health, Harbin Medical University, No. 157 Baojian Road, Nangang District, Harbin 150086, China

Chun-Long Li
Department of General Surgery, The Second Affiliated Hospital of Harbin Medical University, Harbin 150086, China

Li-Na Huang
Liaoning Institute for Food Control, Shenyang 110015, China

Gyanendra Tripathi and Philip G. McTernan
Division of Biomedical Sciences, Warwick Medical School, University of Warwick, Coventry CV2 2DX, UK

Dara A. Al-Disi
Division of Biomedical Sciences, Warwick Medical School, University of Warwick, Coventry CV2 2DX, UK
Department of Community Health Sciences, College of Applied Medical Sciences, King Saud University, Riyadh 11451, Saudi Arabia

Mohammed Alsaif
Department of Community Health Sciences, College of Applied Medical Sciences, King Saud University, Riyadh 11451, Saudi Arabia

Shaun Sabico
Division of Biomedical Sciences, Warwick Medical School, University of Warwick, Coventry CV2 2DX, UK
Biomarkers Research Program, Riyadh Biochemistry Department, College of Science, King Saud University, Riyadh 11451, Saudi Arabia
Prince Mutaib Chair for Biomarkers of Osteoporosis, Biochemistry Department, College of Science, King Saud University, Riyadh 11451, Saudi Arabia

Nasser M. Al-Daghri and Nasiruddin Khan
Biomarkers Research Program, Riyadh Biochemistry Department, College of Science, King Saud University, Riyadh 11451, Saudi Arabia
Prince Mutaib Chair for Biomarkers of Osteoporosis, Biochemistry Department, College of Science, King Saud University, Riyadh 11451, Saudi Arabia

Reem M. Sallam
Obesity Research Center, College of Medicine, King Saud University, Riyadh 11461, Saudi Arabia
Department of Medicine, College of Medicine, King Saud University, Riyadh 11461, Saudi Arabia
Clinical Chemistry Unit, Department of Pathology, College of Medicine, King Saud University, Riyadh 11461, Saudi Arabia

Assim A. Alfadda
Obesity Research Center, College of Medicine, King Saud University, Riyadh 11461, Saudi Arabia
Department of Medicine, College of Medicine, King Saud University, Riyadh 11461, Saudi Arabia

Yiyi Zhang, Dan Liu, Tieyun Zhao and Haoming Tian
Department of Endocrinology and Metabolism, West China Hospital, Sichuan University, Chengdu 610041, China

Wen Liu
Phase I Clinical Research Unit, West China Hospital, Sichuan University, Chengdu 610041, China

Wen-Xing Li
Institute of Health Sciences, Anhui University, Hefei 230601, Anhui, China
State Key Laboratory of Genetic Resources and Evolution, Kunming Institute of Zoology, Chinese Academy of Sciences, Kunming 650223, Yunnan, China

Jing-Fei Huang
State Key Laboratory of Genetic Resources and Evolution, Kunming Institute of Zoology, Chinese Academy of Sciences, Kunming 650223, Yunnan, China
KIZ-SU Joint Laboratory of Animal Models and Drug Development, College of Pharmaceutical Sciences, Soochow University, Kunming 650223, Yunnan, China
Collaborative Innovation Center for Natural Products and Biological Drugs of Yunnan, Kunming 650223, Yunnan, China

Shao-Xing Dai, Jun-Juan Zheng and Jia-Qian Liu
State Key Laboratory of Genetic Resources and Evolution, Kunming Institute of Zoology, Chinese Academy of Sciences, Kunming 650223, Yunnan, China

Jie-Hua Chen, Caiqun Ouyang, Jia Song and Limei Mao
Department of Nutrition and Food Hygiene, School of Public Health and Tropical Medicine, Southern Medical University, Guangzhou 510515, Guangdong, China

Qiang Ding
Department of Nutrition and Food Hygiene, School of Public Health, Tongji Medical College, Huazhong University of Science and Technology, Wuhan 430030, Hubei, China

Wenhong Cao
Department of Nutrition, The Gillings School of Global Public Health, The University of North Carolina at Chapel Hill, Chapel Hill, NC 27599, USA

Daniel König
Department for Nutrition, Institute for Sports and Sports Science, University of Freiburg, Schwarzwaldstr. 175, 79117 Freiburg, Germany
Department of Exercise and Sports Medicine, Centre for Internal Medicine, University Hospital Freiburg, Hugstetterstr. 175, 79106 Freiburg, Germany

Denise Zdzieblik, Aloys Berg and Albert Gollhofer
Department for Nutrition, Institute for Sports and Sports Science, University of Freiburg, Schwarzwaldstr. 175, 79117 Freiburg, Germany

Peter Deibert
Department of Exercise and Sports Medicine, Centre for Internal Medicine, University Hospital Freiburg, Hugstetterstr. 175, 79106 Freiburg, Germany

Martin Büchert
Department of Radiology – Medical Physics, University Medical Center Freiburg, Breisacher Straße 60a, 79106 Freiburg, Germany

Isabel Arrieta-Cruz
National Institute of Geriatrics, Ministry of Health, Periférico Sur No. 2767, Col. San Jerónimo Lídice. Del. Magdalena Contreras, Mexico City 10200, Mexico

Ya Su and Roger Gutiérrez-Juárez
Department of Medicine, Albert Einstein College of Medicine, Yeshiva University, 1300 Morris Park Ave, Bronx, NY 10461, USA

Wen-Chang Chang, James Swi-Bea Wu and Chen-Wen Chen
Graduate Institute of Food Science and Technology, National Taiwan University, Taipei 10672, Taiwan

Po-Ling Kuo and Szu-Chuan Shen
Department of Human Development and Family Studies, National Taiwan Normal University, No. 162, Sec. 1, Heping East Road, Taipei 10610, Taiwan

Hsu-Min Chien
Department of Nursing, Taipei City Hospital, Renai Branch, No. 10, Sec. 4, Renai Road, Taipei 10629, Taiwan

Yuh-Tai Wang
Life Science Center, Hsing Wu Institute of Technology, No. 101, Sec. 1, Fen-Liao Road, Lin-Kou District, New Taipei City 244, Taiwan

María E. Mejía-León and Ana M. Calderón de la Barca
Department Nutrición y Metabolismo, Centro de Investigación en Alimentación y Desarrollo, A.C., Carr. La Victoria, Km. 0.6, Hermosillo, Sonora 83304, Mexico

Marissa Garcia, Julia Shook, Jane Kerstetter and Tania B. Huedo-Medina
Department of Allied Health Sciences, University of Connecticut, Storrs, CT 06269, USA

Jessica D. Bihuniak
NYU Steinhardt, Department of Nutrition and Food Studies, New York University, New York, NY 10003, USA

Anne Kenny
Center on Aging, University of Connecticut Health Center, Farmington, CT06030, USA

Jun Kobayashi, Kazuo Ohtake and Hiroyuki Uchida
Division of Pathophysiology, Department of Clinical Dietetics and Human Nutrition, Faculty of Pharmaceutical Science, Josai University, Saitama 350-0295, Japan

Index

Printed in the USA
CPSIA information can be obtained
at www.ICGtesting.com
LVHW080737221023
761596LV00011B/2162